Gastrointestinal Disease in Primary Care

Gastrointestinal Disease in Primary Care

EDITORS

Lyman E. Bilhartz, M.D., F.A.C.P.

Associate Professor of Medicine
Department of Internal Medicine
Division of Digestive and Liver Diseases
The University of Texas Southwestern Medical Center
Dallas, Texas

Carol L. Croft, M.D.

Assistant Professor of Medicine
Department of Internal Medicine
Division of General Internal Medicine
The University of Texas Southwestern Medical Center
Dallas, Texas

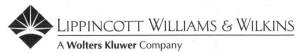

LIPPINCOTT WILLIAMS & WILKINS
A **Wolters Kluwer** Company
Philadelphia · Baltimore · New York · London
Buenos Aires · Hong Kong · Sydney · Tokyo

ACQUISITIONS EDITOR: Timothy Y. Hiscock
DEVELOPMENTAL EDITOR: Leah Ann Kiehne Hayes
MANUFACTURING MANAGER: Kevin Watt
SUPERVISING EDITOR: Mary Ann McLaughlin
COVER DESIGNER: Mark Lerner
PRODUCTION SERVICE: Colophon
COMPOSITOR: Circle Graphics
PRINTER: R.R. Donnelley, Crawfordsville

© 2000 by LIPPINCOTT WILLIAMS & WILKINS
530 Walnut Street
Philadelphia, PA 19106 USA
LWW.com

Printed in the USA

Library of Congress Cataloging-in-Publication Data
Gastrointestinal disease in primary care / editors, Lyman E. Bilhartz, Carol Croft.
    p.   ;   cm.
    Includes bibliographical references and index.
    ISBN 0-683-30444-5 (alk. paper)
    1. Gastrointestinal system—Diseases. 2. Primary care (Medicine)   I. Bilhartz, Lyman.   II. Croft,
Carol.
    [DNLM: 1. Gastrointestinal Diseases.   2. Primary Health Care.   WI 140 G25855 2000]
RC801.G3836 2000
616.3'3—dc21   99-055265

Care has been taken to confirm the accuracy of the information presented and to describe generally accepted
practices. However, the authors, editors, and publisher are not responsible for errors or omissions or for any
consequences from application of the information in this book and make no warranty, expressed or implied,
with respect to the currency, completeness, or accuracy of the contents of the publication. Application of
this information in a particular situation remains the professional responsibility of the practitioner.

The authors, editors, and publisher have exerted every effort to ensure that drug selection and dosage set
forth in this text are in accordance with current recommendations and practice at the time of publication.
However, in view of ongoing research, changes in government regulations, and the constant flow of information relating to drug therapy and drug reactions, the reader is urged to check the package insert for each drug
for any change in indications and dosage and for added warnings and precautions. This is particularly important when the recommended agent is a new or infrequently employed drug.

Some drugs and medical devices presented in this publication have Food and Drug Administration
(FDA) clearance for limited use in restricted research settings. It is the responsibility of the health care
provider to ascertain the FDA status of each drug or device planned for use in their clinical practice.

10 9 8 7 6 5 4 3

Contents

Contributing Authors

David Balis, M.D.
Assistant Professor of Internal Medicine
University of Texas Southwestern Medical Center
5323 Harry Hines Boulevard
Dallas, TX 75235-8889

Lyman E. Bilhartz, M.D., F.A.C.P.
Associate Professor of Medicine
Department of Internal Medicine
Division of Digestive and Liver Diseases
University of Texas Southwestern Medical Center
5323 Harry Hines Boulevard
Dallas, TX 75235-8887

Jay A. Crockett, M.D.
Greenville Colon and Rectal Associates
600 Bear Drive
Greenville, SC 29605

Byron Cryer, M.D.
Assistant Professor of Medicine
University of Texas Southwestern Medical Center
Staff Physician
Department of Gastroenterology
Veterans Administration Medical Center
4500 South Lancaster Road
Dallas, TX 75216

Clark R. Gregg, M.D.
Associate Professor of Medicine
University of Texas Southwestern Medical Center
Chief, Infectious Disease Section
Veterans Administration Medical Center
4500 South Lancaster Road
Dallas, TX 75216

M. Shahbaz Hasan, M.D.
Staff Physician and Assistant Professor,
    General Internal Medicine
Infectious Disease Section
Veterans Administration Medical Center
4500 South Lancaster Road
Dallas, TX 75216

Philip J. Huber, Jr., M.D.
Professor of Surgery
Vice-Chairman, Department of Surgery
University of Texas Southwestern Medical Center
Chairman, Department of Surgery
St. Paul Medical Center
5939 Harry Hines Boulevard
Dallas, TX 75235

Peter J. Kaplan, M.D.
Fellow, Department of Infectious Diseases
University of Texas Southwestern Medical Center
5323 Harry Hines Boulevard
Dallas, TX 75235-9113

Steven L. Leach, M.D.
Assistant Professor of Internal Medicine
University of Texas Southwestern Medical Center
5323 Harry Hines Boulevard
Dallas, TX 75235-8889

David Magee, M.D.
Assistant Professor of Internal Medicine
University of Texas Southwestern Medical Center
5323 Harry Hines Boulevard
Dallas, TX 75235-8887

Naiel N. Nassar, M.D.
Medical Director
Center for AIDS Research, Education, and Services
1500 21st Street
Sacramento, CA 95814

Kevin C. Oeffinger, M.D.
Associate Professor of Family Practice and
   Community Medicine
University of Texas Southwestern Medical Center
5323 Harry Hines Boulevard
Dallas, TX 75235-9067

Shalini Reddy, M.D.
Assistant Professor of Internal Medicine
University of Texas Southwestern Medical Center
5323 Harry Hines Boulevard
Dallas, TX 75235-9113

Michael A. Sheffield, M.D.
Assistant Professor of Medicine
University of Texas Southwestern Medical Center
5323 Harry Hines Boulevard
Dallas, TX 75235-9113

Clifford L. Simmang, M.D.
Assistant Professor of Surgery
University of Texas Southwestern Medical Center
5323 Harry Hines Boulevard
Dallas, TX 75235-9156

Daniel J. Skiest, M.D.
Assistant Professor of Internal Medicine
University of Texas Southwestern Medical Center
5323 Harry Hines Boulevard
Dallas, TX 75235-9113

Helen M. Wood, M.D.
Assistant Professor of Medicine
University of Texas Southwestern Medical Center
Staff Physician
Division of General Internal Medicine
Veterans Administration Medical Center
4500 South Lancaster Road
Dallas, TX 75216

Preface

"I saw blood in the toilet." "My eyes have turned yellow." "My father died of colon cancer." "This heartburn is killing me." "I can't seem to have a bowel movement." "I'm going back to Mexico, and I don't want to get sick again." The primary care provider in the trenches hears these chief complaints and others like them from patients every day. Considering that the gastrointestinal tract encompasses seven organs, two orifices, six sphincters, smooth muscle, epithelia, and glandular tissue, not to mention 100 grams of bacterial flora and a kilogram of food daily, it is not surprising that patients with gastrointestinal disorders present with a myriad of different complaints. The challenge (and fun) for the primary care provider is to listen to the history, let the patients tell you what they are worried about, examine them, formulate a working differential diagnosis and either offer advice, pursue further diagnostic tests, or initiate treatment.

Gastroenterology in Primary Care is designed to guide the primary care provider in the diagnosis and management of the more common disorders affecting the gastrointestinal tract and liver. Diseases were chosen based on their prevalence in the outpatient setting, and, within chapters, the emphasis has been placed on typical clinical presentations, cost-effective diagnostic evaluations, and specific treatment options. Where necessary, pathogenesis of diseases has been presented concisely; technical details of endoscopic and surgical procedures have been omitted entirely.

Each chapter includes a table of contents, a summary of diagnosis, key points, referral information, suggested readings, and a list of commonly asked patient questions. The chapters have been organized in a roughly anatomic arrangement, beginning with disorders of the esophagus and ending with perianal disorders.

We hope you find the book useful and welcome any comments.

LYMAN E. BILHARTZ, M.D., F.A.C.P.
(lyman.bilhartz@email.swmed.edu)
CAROL L. CROFT, M.D.
(carol.croft@email.swmed.edu)

Acknowledgments

The editors wish to express our sincere appreciation to our department chair, Daniel W. Foster, M.D., and our division chiefs, John M. Dietschy, M.D. and W. Gary Reed, M.D., for their provision of "protected time," and to our developmental editor, Leah Hayes.

Gastrointestinal Disease in Primary Care

CHAPTER 1

Gastroesophageal Reflux Disease and Other Esophageal Disorders

Michael A. Sheffield

University of Texas Southwestern Medical Center, Dallas, Texas 75235

DEFINITION

Gastroesophageal reflux (GER), or simply reflux, is the retrograde movement of gastric contents into the esophagus. Heartburn, regurgitation, indigestion, sour mouth, and water brash are all terms used to describe symptoms related to the reflux of gastric contents into the esophagus.

Pathologic reflux develops when the defensive mechanisms of the esophagus are overwhelmed. Symptoms, histologic changes, and complications develop along a common pathway that includes esophageal injury and the response to that injury.

Impact of Disease

Healthy adults frequently suffer transient episodes of reflux, most often while in the upright position after a meal. The most common reason for the use of antacids in the United States is GER. More than 40% of Americans have experienced heartburn at least once within the last month, and 7% have heartburn on a daily basis. Other Western countries report comparable heartburn rates of 5% to 12%.

From this larger population of symptomatic patients, only a minority seek medical advice for their heartburn from their primary care provider. Castell, in his book,

Gastro-Esophageal Reflux Disease, depicted those patients seeking medical attention for their reflux as forming only the midportion and tip of a large, mostly hidden, reflux iceberg. Those who do not seek medical treatment have mild, intermittent symptoms and are presumed to have a low likelihood of developing complications. However, no studies have investigated the complication rate in these patients, and little correlation exists between severity of symptoms and severity of pathology.

Symptomatic patients have a greatly reduced quality of life, similar to that of patients with chronic heart diseases. The frequency of disease and its attendant morbidity require primary care providers to be adept at treating GER and its complications.

Course of Disease

The course of GER is largely unknown. For those patients who present to their health care provider, the course is one of resolutions and relapses. Some develop local complications such as strictures and Barrett's esophagus. Others have extraesophageal complications.

Most patients remain symptomatic without concomitant complications. Because gastrointestinal reflux disease (GERD) is often a relapsing disease, most patients require maintenance therapy to prevent relapses. In a review, Koufmann estimated that 25% of patients have complete resolution of their disease; 50% have a chronic, relapsing course; and 25% have a chronic, often progressive course marked by the development of complications. The course of minimally symptomatic disease, especially when the patient does not seek medical care, is unknown.

Understanding of the Disease

Although descriptions of indigestion and heartburn have existed for a millennium, the current understanding of the disease caused by GER began in 1935. In his classic report, Winkelstein postulated that the esophagitis noted on endoscopy of five index cases was peptic in origin. He ascribed his patients' complaints of heartburn to this "peptic esophagitis." In 1946, Allison clarified further the pathogenesis of peptic esophagitis and introduced the term "reflux esophagitis" into the medical language. Today, the symptom complexes and complications ascribed to GER include both extraesophageal and esophageal manifestations. "Gastroesophageal reflux disease" is now the accepted term that is used to describe any symptoms or histopathologic changes resulting from excessive reflux of gastric contents into the esophagus.

CAUSE

GER is a process that occurs frequently in normal persons as well as those with GERD. The factors that make an individual susceptible to physiologic reflux continue to be defined.

Once thought to be simply the result of an atonic or hypotensive lower esophageal sphincter (LES), the pathogenesis of GERD is now recognized as being multifactorial (Table 1.1). Abnormalities in any of several defensive mechanisms (e.g., the LES, esophageal motility, epithelial resistance) may contribute to GERD in a given patient. Offensive factors such as the composition and quantity of the refluxate may also contribute to GERD. The pathogenicity of the refluxate is probably of limited importance except in certain circumstances.

Anatomically, the functional barrier that prevents reflux of gastric contents into the esophagus has two components, the LES and the crural diaphragm. The LES is a 3- to 4-cm segment of the distal esophagus that is composed of tonically contracted smooth muscle. At rest, the LES pressure in most normal persons is 10 to 30 mm Hg higher than that of the stomach. During the course of a day, the pressure of the LES diminishes after meals but increases with supine lying. The second part of the physiologic barrier to reflux is the crural diaphragm. The role of the diaphragm in preventing reflux in normal persons is minor. Primarily, it increases the resistance to reflux during inspiration or other periods of increased intraabdominal pressure.

Lower Esophageal Sphincter Incompetence

Originally, a hypotensive LES was postulated as the cause of most episodes of GER. However, manometric measurements taken in patients with GERD have not supported this concept. In fact, fewer than one fourth of episodes of reflux are associated with reduced LES pressures.

TABLE 1.1.	Mechanisms Involved in the Pathogenesis of Gastroesophageal Reflux Disease

Lower esophageal sphincter (LES) abnormalities
    Hypotensive LES
    Transient LES relaxation
    Hiatal hernia
Delayed esophageal acid clearance
    Altered esophageal motility
    Diminished saliva
Impaired epithelial resistance to acid
Gastric acid hypersecretion
Bile-acid refluxate

Although a hypotensive LES appears not to be the cause of most reflux episodes, several drugs and foods are known to lessen LES pressure and may place a patient at risk for reflux. According to anecdotal or clinical evidence, several of these agents have been linked to worsened reflux, suggesting that reduced LES pressure is an important contributor to reflux in some circumstances (Table 1.2). Avoidance or removal of these substances forms a part of the management plan for reflux patients.

Transient Lower Esophageal Sphincter Relaxation

Since the discovery that most GERD patients have LES pressures in the normal range, experts have found that transient LES relaxation is the principal contributing factor to reflux. One study noted that 60% to 83% of reflux episodes were associated with transient LES relaxation. Compared with physiologic relaxations induced by swallowing, transient LES relaxations are not initiated by deglutition, are not associated with esophageal peristalsis, and last longer than 10 seconds. However, the presence of transient LES relaxation does not automatically result in reflux. Reports document a rate of reflux associated with transient LES relaxation of 9% to 93%. Although the pathogenesis of these relaxations is not defined, gastric distention and the upright position are known to increase the frequency of transient LES relaxations.

Foods and Drugs Known to Affect Lower Esophageal Sphincter (LES) Tone		TABLE 1.2.
Substances	**Increase LES tone**	**Decrease LES tone**
Drugs	Alpha-agonists	Alpha-antagonists
	Beta-blockers	Beta-agonists
	Cholinergics	Anticholinergics
	Antacids	Theophylline
	Metoclopramide	Somatostatin
	Cisapride	Calcium entry blockers
		Dopamine
		Diazepam
		Progesterone
		Morphine
Foods	Protein	Fat
		Chocolate
		Onion
		Peppermint (carminative)
		Ethanol

Despite the involvement of transient LES relaxations in reflux episodes, no direct correlation between the number of relaxations, the number of reflux episodes, and the development of GERD has been proven. Instead, esophageal damage is related to total acid exposure time.

Hiatal Hernia

The presence of a hiatal hernia further compromises the LES. As mentioned previously, the physiologic barrier to reflux has two parts. The diaphragmatic crura, which forms the second part of the barrier, is compromised in the presence of a hiatal hernia. The role of the diaphragm in preventing reflux is greatest during periods of increased intraabdominal pressure. Therefore, the combination of reduced LES tone and impaired diaphragmatic contraction can lead to significant reflux. A hiatal hernia also delays the clearance of acid from the esophagus, placing the esophagus at further risk by increasing esophageal acid exposure time. However, hiatal hernias are found in 40% to 60% of asymptomatic controls, making them an insignificant finding. Despite the evidence supporting a role for hiatal hernias in reflux, their significance in the pathogenesis of GERD remains controversial.

Delayed Acid Clearance

Once gastric contents have refluxed into the esophagus, a two-step process removes the acid. The first step is the physical removal of most of the gastric refluxate by gravity and peristalsis. The fluid that remains is minimal in volume and, in the second step, is neutralized by bicarbonate-containing salivary fluid. In patients with GERD, the acid clearance time is significantly prolonged.

The abnormality in acid neutralization in patients with GERD is believed to result from abnormal esophageal motility. Compared with controls, patients with GERD have normal saliva volume and bicarbonate content. Because controls and patients with GERD are able to neutralize equivalent amounts of acid, the delayed acid clearance in these patients is probably the result of large, retained volumes of acid refluxate in the esophagus. Esophageal dysmotility increases the volume of acid to be neutralized by the salivary fluid, and clearance time is thereby prolonged.

The incidence and severity of esophagitis are directly proportional to the acid exposure time. The delay in esophageal acid clearance and neutralization appears to be operative in one half of patients with GERD.

Diminished Epithelial Resistance

The newest area of research into the pathogenesis of GERD concerns defense mechanisms and the response to injury of the esophageal epithelium. In rabbit studies, the esophageal epithelium was found to have enzyme systems capable of neutralizing intracellular acid. Theoretically, the epithelium of patients with GERD is unable to appropriately neutralize the acid and is thereby damaged. The response of the epithelium to the acid injury is basal cell hyperplasia. Although it protects the injured esophagus, the proliferation of epithelium may lead to complications, including strictures and metaplasia. The mechanisms underlying epithelial resistance in humans remain largely unknown but are probably important, because the epithelium remains the common link among all causes of esophageal injury.

Refluxate

Finally, the consistency of the refluxed material (refluxate) has been investigated as being pathogenic. Reflux of acid- and pepsin-containing fluid is required for the development of reflux esophagitis, but the question of whether normal concentrations of acid and pepsin are sufficient to cause damage is debated. The composition of gastric fluid and the gastric acid secretory rate do not differ between persons with endoscopic evidence of esophagitis and controls. Conversely, patients with esophagitis resistant to ranitidine treatment have been found to be gastric-acid hypersecretors. In general, experts believe that sufficient exposure to normal amounts of acid and pepsin can result in esophageal damage. Excess acid secretion seems to be important only in refractory cases.

Further complicating the study of the pathogenicity of refluxate is the question of the role of bile acids in causing esophagitis. Bile salts are capable of solubilizing epithelial membranes and exposing the underlying tissue to the refluxate. The most advanced esophagitis is often found in patients with gastroduodenal refluxate containing bile salts. Despite the obvious potential of bile salts to cause esophageal damage, acid and pepsin seem to be required cofactors for the development of esophagitis. Regardless of the composition of the refluxate, the esophageal damage is proportional to the amount and duration of acid exposure.

PATIENT PRESENTATION

History

Classic presentation

The clinical presentation of the stereotypic patient with GER is well known. Such patients are mildly obese smokers who complain of postprandial, retrosternal burning that is worst after large meals containing fatty or spicy foods. They note that they more frequently have heartburn after imbibing ethanol or eating chocolate. Their heartburn increases with recumbency and

bending over and is ameliorated by antacids. Such typical presenting features are found in two thirds to three fourths of patients with GER.

The hallmarks of GERD are heartburn (pyrosis) and acid regurgitation, but these symptoms are present in fewer than 70% of patients with abnormal 24-hour pH monitoring results. Heartburn is described as a retrosternal burning that moves from the stomach into the neck and is typically described by a sweeping motion of the open hand. Together, heartburn and regurgitation have proved to be the only symptoms that helped distinguish control subjects from patients with reflux.

Other typical symptoms of GERD include dysphagia, odynophagia, water brash, and belching (Table 1.3). Water brash is the sudden appearance of a salty or sour fluid emanating from the salivary glands in response to intraesophageal acidification.

Atypical presentations

The remaining patients present with symptoms that are more difficult to relate to abnormal reflux (Table 1.3). Patients may complain of chest pain, chronic cough, hoarseness, wheezing, dyspnea, or globus, instead of heartburn and regurgitation.

In one study, atypical presentations were found in 15% of patients subsequently found to have GERD. Because many patients with atypical reflux symptoms go undiagnosed, the frequency of atypical symptoms is likely to be much higher. For example, GERD was found to be the cause in 20% to 50% of cases of noncardiac chest pain by pH monitoring, and it was present in up to 80% of adult asthmatics. Furthermore, asymptomatic patients must be included in the atypical group. For example, one third of patients with Barrett's esophagus (see discussion in next section) have no symptoms

TABLE 1.3.	Symptoms Commonly Ascribed to Gastroesophageal Reflux
Typical symptoms	**Atypical symptoms**
Heartburn	Chest pain
Regurgitation	Cough
Dysphagia	Wheezing
Odynophagia	Dyspnea
Water brash	Hoarseness
Belching	Throat clearing
Epigastric pain	Globus sensation
	Halitosis
	Asymptomatic

on acid perfusion testing. These findings suggest that patients may have severe pathology with minimal symptoms, or severe symptoms with minimal pathology.

Physical Examination

The physical examination of the patient with GERD is largely unrevealing. Most patients have a normal examination or mild epigastric tenderness on palpation of the abdomen. Complications such as asthma are similarly evident on examination in patients with and without GERD, i.e., a prolonged expiratory phase with wheezes. The utility of the examination is to exclude other disease states.

Complications

Most patients with GERD have no complications from the reflux of acid into the esophagus. Patients with complications can have either esophageal or extraesophageal complications, or both (Table 1.4). As stated previously, the severity of symptoms bears little or no relation to the likelihood of having esophageal complications. Also, the atypical symptoms associated with extraesophageal complications may be the predominant manifestations of GERD, rather than the more typical heartburn and regurgitation. In addition to the usual medical and surgical therapies, these complications often require additional interventions.

Esophagitis

Esophagitis is the most common complication of GERD. It is found in 2% to 4% of the general population, with two thirds or more of these persons having mild to moderate changes only.

Esophagitis can range from minimal changes seen only on histologic specimens to severe ulcerations and

TABLE 1.4. Esophageal and Extraesophageal Complications of Gastroesophageal Disease

Esophageal complications	Extraesophageal complications
Esophagitis	Laryngitis
Esophageal hemorrhage	Laryngeal carcinoma
Esophageal stricture	Tracheal stenosis
Barrett's esophagus	Asthma
Esophageal adenocarcinoma	Aspiration pneumonitis
	Chronic cough and hiccoughs
	Dental caries

even perforation. Furthermore, 20% of patients with esophagitis have complications such as ulcer, hemorrhage, stricture, or Barrett's esophagus. Erosions of even mild esophagitis are often associated with complaints of odynophagia. If the erosions deepen to an esophageal ulcer, the odynophagia may progress to complaints of ulcer-like pain. Gross gastrointestinal bleeding and iron deficiency anemia are rare manifestations of esophagitis. The development of strictures and Barrett's esophagus results from the esophageal response to injury.

Esophageal stricture

An esophageal stricture can complicate further the course of GERD with esophagitis. Strictures develop as part of the epithelial response to recurrent injury and inflammation from repeated episodes of reflux. Approximately 10% of patients with severe esophagitis develop a stricture; the prevalence increases with age and duration of reflux. Patients with strictures complain of progressive dysphagia, first to solids and then to liquids. Elderly patients with strictures may be evaluated for unexplained weight loss before the abnormality is discovered. The stricture is made of scar and is worsened by overlying spasm and edema. Esophageal dysmotility and LES hypotonia are often noted after a stricture develops, further worsening GERD.

Barrett's esophagus

The replacement of esophageal squamous epithelium with metaplastic columnar epithelium similar to that of intestinal mucosa is known as Barrett's esophagus or metaplasia; it occurs in response to severe, chronic GER. It is the most feared of the complications of GERD because it is generally regarded as a premalignant condition in the development of esophageal adenocarcinoma.

The tissue is believed to develop from multipotent stem cells after the overlying squamous epithelium has been denuded by recurrent acid injury. Instead of differentiating into squamous epithelium, the stem cell produces columnar epithelium in the face of repeated acid exposure. The risk for development of adenocarcinoma in the abnormal epithelium is debated but is generally accepted to be approximately 10%. Esophageal adenocarcinoma develops almost exclusively in Barrett's metaplasia. Adenocarcinoma of the esophagus recently has replaced squamous cell carcinoma as the most common esophageal malignancy among Western white men, and its incidence continues to increase at logarithmic rates. The need for effective treatment of patients with GERD and metaplasia cannot be overstated.

Extraesophageal manifestations

The complications of GERD extend beyond the esophagus. The extraesophageal manifestations principally affect the respiratory tract because of its anatomic proximity and shared innervation (Table 1.4). Often, the complications are not associated with the symptoms of heartburn or regurgitation.

Asthma   More than 15 million Americans have asthma, and the incidence continues to increase. The role of GERD in nonallergic or intrinsic asthma is widely debated. Simply put, the prevalences of GERD and asthma are sufficiently great that the occurrence of both diseases in a single person is also common. The question of causality is therefore somewhat controversial. Although the prevalence of esophagitis in the general public is 2% to 4%, it is up to 40% in asthmatics, and abnormal reflux occurs in 34% to 89% of asthmatics. The increased prevalence of GERD in asthmatics compared with the general public suggests a role of reflux in the pathogenesis of intrinsic asthma. Further support for the hypothesis that GERD may contribute to the development of asthma is the fact that bronchospasm can be induced either by aspiration of acid material into the lungs or by a vagal reflex caused by esophageal acidification.

A more direct role for GERD in the pathogenesis of asthma is supported by two studies in which antireflux therapy improved measures of asthma. In a study of patients with asthma and GERD, 50% had no symptoms of asthma at 6 years after surgery for relief of their reflux. Harding et al., in a prospective, open, uncontrolled trial, gave 30 patients with symptomatic reflux 3 months of omeprazole therapy and then assessed them for the severity of their asthma. Almost three fourths of patients had clinical improvement at the end of the study. Those who responded had either frequent regurgitation or documented proximal esophageal acidification with their reflux. The study was not of sufficient power to demonstrate an objective improvement in pulmonary function testing.

Otolaryngologic complications   Patients who reflux acid into the proximal esophagus are at risk for otolaryngologic complications in addition to asthma. As few as 20% of these patients have heartburn, and fewer still have esophagitis on endoscopy. The complications that have been linked to GER are believed to be caused by either laryngeal or pharyngeal mucosal injury resulting from contact with acid refluxate. Furthermore, acid usually must reach the proximal esophagus for the patient to be at risk. Because typical reflux symptoms are commonly absent, the diagnosis of GERD-related otolaryngologic conditions such as hoarseness is difficult.

LARYNGITIS   Instead of heartburn, the patient with reflux laryngitis complains of chronic cough, dysphonia, excessive throat clearing, sore throat, or a globus sensation. Despite a diagnostic search or empiric therapy for causes such as infection or allergy, the patient remains symptomatic and often is referred to an otolaryngologist for diagnostic laryngoscopy. Findings at that time include granulomas, ulcerations, and edema of the vocal cords. The injury is isolated to the posterior third of the vocal cords and surrounding tissue, an almost pathognomonic finding.

Reflux laryngitis seems to be associated with the development of squamous cell carcinoma of the larynx, especially in nonsmokers. Case series describe several nonsmokers with GERD and laryngitis who developed laryngeal cancer. Although smoking and alcohol remain the primary risk factors for the appearance of laryngeal cancer, lesions of reflux laryngitis have been observed prospectively as they evolved into malignant lesions in the absence of smoking or alcohol. Many experts believe that a link between the lesions of reflux laryngitis and cancer exists.

TRACHEAL STENOSIS   In adults, almost all cases of subglottic tracheal stenosis occur in patients who have been intubated for longer than 48 to 72 hours. Laryngeal mucosal injury begins to develop with prolonged intubation. Further injury by acid contact is believed to contribute to the continuum of injury, inflammation, and repair that results in the development of stenosis. Esophageal pH recordings in supine, intubated patients show frequent proximal acidification, suggesting a role for GER in the development of tracheal stenosis. No prospective trials addressing the protective effect of acid suppression in preventing tracheal stenosis have been performed. But, given the association, patients who develop tracheal abnormalities after intubation should be evaluated for GERD.

DIAGNOSIS

The diagnosis of the classic patient described in the preceding section is straightforward. Most patients present with features typical of GERD and can be treated empirically, but certain subsets of patients require diagnostic testing. Patients who should undergo diagnostic testing are those who present with features atypical for GERD, fail to respond to initial therapy, are believed to have complications of GERD, or are being considered for antireflux surgery. Patients who present with heartburn complicated by odynophagia, bleeding, or dysphagia need further diagnostic workup, including endoscopy, to evaluate for the presence of esophagitis.

Laboratory Tests and Radiologic Studies

Five principal tests are used in the diagnosis of GERD (Table 1.5). Because no single test provides all the needed information and no test is 100% accurate, the health care provider must choose the appropriate testing modality based on clinical impression and the patient's symptoms. Tests are best placed into two categories: One group of tests proves that reflux occurs, and the other shows that esophageal injury has occurred. Table 1.6 gives the indications for each test.

Empiric trial of therapy

In patients with mild to moderate symptoms typical for GER and no evidence of a complication, a trial of aggressive acid suppression should be the first "diagnostic test." Although the patient may not respond to therapy for several weeks, the trial of acid suppression is without significant clinical harm.

The sensitivity of a trial of omeprazole as a diagnostic test for GER was calculated in one study. Patients were given omeprazole, 40 mg by mouth twice daily for 7 days. A 75% decrease in symptoms was considered a positive test for GER. By these criteria, the omeprazole trial had an 83% sensitivity for diagnosis of reflux, with esophageal pH monitoring as the gold standard. Lesser doses of omeprazole had diminished sensitivity.

Barium esophagogram

The air-contrast or double-contrast barium esophagogram is the only test used routinely for diagnosis of both reflux and esophagitis. It is also the only study not requiring a specialty referral, a fact that probably con-

TABLE 1.6.

Recommended Initial Studies Based on Symptoms in Patients with Gastroesophageal Reflux Disease

Symptoms	Initial test
Heartburn	Empiric trial of PPI or H2RA[a]
Dysphagia	Barium esophagogram
Odynophagia	EGD with biopsy
Chest pain	pH monitoring with symptom diary
Asthma	pH monitoring—distal and proximal
Hoarseness	Laryngoscopy

PPI, proton pump inhibitors; H2RA, histamine receptor antagonist; EGD, esophagogastroduodenoscopy
[a] Decreased sensitivity with the use of H2RA

tributes to its continued popularity. Although of limited utility to the majority of patients with GERD, the barium esophagogram is important in the evaluation of patients with GERD complicated by dysphagia.

Traditionally, the barium esophagogram was used to diagnose sliding hiatal hernia, once thought to be a congener for GERD. However, more recent evidence suggests that these lesions are found frequently in healthy individuals. Therefore, the specificity of the barium esophagogram is limited.

The sensitivity of the barium esophagogram for demonstrating GERD has been estimated to be only 25% to 62%. Maneuvers such as the water-siphon test can increase the sensitivity, but at the cost of increasing the number of false-positive studies, and they are no longer recommended. The accuracy in diagnosing esophagitis is suboptimal, because the characteristics of the test make it sensitive only for moderate to severe esophagitis. Although the accuracy of diagnosing severe esophagitis approaches 90%, that for mild esophagitis is only 25%. With the understanding that most esophagitis is of a mild grade, the usefulness of the barium esophagogram is diminished further.

Despite the limited sensitivity and specificity of the barium esophagogram as a diagnostic test for either reflux or esophagitis, it is useful in the evaluation of patients presenting with complaints of dysphagia. Such patients should have an esophagogram, including a solid bolus study, as a part of their initial evaluation. Findings can include compressive intrinsic or extrinsic masses, rings, strictures, and esophageal dysmotility. If a stricture is detected, endoscopy with biopsy to exclude malignancy is required.

TABLE 1.5.

Diagnostic Tests Used in the Evaluation of Gastroesophageal Reflux Disease

Tests to prove gastroesophageal reflux	Tests to prove esophagitis
Ambulatory pH monitor	Barium esophagogram
Barium esophagogram	Esophagoscopy with biopsy
Scintigraphy	Acid perfusion tests
Manometry	
Omeprazole trial	

Scintigraphy

Scintigraphy, which is sparingly used, is a nuclear test designed to demonstrate reflux. A mixture of saline and technetium Tc 99m sulfur colloid is introduced into the patient's stomach, and abdominal pressure is applied. Radioactivity is then measured over the chest. A positive test is one in which technetium is detected in the chest.

The sensitivity of the test is similar to that of the esophagogram, with an average of 68% and a range in clinical trials of 11% to 90%. In children the test has a sensitivity of 56% to 80%, and it is used more often in young patients. Given the lack of improved sensitivity and the inability to show mucosal or motility abnormalities, scintigraphy is not as useful as the esophagogram in the evaluation of GERD.

Manometry

The use of esophageal manometry in confirming or making the diagnosis of GERD is not indicated. The benefit of esophageal manometry is in the evaluation of esophageal motility disorders, in the preoperative evaluation of patients before antireflux surgery, and in the correct positioning of pH probes in the esophagus.

Richter and Castell reported in a review that the finding of an LES pressure of less than 10 mm Hg had a sensitivity of 58% and a specificity of 84% for GERD. The more specific cutoff of less than 6 mm Hg was rarely found.

Fifty percent of patients with mild to severe esophagitis have abnormal motility on manometric evaluation, suggesting that altered peristalsis contributes to the pathogenesis of GERD.

pH monitoring

Introduced into clinical practice in the late 1960s, ambulatory pH monitoring has become the gold standard for demonstrating GER. The procedure is well tolerated and involves placing a probe to within 5 cm of the manometrically determined LES and recording the esophageal pH while the patient carries out the usual daily activities. Frequently, the patient maintains a diary of symptoms concomitantly. An episode of reflux occurs when the pH falls to less than 4. Six different measurements are usually recorded during testing. They are percentage of time with pH-defined reflux while the patient is in the upright position; percentage of time with reflux while supine; percentage of total time with reflux; number of reflux episodes; number of reflux episodes lasting longer than 5 minutes; and longest reflux episode. Using the first three measurements of percentage of time spent in reflux, sensitivities and specificities for

detecting GERD of greater than 85% and 95%, respectively, have been reported. One study of 90 patients demonstrated a sensitivity, specificity, and accuracy of 96% for diagnosis of GERD.

Other work has cast doubt on the apparently extraordinary accuracy of this test. Among patients with endoscopic evidence of reflux esophagitis, 23% to 29% had normal pH monitoring tests. Despite these doubts and the requirement for referral to a gastroenterologist, ambulatory pH monitoring is considered to be the single best test to diagnose GERD. Monitoring is of particular use in patients for whom therapy has failed and in patients who have unusual symptoms of GERD.

The American Gastroenterological Association recommends the use of ambulatory pH monitoring for patients who do not have endoscopic esophagitis and are being considered for antireflux surgery, patients with refractory symptoms including chest pain and otolaryngologic manifestations, and patients with continued symptoms after antireflux surgery.

Esophagogastroduodenoscopy

As a test for GERD, esophagogastroduodenoscopy (EGD) is unique in that it provides a direct view of the esophageal mucosa; for this reason, it is the principal test to determine whether the mucosa remains intact. If a stricture, mass effect, or Barrett's esophagus is suspected because of results of a barium esophagogram, EGD is mandatory. The American College of Gastroenterology recommends an EGD for patients who do not respond to acid suppression or who experience a recurrence of symptoms after discontinuation of therapy.

The sensitivity of EGD for detecting GERD is limited by the fact that as few as one third of all patients with reflux develop any of the mucosal changes of esophagitis. Among patients who present to their physician with reflux, the rate of esophagitis is 50% to 65%. Overall, the sensitivity of EGD for detecting pathologic reflux is 62% and is improved by mucosal biopsy. The specificity approaches that of pH monitoring.

EGD is particularly useful in excluding other diagnostic considerations, especially in immunocompromised patients, such as those with human immunodeficiency virus (HIV) infection and those who are receiving chemotherapy. Mucosal inspection allows the physician to look for evidence of fungal and viral infections that could mimic or worsen the symptoms of acid reflux. Using a grading system to quantify the severity of esophageal injury, gastroenterologists find most esophagitis to be mild to moderate in severity.

To summarize, EGD should not be used routinely as the initial study to diagnose reflux because it has limited sensitivity. However, if mucosal complications are suspected or if the patient's condition fails to respond to therapy, referral for EGD is recommended.

Bernstein's test

The acid perfusion test to detect esophagitis was developed by Bernstein and Baker in 1958. The test requires that a nasogastric tube be placed into the distal esophagus. Normal saline is infused for 15 minutes, after which a 0.1 N HCl solution is infused. The rate of infusion is 6 mL per minute; this is continued until retrosternal pain is produced or until 45 minutes has elapsed.

The sensitivity and specificity of this test are limited. Studies have shown a sensitivity that ranges from 32% to 80% and a specificity of 50% to 60%. A positive test suggests that the symptoms produced are esophageal in origin but not necessarily that they are caused by acid reflux.

The acid perfusion test is used primarily in the diagnosis of noncardiac chest pain in patients with a normal EGD; however, compared with 24-hour pH monitoring, its sensitivity is only 59%. The use of acid perfusion tests should be limited, because more accurate tests are available to detect esophageal injury.

Differential Diagnosis

The esophagus performs a complicated and integrated function in transporting a bolus from the mouth to the stomach. However, the response of the mucosa to injury is limited. The finding of esophagitis on barium studies or by EGD cannot be assumed to be the result of acid reflux. As many as 10% to 25% of cases of esophagitis have a cause of injury other than peptic acid (Table 1.7).

Typical infectious causes of esophagitis include *Candida* spp., herpes simplex viruses, cytomegalovirus, and

Differential Diagnosis of Esophagitis	TABLE 1.7.

Infectious causes
  Cytomegalovirus
  Herpes simplex virus
  Candida spp.
  Human immunodeficiency virus
Contact injury
  Pill-induced (quinidine, potassium chloride, doxycycline, alendronate)
  Lye
Bile-acid reflux or alkaline reflux
Radiation injury

Summary of Diagnosis

- The diagnosis of GERD involves two separate paths of investigation. One objective is to demonstrate that reflux of gastric acid is occurring; the other is to show esophageal injury resulting from this exposure. The strategy of additional testing must be individualized and the order of tests adapted to the patient.
- Only those patients with less typical symptoms (e.g., hoarseness, dyspnea, cough) should undergo early testing. For these patients, 24-hour pH monitoring is the most accurate single test.
- All other patients should be given an acid suppression regimen for 6 to 8 weeks before further testing is undertaken.
- Even in patients with less typical presentations in whom reflux is suspected, an empiric trial of acid suppression can be performed before further diagnostic testing is pursued.

HIV. These causes are usually determined by histologic or microbiologic evaluation.

Iatrogenic causes of esophagitis include radiation and contact injury from pills. Common offending agents include potassium preparations, alendronate, tetracyclines, and quinidine. Radiation esophagitis occurs in patients who have received a dose of at least 6,000 rads to the mediastinum; the typical patient has chronic inflammatory changes on biopsy and reports a history of radiation for a lymphoma or lung cancer.

Also included in the differential for acid-reflux–induced esophagitis is alkaline reflux. Estimates suggest that 10% to 30% of patients who have undergone gastrectomy or partial gastrectomy have alkaline reflux as documented by pH monitoring. As discussed previously, the role of bile acids in promoting esophageal injury is unclear. Histologically and grossly, the alkaline esophagitis is indistinguishable from peptic esophagitis.

Typically, patients with one of these less-typical causes of esophagitis fail to respond to an empiric trial of acid suppression or, on clinical evaluation, have findings that suggest a nonpeptic cause of their symptoms. Appropriate evaluation can lead to the diagnosis.

MANAGEMENT

Heartburn and indigestion have plagued humankind for thousands of years. Management has included the use of everything from seminal fluid and baby urine to coral powder and milk. In 1915, Sippey introduced the hourly ingestion of milk and antacids as the standard care for peptic diseases. Treatment of GERD followed these recommendations plus lifestyle modifications until strong acid suppressors were developed in the 1970s. The management of reflux is problematic because of the incidence of disease, the recognition that severity of symptoms does not correlate with severity of histologic changes or development of complications, and the typically chronic and relapsing course.

An uncontrolled clinical trial in which patients with GERD receiving conservative therapy were monitored for 17 years gives some suggestion of the course in patients who are symptomatic. Only 12% of patients in the study were asymptomatic at the end of the study, whereas 12% had developed Barrett's esophagus. Also, 66% had histologic changes consistent with or ambulatory 24-hour pH monitoring that demonstrated ongoing pathologic reflux. Reflux is a chronic, relapsing disease that requires ongoing therapy.

The goals of treatment are to relieve symptoms, to heal mucosal injury, and to prevent complications. In theory, effective therapy could be directed at correcting any of the physiologic abnormalities contributing to pathologic reflux. In practice, only acid suppression has been consistently effective in achieving these goals.

Treatment

Therapy is divided into three phases. Phase I therapy involves lifestyle modifications and acid neutralization. Phase II therapy is pharmacologic therapy designed to suppress acid production or improve esophageal motility. Finally, if more conservative treatments fail, phase III therapy, antireflux surgery, can be offered. In general, patients require aggressive therapy both to achieve remission of symptoms and to maintain control.

Phase I: Lifestyle modifications and acid neutralization

Most of the patients who do not seek medical advice regarding their reflux use some form of acid neutralization as therapy. In addition, through trial and error, many avoid foods and medicines that worsen their symptoms.

The cornerstone of therapy in more symptomatic patients begins similarly with lifestyle modifications, education, and acid neutralization. Typically, GERD can be managed by these conservative measures alone only patients without reflux esophagitis.

The following phase I treatments are recommended.

Body position Elevate the head of the bed 2 to 6 inches with blocks, bricks, or wood, or use a foam wedge to support the upper half of your body when supine. Do not use pillows for head elevation, because you may slide down during the night.

The rationale behind this recommendation is that most reflux patients have pathologic reflux in the supine position, according to pH monitoring. The frequency of reflux should decrease in a more upright position. Also, the duration of acid exposure should decrease, because gravity assists with acid clearance. Studies confirm these findings. In patients with reflux esophagitis, the addition of instructions to raise the head of the bed was found to have an additive effect on symptoms in patients being treated with ranitidine.

Postprandial recumbency Do not lie down for at least 2 hours after a meal.

This recommendation is based on the purported benefits of gravity on esophageal acid exposure and clearance and on the more frequent occurrence of reflux in the postprandial setting, probably because of gastric distention. Because pathologic reflux also occurs more often in the supine position, the rationale for not assuming a recumbent position after meals is self-evident. Despite the lack of clinical trials to support this theory, the recommendation remains a standard for patients with GERD.

Dietary modifications Avoid foods that worsen reflux symptoms or that have been demonstrated objectively to worsen reflux.

Frequently, patients identify specific foods or types of foods that worsen heartburn and regurgitation. Symptoms may be worsened either by increased esophageal exposure to acid or by direct irritation of damaged esophageal mucosa.

Foods to be avoided are listed in Table 1.8. Chocolate has been proven to increase acid exposure and to

TABLE 1.8.	Mechanisms for Worsening of Gastroesophageal Reflux Disease by Selected Foods and Drinks

Decrease LES tone	Increase acid exposure	Irritate mucosa
Fat	Fat	Tomatoes
Chocolate	Chocolate	Citric acids
Coffee	Onions	Coffee
Carminatives	Carminatives	Tea
Ethanol	Ethanol	Cola

decrease LES tone. Similarly, the carminatives found in peppermint and spearmint have been shown to decrease LES tone and to worsen symptoms of GERD. Meals with higher fat content have been shown to decrease LES tone and increase acid exposure, but they may be more important in promoting reflux in patients without pathologic reflux. By an unknown mechanism, onions increase esophageal acid exposure; this may explain in part the well-known association of spicy foods with worsened heartburn. Ethanol ingestion should be discouraged because it lowers LES tone, impairs esophageal motility, and increases esophageal acid exposure.

Although frequently cited as exacerbating GERD, coffee has been found to have a variable effect on LES tone when studied with manometry. Instead, coffee may worsen symptoms by directly irritating damaged esophageal mucosa. Other substances to be avoided that seem to have a direct irritative effect include citric juices, tomatoes, and colas. Patients should be instructed to note foods that worsen their reflux symptoms and to avoid them in the future.

Smoking cessation   Stop or decrease smoking.

The data to support this recommendation are limited. LES pressure falls and the frequency of reflux episodes increases with smoking; however, the total acid exposure time in smokers is not different from that in nonsmokers. Furthermore, in patients with esophagitis, cessation of smoking does not reduce acid exposure time but does reduce the frequency of abnormal reflux episodes. Despite the lack of convincing evidence, the recommendation to stop smoking remains a cornerstone of therapy because of its other health benefits.

Weight loss   Lose weight if you are obese.

Obesity increases intraabdominal pressure and overwhelms the LES, leading to increased reflux. Because LES tone has not been demonstrated consistently to be reduced in manometric studies of obese patients with GERD, the increase in reflux episodes is believed to be caused by the increased intraabdominal pressure.

Similar arguments can be made to support the recommendations to avoid tight-fitting garments and bending over at the waist.

Meal-size reduction   Avoid consuming large meals.

LES relaxation is more common when the stomach is distended, and reflux episodes are increased. The pathophysiology most likely involves both LES relaxation and increased abdominal pressure with gastric distention. Although no clinical trials have addressed this

issue directly, most physicians recommend reducing the size of meals to avoid gastric overdistention.

Antacids and alginates   Take antacids at bedtime and 1 and 3 hours after each meal.

Before the advent of histamine receptor antagonist therapy, antacids and alginates were the mainstays of therapy for symptomatic reflux. Antacids and, to a lesser degree, alginates continue to be used widely by patients, especially the majority who do not seek medical advice. Both antacids and alginates have been shown to be superior to placebo for symptomatic relief. Also, the combination of antacid and alginate is more effective than placebo or either agent alone in relieving the symptoms of GERD.

More objective results (e.g., healing of esophagitis) have been difficult to demonstrate; however, the addition of antacids or alginates to more aggressive therapy continues to be routinely advised. Patients who are minimally symptomatic should be advised to use antacids or alginates, or both, for symptom breakthrough as part of phase I therapy.

Phase II: Pharmacologic therapy

When lifestyle modifications and use of conservative therapies such as antacids and alginates proves unsuccessful, most patients seek medical advice. These patients should be educated and instructed on phase I therapies, but often they require more aggressive pharmacologic treatment for the relief of symptoms and healing of esophageal damage.

As discussed previously, many factors are involved in the pathogenesis of reflux; esophageal damage is most directly related to acid exposure time. Transient LES relaxations, impaired esophageal acid clearance, and reduced epithelial defense mechanisms are all important. Therapies that improve each of these factors have been tested with varied, often disappointing, results. On the other hand, despite the lack of scientific evidence suggesting a role for abnormal acid secretion in the development GERD in most cases, acid suppression is currently the most effective medical treatment. Three classes of agents are currently prescribed for the treatment of GERD: histamine receptor antagonists, prokinetic agents, and proton pump inhibitors.

Histamine receptor antagonists   Since the development and introduction of histamine receptor antagonists in the 1970s, acid suppression has become the principal means of treating peptic diseases, including GERD. Histamine receptor antagonists work to reduce gastric acid production by blocking the histamine receptors located on the basolateral surface of the parietal cells in the stomach. This reversible blockade prevents histamine's activation of the parietal cells and reduces acid production. No effect on LES tone or esophageal acid clearance has been demonstrated with any of these agents. Currently four agents are available for use in the management of GERD (Table 1.9); they are equally effective when equivalent doses are used.

Although histamine blockers have been widely used in the treatment of GERD, the evidence supporting their use has been conflicting. Trials to establish the effective dose of histamine receptor antagonists for treatment of peptic ulcers were performed in the 1970s, but similar trials for the treatment of GERD were not performed. Early studies of histamine receptor antagonists in GERD used doses that were effective for the treatment of duodenal and gastric ulcers and were disappointing. Subsequently, higher doses of these agents were used in clinical trials with improved efficacy, although the rate of healing of esophagitis did not approach that of ulcer healing. In general, symptom relief was achieved in 32% to 82% of patients treated with various doses of histamine receptor antagonists, and esophageal healing was documented in 0% to 83%. Studies have shown a 60% rate of response and 50% rate of healing with use of histamine receptor antagonists.

At a minimum, the doses required for esophageal healing are on the order of 1,200 to 1,600 mg per day of cimetidine (or equivalent), taken in two or three divided doses. Doses of ranitidine as high as 300 mg four times a day have been safely used in trials to effect esophageal healing in a statistically superior manner when compared with conventional doses of ranitidine. Taken as a whole, the use of histamine receptor antagonists is effective, but high doses may be required for effective therapy.

Prokinetic agents   The use of prokinetic agents has not been as rewarding as would be suggested by the obvious role of dysmotility in the pathogenesis of GERD. Their use in the treatment of GERD should be that of a second- or third-line agent, or they may be used in conjunction with histamine receptor antagonists. Cisapride, because of its efficacy and low side-effect profile, is probably the drug of choice when a prokinetic agent is selected.

BETHANECHOL   This agent acts directly at the muscarinic receptor and is not hydrolyzed by the cholinesterases in the synaptic space. The effects at the esophageal level are to increase LES resting tone and to enhance esophageal peristalsis. Clinical trials have been few in number; however, at a dose of 25 mg by mouth four times a day, symptoms of GERD are reduced, and esophagitis begins to heal in 4 weeks. Also, at least one trial has shown bethanechol to be as effective as cimetidine in relieving symptoms and healing esophageal tissue. Side effects such as abdominal cramping, diarrhea, and blurry vision are infrequent and are well tolerated at the doses used for reflux.

METOCLOPRAMIDE   This motility agent also increases the LES tone. Although the mechanism of action of metoclopramide is not known entirely, much of its action is attributed to antagonism of the dopamine pathway. The improvement in gastric emptying seen with the use of this drug is probably the principal mechanism responsible for its efficacy in the treatment of GERD.

Three trials have documented symptomatic improvement without concomitant esophageal healing. When metoclopramide was combined with a histamine H2 receptor antagonist, esophageal healing was significantly improved in one trial, but not in another. In addition, the side effects of metoclopramide make it an unfavorable agent for long-term use. Side effects, including lethargy, fatigue, confusion, and extrapyramidal motor abnormalities, develop in 10% to 30% of patients taking metoclopramide. The combination of inconsistent efficacy and unfavorable side-effect profile restricts the use of metoclopramide to only a few patients, principally those with documented impairment of gastric emptying.

CISAPRIDE   This relatively new agent also works as a promotility agent and enhances both LES tone and gastric emptying by improving acetylcholine release in the myenteric nerves. Esophageal peristalsis is strengthened, thus reducing exposure time to esophageal acid. Symptoms of nocturnal heartburn were reduced by the administration of cisapride alone in one trial. Other trials have shown equal efficacy to the histamine receptor antagonists in healing and symptom relief.

Although the side-effect profile of cisapride is much better than that of metoclopramide, it has significant

TABLE 1.9.   Histamine Receptor Antagonists and Equivalent Doses Used to Treat Gastroesophageal Reflux Disease

Histamine antagonist	Dose (mg/day)[a]
Cimetidine	1,200–1,600
Ranitidine	300
Nizatidine	300
Famotidine	40

[a] Administered in divided doses two or three times daily.

drug-drug interactions that should be reviewed before it is administered.

Proton pump inhibitors   The most effective acid suppressors are the class of drugs known as proton pump inhibitors. These agents diminish gastric acid production by irreversibly binding and permanently inhibiting the apical or secretory surface H+, K+-adenosinetriphosphatase on the gastric parietal cell. These agents effectively reduce acid production by 95%, compared with the 60% to 70% reduction provided by histamine receptor antagonists. Both basal and stimulated acid production are reduced. Currently, omeprazole and lansoprazole are available for use in the United States.

Clinical trials have established the proton pump inhibitors as the single most effective agent for use in the treatment of GERD. In placebo-controlled trials, healing rates of 74% to 88% at 8 weeks and symptom response rates of 80% to 82% were documented. In comparison trials of histamine receptor blockers and omeprazole, omeprazole consistently was more effective at healing esophagitis and relieving symptoms; 74% to 96% of the patients who received omeprazole were completely healed at 8 to 12 weeks, compared with 28% to 66% of those who received histamine receptor antagonists. Also, omeprazole effectively healed esophagitis resistant to histamine receptor antagonists 90% of the time. Similarly, lansoprazole therapy resulted in healing of almost 90% of patients with ranitidine-resistant esophagitis, confirming that the benefits apply to the class of proton pump inhibitors.

The principal concern with these drugs is the possibility of inducing gastric cancer. Gastric acid production is reduced to almost zero, and as a result, gastrin levels rise to 2 to 4 times normal. In theory, the hypergastrinemic state could lead to the development of a gastric carcinoid. In practice, after 10 years of use of proton pump inhibitors, no cases of gastric carcinoid have been reported, except in patients with multiple endocrine neoplastic syndromes. In addition, atrophic gastritis has been linked to the development of gastric adenocarcinoma. Although more than 30% of patients taking omeprazole experienced atrophic gastritis, only those patients with Helicobacter pylori infection seemed to be at risk for gastric adenocarcinoma. Because proton pump inhibitors are singularly effective and well tolerated, they have become first-line therapy for patients with moderate to severe reflux or esophagitis.

Phase III: Antireflux surgery

No consensus exists on who should be offered surgery; however, for patients with severe complications and re-

fractory symptoms, antireflux surgery is an option (Table 1.10).

Patients who continue to have debilitating symptoms or complications of GERD despite aggressive medical therapy with proton pump inhibitors should be considered for an open or laparoscopic fundoplication, with laparoscopic interventions now the preferred method. At surgery, a portion of the cardia is mobilized and wrapped around the distal esophagus to construct a new LES.

In trials of open fundoplication versus phase I therapy or phase II therapy, a significant improvement in esophageal healing and symptom scores was demonstrated in the surgical arm. Although trials comparing laparoscopic fundoplications with aggressive medical therapy are lacking, the short-term success rate in two trials of laparoscopic antireflux surgery was greater than 90%. The long-term success of antireflux surgery is less clear. In a cohort of patients who underwent antireflux laparoscopic procedures and were monitored for up to 5 years, use of medications returned to preoperative levels within 3 years of having the procedure.

Complications are relatively infrequent but include the gas bloat syndrome (described as an inability to belch), dysphagia, splenic trauma, vagal injury, and gastric ulceration. The incidence of dysphagia is reduced by excluding patients with esophageal motor abnormalities demonstrated on preoperative manometric studies.

Indications and Contraindications for Antireflux Surgery   **TABLE 1.10.**

Indications

Anatomically or mechanically defective LES

Failure to heal esophagitis with prolonged PPI therapy (<5% of patients)

Esophageal bleeding or perforation

Refractory extraesophageal complications including asthma and laryngitis

Patient preference, especially in young, healthy patients

Relative contraindications

Patients with substantial comorbid conditions, especially pulmonary disease

Esophageal dysmotility by manometry

Symptoms not known to be conclusively the result of GERD

Lack of surgical expertise with either open or laparoscopic procedures

---

LES, lower esophageal sphincter; PPI, proton pump inhibitors; GERD, gastroesophageal reflux disease.

Follow-Up

GERD is a disease marked by the regular occurrence of relapses in most patients. The concept that maintenance therapy is needed to control symptoms at a reasonable level and to prevent further complications has been accepted as the standard. What is not as clear is the level of maintenance therapy that is required.

In 20% of patients, most with minimal to mild symptoms and no esophageal damage, antacids, alginates, and lifestyle modifications are all that is required. The role of over-the-counter histamine receptor antagonists in such patients has not been established.

For most patients, more aggressive therapy is required for both initial treatment and maintenance. In general, maintenance therapy resembles the therapy used to gain control of symptoms. If a proton pump inhibitor was used to control symptoms and heal esophageal injuries, then it will probably continue to be needed in the maintenance phase. Alternate-day and weekend omeprazole regimens have been ineffective in maintaining remission. Once-daily use of histamine receptor antagonists is similarly ineffective.

The concept of reduced therapy, as in the maintenance phase of peptic ulcer disease, is not valid in these patients.

Treatment of Complications

Esophagitis

If mild esophagitis is noted, management can be achieved with histamine receptor antagonists alone. However, if moderate to severe esophagitis, ulcer, or hemorrhage is noted, the use of proton pump inhibitors is indicated. As discussed previously, the disease is likely to relapse once therapy is discontinued. Maintenance therapy at levels of acid suppression that approach those of the initial therapy is generally required. If esophagitis fails to heal with the use of high-dose proton-pump inhibitors, antireflux surgery is recommended.

Esophageal strictures

The management of benign strictures requires both aggressive acid suppression and esophageal dilation. This conservative medical management is usually effective, although patients may undergo repeated dilations for recurrence of the stricture.

Antireflux surgery and esophageal dilation are also effective in managing esophageal strictures. Esophageal dilation with solid or pneumatic balloon dilators is effective approximately 75% of the time in relieving dysphagia. About 60% of patients with a stricture require repeated dilations for stricture recurrence at an average interval of 1 year. After dilation, stricture recurrence can be reduced by the use of proton pump inhibitors to prevent further esophageal injury.

Barrett's esophagus

The treatment of patients with metaplastic epithelium requires aggressive acid suppression and endoscopic surveillance.

The reflux resulting in Barrett's metaplasia should be regarded as severe, and proton pump inhibitors should be used routinely in addition to the usual lifestyle modifications. The need to document acid suppression and reduced esophageal acid exposure has not been proven. The use of lansoprazole in one trial resulted in a decrease in the area of metaplasia but did not cause complete healing of the metaplasia. Photodynamic ablation after porphyrin administration has been combined with acid suppression to effect squamous reepithelialization. Despite these advances, only esophagectomy results in complete removal of the metaplastic epithelium and abolishes the risk of subsequent adenocarcinoma.

The second part of treatment is endoscopic surveillance for dysplastic changes in the metaplastic epithelium. In a study of patients with high-grade dysplasia, one third developed esophageal adenocarcinoma over the next 5 years. The goal of surveillance is to detect dysplastic lesions and resect the injured esophagus to prevent the development of subsequent malignancy.

Table 1.11 contains the guidelines of the World Health Organization for the endoscopic management of Barrett's esophagus. The required frequency of endoscopic surveillance in cases of nondysplastic epithelium is debated and should be determined in consultation with a gastroenterologist.

Extraesophageal manifestations

Asthma   Although GERD has not been established clearly as a cause of asthma, patients with refractory asthma and GERD should be considered for therapy with proton pump inhibitors or antireflux surgery. To assess the response to therapy, esophageal pH monitoring should also be considered.

Laryngitis   Therapy for the laryngitis requires aggressive acid suppression, usually with proton pump inhibitors. Trials have demonstrated healing of the vocal cord injury with prolonged acid suppression.

REFERRAL

From the preceding discussion, it is clear that most patients with GERD can be managed by a primary care

World Health Organization Guidelines for the Endoscopic Surveillance of Barrett's Esophagus   **TABLE 1.11.**

1. Have an expert in gastrointestinal pathology review questionable samples.
2. No dysplasia
   Repeat endoscopy with biopsy every 18 to 24 months.
3. Low-grade dysplasia
   Treat patient with 12-wk course of PPI and repeat EGD with biopsy.
   If dysplasia persists, repeat EGD with biopsy annually; if not dysplastic after review by expert, resume surveillance as with no dysplasia.
4. High-grade dysplasia
   If good surgical candidate, refer for esophagectomy to experienced surgeon.
   If poor surgical candidate, refer for photochemical ablation.

PPI, proton pump inhibitors; EGD, esophagogastroduodenoscopy.

physician. Some patients require specialist care to manage, diagnose, or treat their reflux.

Referral to a gastroenterologist should be given to those patients who need endoscopy. Indications for endoscopy include diagnosis of atypical GERD, diagnosis and management of peptic complications such as stricture, and evaluation and treatment of patients with refractory GERD.

All patients with a prior history of Barrett's metaplasia should be seen in conjunction with a gastroenterologist.

Referral to an otolaryngologist or pulmonologist is appropriate when extraesophageal complications of GERD are suspected.

Finally, for the patient who does not wish to take medications or the patient with reflux and complications refractory to proton pump inhibitors, consultation with both a gastroenterologist and a general surgeon to coordinate care is appropriate.

KEY POINTS

- Reflux of gastric contents into the esophagus is a common problem that leads thousands of patients to present to their primary care physician annually.

- Although typically a benign disease that primarily impairs the quality of life of the patient, GERD has

the potential to impart significant morbidity and mortality to some. For this reason, the health care provider must become adept at diagnosing and treating the disease and its complications. Most often, diagnostic tests beyond empiric therapy are not needed.

- Because most reflux is mild to moderate in severity, patients can be managed most simply with histamine receptor antagonists or proton pump inhibitors. In addition, the competent health care provider should provide lifestyle modification instructions to all patients.

- Careful follow-up detects those patients whose disease is refractory or who develop complications, such as esophagitis and stricture. It is this group of high-risk patients who most often need referral to specialists for further care.

- The chronicity of the disease, like that of many common health problems (e.g., hypertension), necessitates prolonged therapy. However, with aggressive and effective management, most patients have a significant improvement in quality of life and avoid the complications of reflux.

COMMONLY ASKED QUESTIONS

How long do I have to take this medicine before my heartburn gets better?
You need to take it for at least 2 weeks before you can know if it is going to work. After 2 weeks, I may continue you at the same dose or I may increase the dose. If you are not better after 6 to 8 weeks, I will refer you for an endoscopy or EGD.

Will I have to take this medicine for the rest of my life?
I'm not sure at this point. If your symptoms resolve, I will have you take the medicine for at least 8 weeks before stopping. After stopping their medicine, some patients never have their symptoms again, but many have a relapse later. If you relapse, you are likely to need indefinite therapy to control your disease.

What can I do if I get a bad case of heartburn while I am on this medicine?
You can take one of the over-the-counter antacids. Those medicines tend to work in a few minutes and will not interfere with your prescribed medicine. I do not want you to take any of the over-the-counter acid blockers.

When should I be worried that my reflux is not getting better?
As discussed, I think you will start feeling better in about 2 weeks; if you do not, I need you to call me. Also, if you develop problems swallowing food or liquids or have pain with swallowing, you need to call me.

Do I need any tests to confirm that I have reflux?
No, your response to the acid suppressor is enough of a test. I will order other tests if you do not get better or if you get new symptoms such as difficulty or pain on swallowing.

SUGGESTED READINGS

Allison PR. Peptic ulcer of the esophagus. J Thor Surg 1946;15:308–317.

Bernstein LM, Baker LA. A clinical test for esophagitis. Gastroenterology 1958;34:760–781.

Castell DO. Pathogenesis, diagnosis, therapy. In: Castell DO, Wu WC, Ott DJ. Gastro-esophageal reflux disease. New York: Futura Publishing Company, 1985:3–9.

DeMeester TR, Bonavina L, Albertucci M. Nissen fundoplication for gastroesophageal reflux disease. Ann Surg 1986;204:9–20.

Dent J, Dodds WJ, Hogan WJ, et al. Factors that influence induction of gastroesophageal reflux in normal human subjects. Dig Dis Sci 1988;33:270–275.

DeVault KR, Castell DO. Guidelines for the diagnosis and treatment of gastroesophageal reflux disease. Arch Intern Med 1995;155:2165–2173.

Harding SM, Richter JE, Guzzo MR, Schan CA, Alexander RW, Bradley LA. Asthma and gastroesophageal reflux: acid suppressive therapy improves asthma outcome. Am J Med 1996;100:395–405.

Hewson EG, Sinclair JW, Dalton CB, Richter JE. Twenty-four-hour esophageal pH monitoring: the most useful test for evaluating noncardiac chest pain. Am J Med 1991;90:576–583.

Ireland AC, Holloway RH, Toouli J, Dent J. Mechanisms underlying the antireflux action of fundoplication. Gut 1993;34:303–308.

Isolauri J, Luostarinen M, Isolauri E, et al. Natural course of gastroesophageal reflux disease: 17–22 year follow-up of 60 patients. Am J Gastroenterol 1997;92:37–42.

Kamel PL, Hanson D, Kahrilas PJ. Prospective trial of omeprazole in the treatment of posterior laryngitis. Am J Med 1994;96:321–326.

Klauser AG, Schindlebeck NE, Muller-Lissner SA. Symptoms in gastro-oesophageal reflux disease. Lancet 1990;335:205–208.

Koufmann JA. The otolaryngologic manifestations of gastroesophageal reflux disease (GERD): a clinical investigation of 225 patients using ambulatory 24-hour pH monitoring and an experimental investigation of the role of acid and pepsin in the development of laryngeal injury. Laryngoscope 1991;101:1–64.

Kuipers EJ, Lundell L, Klinkenberg-Knol EC, et al. Atrophic gastritis and Helicobacter pylori infection in patients with reflux esophagitis treated with omeprazole or fundoplication. N Engl J Med 1996;334:1018–1022.

Richter JE, Castell DO. Gastroesophageal reflux: Pathogenesis, diagnosis, and therapy. Ann Int Med 1982; 97:93–103.

Sampliner RE, Jaffe P. Malignant degeneration of Barrett's esophagus: the role of laser ablation and photodynamic therapy. Dis Esophagus 1995;8:104–108.

Schindlebeck NE, Klauser AG, Voderholzer WA, Muller-Lissner SA. Empiric therapy for gastroesophageal reflux disease. Arch Intern Med 1995;155:1808–1812.

Sontag SJ. Gastroesophageal reflux disease. Aliment Phamacol Ther 1993;7:293–312.

Winkelstein A. Peptic esophagitis: a new clinical entity. JAMA 1935;104:906–908.

CHAPTER 2

Peptic Ulcer Disease and the Treatment of *Helicobacter pylori* and NSAID Ulcers

Byron Cryer
University of Texas Southwestern Medical Center and Veterans Administration Medical Center, Dallas, Texas 75216

DEFINITION

A peptic ulcer is a mucosal break of the stomach or duodenum; the term includes both the gastric ulcer and the duodenal ulcer. The manner in which an ulcer manifests symptomatically and its natural history vary according to whether the cause of the ulcer is related to *Helicobacter pylori* or to ingestion of nonsteroidal antiinflammatory drugs (NSAIDs). Therapeutic approaches differ depending on which of these is responsible for the ulcer.

Peptic ulcer disease (PUD) is widely prevalent and affects 10% of the population worldwide at some point in their lives. In the United States, the lifetime prevalence of PUD is about 12% in men and 9% in women, although most of those presentations are asymptomatic. At any point in time, the prevalence of *symptomatic* PUD is about 2%. As seen in Figure 2.1, both gastric and duodenal ulcer incidences increase with advancing age. There are also gender differences; duodenal ulcers are much less common in women, although their incidence is increasing.

CAUSE

In general, gastrointestinal mucosal homeostasis can be maintained by a balance between mucosal defensive

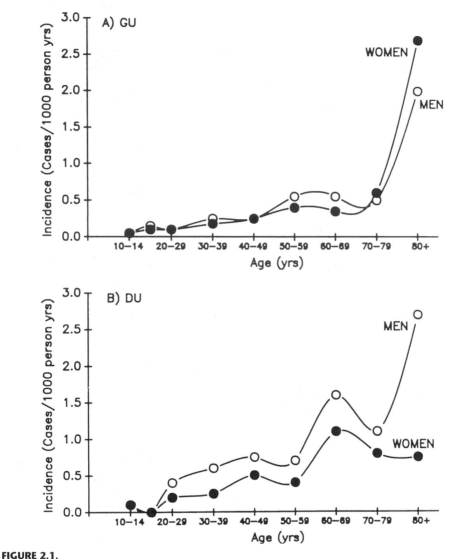

FIGURE 2.1.
(**A**) Gastric ulcer (GU) incidence as a function of age for men and women. (**B**) Duodenal ulcer (DU) incidence as a function of age for men and women. (Adapted from Cryer B, Feldman F. Peptic ulcer disease in the elderly. Semin Gastrointest Dis 1994;5: 166–178.)

mechanisms such as mucus and bicarbonate secretion and aggressive factors such as acid and pepsin secretion. As implied by the name "peptic ulcer," it was originally thought that gastric acid and pepsin secretion were the principal components responsible for the pathogenesis of gastric and duodenal ulcers. However, most duodenal ulcer patients are not hypersecretors of acid, although some people with duodenal ulcers make excessive amounts of gastric acid. Gastric acid is required for peptic ulcer formation, but acid alone rarely causes ulcers. A revised hypothesis for the pathogenesis of PUD is shown in Figure 2.2.

The most common causes of PUD are infection with the bacterium *H. pylori* and use of NSAIDs. Approximately 90% of patients with PUD are infected with *H. pylori* or are taking an NSAID, or both. Through separate mechanisms, as discussed later, *H. pylori* and NSAIDs increase susceptibility to ulceration by compromising mucosal defense mechanisms. The introduction of noxious agents, such as smoking or other corrosive substances, or persistent exposure to endogenous noxious substances such as gastric acid or pepsin, in combination with reduced mucosal defenses, creates a milieu that increases the likelihood of ulceration.

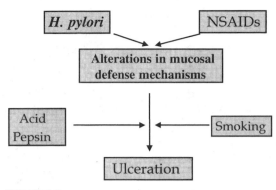

FIGURE 2.2.
Current concept for pathogenesis of peptic ulcer disease.

Helicobacter pylori–Related Ulcers

H. pylori is a gram-negative spiral bacterium that infects gastric-type human epithelium. It is probably the most common chronic bacterial infection in humans. A summary of the current understanding of the pathogenesis of *H. pylori* induced duodenal ulcer is shown in Figure 2.3.

Most patients with gastric colonization by *H. pylori* never develop an ulcer and remain asymptomatic. The lifetime risk for development of a gastric or duodenal ulcer in an asymptomatic, *H. pylori*–infected person who is otherwise healthy is about 15% (1 in 6). Why some of these people develop PUD and others remain healthy is not completely known. Host factors, bacterial factors, or a combination may be involved. It has been suggested that the strains of *H. pylori* from duodenal ulcer patients produce a cytotoxin that increases susceptibility to ulceration. *H. pylori*–infected persons without PUD may have bacterial strains that are nonpathogenic and genetically different from those in ulcer patients. These speculations, however, are controversial.

The claim that *H. pylori* is a cause of PUD is based on two lines of evidence. First, patients with peptic ulcers (duodenal or gastric) have a substantially higher prevalence of *H. pylori* infection compared with age-matched controls. At least 90% of patients with duodenal ulcers have evidence of *H. pylori*, and 50% to 80% of patients with gastric ulcers are infected. Second, when duodenal ulcers are healed by eradication of *H. pylori*, rates of recurrent ulcers are less than 10 %, much lower than when ulcers are healed with acid-suppressive therapy but *H. pylori* is not eradicated. This dramatic reduction in recurrence of peptic ulcer provides the best evidence that *H. pylori* is a major etiologic factor in the development of PUD. These data have led to the recommendation that all ulcer patients undergo testing and treatment for the infection.

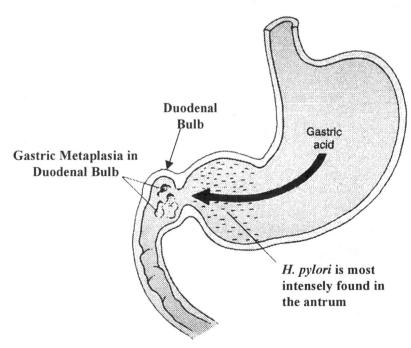

FIGURE 2.3.
Proposed pathogenesis of *Helicobacter pylori*–induced duodenal ulcer.

Incidence

In the United States, up to 60% of asymptomatic people older 60 years of age have evidence of having acquired the infection at some point in their lives. Younger subjects have much lower infection rates; for example, those younger than 30 years have a prevalence rate of 10% to 20%. The risk of *H. pylori* infection is declining in developed countries, as is the risk of PUD. In some Latin American countries, such as Peru and Columbia, the incidence of *H. pylori* infection in asymptomatic adults is as high as 90%. Rates of *H. pylori* infection increase with lower socioeconomic conditions and are higher in African-Americans and Hispanics in the United States.

Method of transmission

Transmission of *H. pylori* appears to occur by direct, person-to-person contact. Fecal-oral, oral-oral, and gastric-oral routes of transmission have been postulated.

Inflammatory response

The organism causes chronic active gastritis, which predominantly affects the gastric antrum but also less intensely affects the gastric body. *H. pylori* is a true pathogen: It elicits a local inflammatory response and a systemic immune response. The exact pathogenic mechanisms by which mucosal infection with *H. pylori* leads to mucosal inflammation and, in some persons, to ulceration are unknown. One hypothesis is that after mucosal colonization by *H. pylori*, inflammation ensues, possibly in response to some chemotactic factors or toxins that are elaborated by the organism. The inflammatory response alone, or in combination with toxins or other damaging agents elaborated by *H. pylori*, may weaken mucosal resistance, thereby increasing the predisposition for ulceration.

Duodenitis

H. pylori can also colonize the duodenal bulb and cause duodenitis. However, *H. pylori* adheres only to ectopic gastric tissue present in the duodenum; this phenomenon, called gastric metaplasia, occurs in approximately 30% of the population. The suspected sequence of events through which gastric metaplasia occurs are shown in Figure 2.4. The current hypothesis is that duodenal gastric metaplasia develops in response to duodenal acid exposure, leading to direct epithelial damage or secondary inflammation. These injured duodenal areas may heal by acquiring gastric epithelium, which may better adapted than duodenal epithelium for acid exposure. After gastric metaplasia has occurred, these areas provide a site for *H. pylori* adherence because there are specific adhesins for *H. pylori* on gastric epithelial cells. Gastric metaplasia can occur in subjects who have not yet been infected with *H. pylori*. When *H. pylori* does colonize gastric metaplastic tissue in the duodenum, it increases the risk for duodenal ulcer.

Increased release of gastrin

H. pylori infection can also result in increases in serum gastrin, an agent that stimulates parietal cell growth and secretion of gastric acid. The degree of acid production resulting from the increased gastrin release is variable

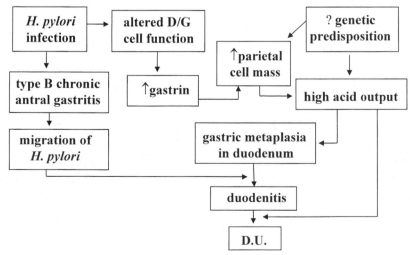

FIGURE 2.4.
Model for development of gastric metaplasia in the duodenal bulb.

and is determined by the subject's sensitivity to gastrin. Patients with duodenal ulcers are characterized by a high sensitivity to gastrin, which explains their marked acid hypersecretion in response to *H. pylori*–induced hypergastrinemia. The specific process by which *H. pylori* causes hypergastrinemia is as follows: Gastrin (produced by antral G cells) is normally inhibited by somatostatin (produced by antral D cells); *H. pylori* infection impairs somatostatin release, thus disinhibiting gastrin.

Ulcers Induced by Nonsteroidal Antiinflammatory Drugs

After *H. pylori*, NSAIDs are the most common cause of PUD. Among patients who take NSAIDs, the incidence of gastric inflammation is no higher than that observed in age-matched controls. Because experimental administration of an NSAID almost never results in histologic gastritis, NSAID use per se is not believed to induce histologic gastritis. However, NSAID exposure frequently causes multiple erosions and hemorrhages of the stomach. These lesions are very commonly seen on endoscopy in persons who take NSAIDs and are asymptomatic. Because these diffuse erosions and hemorrhages are not associated with an increase in histologic inflammation, *gastropathy* is the preferred term to describe the erosive and hemorrhagic gastric effects of NSAIDs.

Epidemiology

It is currently estimated that 33 million Americans commonly use NSAIDs. The major significant adverse effect of NSAIDs is gastrointestinal ulceration. Between 1% and 4% of persons exposed to NSAIDs develop a clinically serious adverse gastrointestinal complication, such as a perforated, bleeding, or obstructing ulcer. Although these percentages are relatively small, the widespread use of NSAIDs results in a considerable number of NSAID-induced ulcer complications every year.

Method of ulceration

There are two principal pathogenic mechanisms by which NSAIDs cause ulceration: reduction of gastrointestinal mucosal prostaglandins and local, topical injury to surface epithelial cells. The former mechanism is the more prevalent.

Prostaglandins, fatty acids produced by almost all of the body's cells, protect against injury in the gastrointestinal tract. NSAIDs inhibit cyclooxygenase (COX), the rate-limiting enzyme in prostaglandin synthesis. Therefore NSAIDs reduce gastroduodenal mucosal

prostaglandin concentrations, resulting in the loss of a major mechanism for protection against mucosal injury and increasing the susceptibility for ulceration. Two COX isoforms exist, COX-I and COX-2. COX-I is the predominate isoform present in the gastrointestinal tract; COX-2 is primarily present at sites of inflammation. In general, NSAIDs that inhibit primarily COX-2 cause less of a reduction in gastrointestinal prostaglandins and probably are associated with lower rates of NSAID-induced ulcers.

Other Causes of Peptic Ulcer Disease

Most cases of PUD are caused by either *H. pylori* or NSAIDs; by some reports they account for up to 90% of ulcers. However, an increasing number of cases are reported that are unrelated to either of causes. In one epidemiologic study, 40% of patients with gastric ulcer, duodenal ulcer, or both tested negative for *H. pylori* and had no reported history of NSAID use. Moreover, some patients are known to have recurrent PUD even after effective anti–*H. pylori* therapy.

Other causes of gastric or duodenal ulcers are listed in Table 2.1. In cases of *H. pylosri*–negative ulcer disease in a patient without a history of NSAID use, these other causes should be considered.

Causes of Gastric or Duodenal Ulcers **TABLE 2.1.**

Very common
  Helicobacter pylori infection
  Nonsteroidal antiinflammatory drugs
Less common
  Gastric malignancy (adenocarcinoma or lymphoma)
  Stress ulceration
  Viral infection (herpes simplex virus type 1 or cytomegalovirus)
Uncommon or rare
  Zollinger-Ellison syndrome
  Cocaine use
  Crohn's disease
  Systemic mastocytosis
  Myeloproliferative disorders with basophilia
  Idiopathic (non–*H. pylori*) hypersecretory duodenal ulcer
  Abdominal radiotherapy
  Hepatic artery infusion of 5-fluorouracil

Malignancy

The possibility of malignancy should always be considered, especially for gastric ulcers. Any gastric ulcer documented by upper gastrointestinal barium study should be endoscopically biopsied.

Ulcers associated with the Zollinger-Ellison syndrome, which is caused by gastrin-secreting islet cell tumors (gastrinomas) driving excessive secretion of gastric acid, are also considered a form of peptic ulcer.

Gastrointestinal ulcers also may occur after abdominal radiotherapy or chemotherapy with hepatic artery infusion of 5-fluorouracil.

Stress ulcers

Stress ulcers usually are gastric ulcers occurring in critically ill patients in intensive care units. These gastric ulcers are typically multiple and shallow and have a tendency to manifest with hematemesis or melena. The cause of stress ulcers is thought to be mucosal ischemia secondary to reduced mesenteric vascular perfusion associated with severe illness.

Viruses

Viral agents, such as herpes simplex type I and cytomegalovirus (CMV), should be suspected in immunocompromised patients and those who have undergone organ transplantation. CMV has been reported in association with PUD in nonimmuncompromised hosts after blood transfusion and in persons with no known predisposing factors.

Cocaine

Gastric, duodenal, and more distal intestinal ulcers have been reported in users of crack cocaine or intranasal cocaine. In these instances, cocaine-induced mesenteric ischemia is the suspected pathophysiologic basis for ulceration.

Crohn's disease and other diseases

Crohn's disease can be associated with ulcers in any gastrointestinal location from the mouth to the anus. However, gastroduodenal ulceration secondary to Crohn's disease is uncommon. When Crohn's disease does involve the stomach and duodenum, it is associated almost always with concurrent terminal ileal disease. Other, less common diseases that are associated with the hypersecretion of gastric acid and that cause gastrointestinal ulcers are systemic mastocytosis, myeloproliferative disorders associated with basophilia, and idiopathic (non–*H. pylori*) hypersecretory duodenal ulcers.

Putative Risk Factors or Causes

Cigarette smoking

In the absence of NSAIDs or *H. pylori*, cigarette smoking does not seem to be a primary risk factor for PUD. However, epidemiologic studies indicate that smokers are at increased risk for both duodenal and gastric ulcers and that this risk is proportional to the amount smoked. Furthermore, smoking impairs ulcer healing, promotes recurrences, and is associated with higher death rates from ulcer disease compared with rates in nonsmokers.

Alcohol

Data suggesting that alcohol is a cause of ulcer disease come mostly from animal studies, in which high concentrations of alcohol were observed to cause gastrointestinal mucosal injury. In humans, the incidence and prevalence of PUD are increased in patients with cirrhosis. However, these relationships appear to correlate with cirrhosis rather than with ethanol consumption. In human studies of volunteers experimentally given high concentrations of alcohol, acute hemorrhage and erosions were observed. There are no convincing data, however, that chronic alcohol use causes chronic peptic ulcer, especially with the ethanol concentrations experienced in social drinking.

Corticosteroids

Evidence suggests that corticosteroids alone do not increase the risk of PUD. However, when corticosteroids are taken in combination with NSAIDs, the risk of PUD is greatly increased over the risk with NSAIDs alone.

Diet

Although many foods, beverages, and spices cause dyspepsia, there is no evidence that any specific food causes ulcers. Moreover, there is no good evidence to suggest that a bland diet or a dairy-rich diet is useful in the treatment of peptic ulcers.

Psychological status

The role of psychological factors in PUD remains controversial. In contrast to earlier hypotheses regarding the impact of psychological profiles on ulcer pathogenesis, there is no typical personality that predisposes to PUD. However, chronic anxiety and psychological stress may be factors that exacerbate ulcer activity.

Hyperpepsinogenemia

In the older literature, PUD in childhood and familial clusterings of ulcers were believed to reflect an inherited form of hyperpepsinogenemia. However, in light of what is now known about *H. pylori*, most of these cases were probably consequences of high rates of *H. pylori* transmission within families and organism acquisition during early childhood. Among children with duodenal ulcer, *H. pylori* is found in more than 80%, compared with a 10% seroprevalence in children without ulcer disease.

PATIENT PRESENTATION

Typical clinical presentations of PUD are shown in Table 2.2. Although the listed symptoms are classic manifestations of PUD, there is wide variation in the clinical presentation.

History

The uncomplicated peptic ulcer most commonly manifests with abdominal pain. The pain is usually in the epigastrium (upper middle portion of the abdomen), is rhythmic in nature, and often is described as burning, sharp, or gnawing. However, it may also be characterized as vague abdominal discomfort; nausea; a deep, ill-defined, boring or aching pain; abdominal pressure or fullness; or a hunger sensation. The pain occurs 1 to 3 hours after meals, at night, or at other times when the stomach is empty. At times, it awakens the patient from sleep. Food and antacids usually relieve the pain of uncomplicated ulcers for a short period. However, the pain usually returns in 30 to 60 minutes.

Episodes of pain may persist for several days to weeks or months. Patients commonly have a history of self-treatment with antacids, frequent and long-standing use of histamine (H2)–receptor antagonists, and/or cigarette smoking. Although symptoms tend to be recurrent and episodic, ulcers often recur in the absence of pain. Periods of remission usually last from weeks to years and are almost always longer than the episodes of pain. In some patients, however, the disease is more aggressive, with frequent and persistent symptoms or development of complications.

Children

Children with PUD present with atypical manifestations, such as higher rates of nocturnal pain and increased initial presentations with gastrointestinal bleeding.

The elderly

The increasing incidence of PUD with advancing age reflects an increased prevalence of *H. pylori* infection and NSAID consumption with age. Elderly patients have increased initial PUD presentations of complicated ulcers (bleeding and perforated) that previously were asymptomatic. This phenomenon is probably attributable to the greater use of NSAIDs in this population. In addition to increased NSAID consumption with age, older age itself is thought to increase the risk for NSAID-induced ulcer complications. Therefore, the decision to prescribe NSAIDs for older patients should be carefully considered. The high PUD morbidity and mortality in older populations probably reflects the increased number of comorbid diseases as well as increased numbers of ulcer complications.

Pregnant women

The observation that the seroprevalence of *H. pylori* in pregnant women is no different than in the general population suggests that ulcer prevalence should be the same in pregnant and nonpregnant women. However, epidemiologically, PUD is reported less frequently in pregnant women than in age-matched female controls.

One explanation for this finding may be decreased evaluations of symptoms of PUD in pregnant women, rather than an actual decrease in disease incidence. In these patients, there is a tendency to treat upper gastrointestinal symptoms empirically rather than to perform diagnostic tests such as barium x-ray or endoscopic studies. The symptoms of PUD in pregnant women are no different than ulcer symptoms experienced by nonpregnant ulcer patients. However, the dyspepsia of PUD during pregnancy may be confused with or attributed to other gastrointestinal problems that are common during pregnancy, such as nausea, vomiting, or gastroesophageal reflux disease (GERD) (see Differential Diagnosis).

Physical Examination

On physical examination, epigastric tenderness is the most frequent finding. The area of tenderness is usually in the midline, often midway between the umbilicus and the xiphoid process. In approximately 20% of patients, the tender area is to the right of midline.

Presentation of Uncomplicated Peptic Ulcer Disease	TABLE 2.2.

Burning, sharp, or deep epigastric pain 1 to 3 hours after eating

Vague abdominal discomfort or nausea rather than pain

Relief of symptoms by eating or taking antacids

Occurrence of symptoms when the stomach is empty or at night

History of self-treatment with antacids, frequent and longstanding use of H_2-receptor antagonists, and/or cigarette smoking

Symptoms recurring over months or years

Epigastric tenderness on palpation (with active symptomatic ulcers)

Complications

In many persons, peptic ulceration is asymptomatic, and the first presentation is with a complication. This type of clinical presentation of PUD is particularly prevalent in elderly patients.

The most common ulcer complications are bleeding, perforation, and obstruction.

Bleeding

Bleeding ulcers are commonly manifested by black stools. Rarely, peptic ulcers chronically bleed, causing severe iron deficiency anemia or occult blood in the stools.

Perforation

Severe, sudden abdominal pain, often associated with shock, suggests acute perforation of an ulcer, complicated by peritonitis. On examination, a perforated ulcer usually manifests as a rigid, board-like abdomen, typically with generalized rebound tenderness. Auscultation of the abdomen initially may reveal hyperactive bowel sounds; with clinical progression, these may diminish or disappear.

Obstruction

The principal symptoms of obstruction are nausea, vomiting, and early satiety. The vomiting tends to occur 30 to 60 minutes after a meal. Patients with obstruction frequently remain satiated for many hours after a meal. Ulcers that cause obstruction usually are located in the pyloric channel or duodenal bulb, areas where the gastrointestinal lumen naturally narrows to small diameters. With acute ulceration, there is local swelling in these narrowed areas, leading to gastric outlet obstruction and delayed passage of gastric contents. On examination, patients with gastric outlet obstruction caused by a pyloric channel or duodenal ulcer may have a succussion splash produced by retained fluid and air within a distended stomach. As the acute ulceration is treated, the swelling resolves and the obstructive symptoms in many instances subside.

DIAGNOSIS

The primary indication for testing for *H. pylori* infection is to identify cases one would treat.

If early endoscopy is not called for (as discussed later in this section) in the dyspeptic patient, NSAIDs should be stopped if they are being taken. If there is no current NSAID use, or if symptoms persist after cessation of NSAIDs, the possibility of an *H. pylori* infection should be evaluated by a serologic test. If the test is positive, *H. pylori* infection should be treated. If *H. pylori* infection

is not present by serology, empiric therapy for nonulcer dyspepsia should be given, and symptoms persisting after empiric therapy should be evaluated by endoscopy.

Reasonable clinical scenarios indicating a need to test for *H. pylori* include the following:

- History of PUD or ulcer complication
- Family history of gastric cancer in a first-degree relative
- Dyspepsia evaluation in a patient suspected to have PUD (Fig. 2.5 provides an algorithm for the workup of dyspeptic patients)

The decision to test for the organism should be based on the assumption that the patient will be treated if test results are positive. As discussed earlier, the diagnosis of PUD during pregnancy is difficult owing partly to the overlap in symptoms with GERD and partly to a reluctance to perform diagnostic procedures on pregnant patients. Many of the medicines used in *H. pylori* eradication regimens have adverse fetal effects; therefore, there is no reason to evaluate for *H. pylori* during pregnancy, because it would not be prudent to prescribe some of the medicines required to treat the infection.

Given the number of tests available to assess for *H. pylori*, the choice of an appropriate diagnostic test can be confusing. One approach that may be useful is shown in Table 2.3.

Endoscopic Studies

The first clinical decision to make when there is a high suspicion of PUD is to determine whether endoscopy should be performed as the initial diagnostic test. Any positive findings on endoscopy should be specifically treated; if the endoscopy is negative, the patient should be empirically treated for nonulcer dyspepsia.

The decision regarding endoscopy is based on whether the patient has any findings that might suggest the possibility of gastric malignancy or an ulcer complication (i.e., "alarm features"). These features are listed in Table 2.4 and include new-onset symptoms after the age of 50 years, anorexia, dysphagia, gross or occult gastrointestinal bleeding, unexplained anemia, weight loss, significant vomiting, or a upper gastrointestinal barium study with findings suspicious for cancer. If any of these alarm symptoms are present, the patient should be referred for early endoscopy (Fig. 2.5).

Laboratory Tests

A variety of tests are available to diagnose *H. pylori*. They can be divided into those that do not require endoscopy (noninvasive tests) and those that do require endoscopy

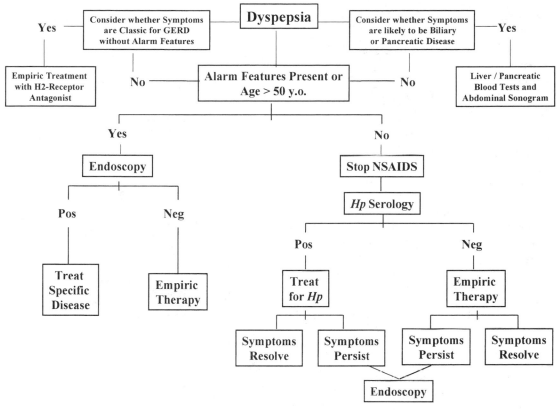

FIGURE 2.5.

Algorithm for evaluation of dyspepsia.

(invasive tests). All of these tests have reasonably high sensitivity and specificity, but they differ in cost and in the clinical scenarios in which each might be appropriately used. The available diagnostic tests, along with their sensitivities, specificities, and costs, are shown in Table 2.5. Estimated costs for the invasive tests do not include the cost of endoscopy. When endoscopic costs are considered, the invasive tests become extremely expensive methods to test for *H. pylori*.

Serologic tests

A number of serologic tests that detect antibodies to *H. pylori* have been approved by the U.S. Food and Drug Administration. These tests are most useful for screening

Use of Diagnostic Tests for Detection of *Helicobacter pylori* Infection	**TABLE 2.3.**
Clinical setting	**Diagnostic test**
New ulcer, recurrent ulcer, or history of peptic ulcer disease	Serology or urea breath test
Complicated peptic ulcer disease	Endoscopy with histology
Follow-up after *H. pylori* therapy	Wait 4 wk, then urea breath test or endoscopy for histology
Patient undergoing endoscopy for another indication	Rapid urease testing or histology
Compliant patient with several treatment failures	Endoscopy, histology, culture and susceptibility testing

TABLE 2.4.	Alarm Features: Indications for Early Endoscopy

New-onset symptoms after 50 years of age
Anorexia
Dysphagia
Gross or occult gastrointestinal bleeding
Unexplained anemia
Weight loss
Significant vomiting
Upper gastrointestinal barium study suspicious for cancer

TABLE 2.5. Diagnostic Tests for *Helicobacter pylori* Infection

Test	Sensitivity (%)	Specificity (%)	Estimated cost ($)
Noninvasive tests			
Antibody tests			
Office	90	90	15
Laboratory	90	95	75
Urea breath test	95	98	200
Invasive tests			
Rapid urease tests	90	98	10[a]
Histology	95	99	150[a]
Culture	80	100	150[a]

[a] Does not include cost of endoscopy.
Estimates provided by the American Digestive Health Foundation, Inc., Bethesda, MD., 1996. From Soll AH.

of patients who are of unknown *H. pylori* status and who have not been previously treated with anti–*H. pylori* therapies.

All of the available serologic tests measure serum immunoglobulin G (IgG) and are sensitive, specific, and relatively inexpensive. No available test assesses IgA or IgM because both are relatively poor predictors of the presence or absence of *H. pylori* infection. Office-based serum antibody tests are slide kits that yield rapid results and are easy to perform. Their accuracy is almost as good as that of the laboratory-based (send-out) tests. Further, the office-based tests have a much lower cost. Office-based serologic kits that use whole blood rather than serum are also available, but they are not as accurate as antibody tests that use serum. Preliminary results from saliva and urine antibody tests suggest that their sensitivity and specificity are inferior to those of the serum IgG antibody tests.

Urea breath tests

One unique aspect of *H. pylori* is that it possess the enzyme urease, which helps it adapt to the hostile gastric environment. Urease metabolizes urea to ammonia and carbon dioxide. Because urease activity is not normally present in the human stomach, its presence is a sensitive and specific indicator of the presence of *H. pylori*. Two tests for *H. pylori*, the urea breath test and the rapid urease assay, indirectly test for the presence of *H. pylori* through assessment of urease activity.

Diagnosis of *H. pylori* by the urea breath test is based on urease metabolism of ingested urea. A urea solution labeled with either carbon 13 or carbon 14 is taken by mouth; 13C is a nonradioactive carbon isotope, and 14C is radioactive. If *H. pylori* is present, urea is metabolized to ammonia and carbon-labeled carbon dioxide. The labeled carbon dioxide is then excreted in breath, collected, and quantified. Both the 13C and the 14C tests are currently clinically available. The breath test is an excellent

noninvasive test, both for identifying the presence of active infection and for confirming the eradication of the organism 1 month or longer after antibiotic therapy.

Rapid urease tests

Another indirect test for *H. pylori*, the rapid urease test, is also based on metabolism of urea by urease. In this test, an endoscopically obtained mucosal biopsy specimen is inoculated into a well that contains urea and a pH-sensitive dye. If urease is present in the biopsy sample, urea in the medium is converted to ammonium ion ($NH4+$), which raises the pH and causes a color change. Although the accuracy of this test is high, it requires endoscopy and therefore is expensive. Its usefulness is speed: It can provide an answer regarding *H. pylori* status in minutes to several hours, generally before a histologic evaluation would be reported by a pathologist. Also, the cost of the rapid urease test is usually much lower than fees to have a biopsy processed for histology and evaluated by a pathologist. The greatest use of the rapid urease test is for patients who are already undergoing upper endoscopy for another indication, during which a biopsy can be obtained for this test at little additional cost (approximately $10).

Histology

Mucosal biopsy and histologic examination of the specimen for the presence of *H. pylori* and/or gastritis is the "gold standard" test for the assessment of *H. pylori*. To maximize the diagnostic yield, it is recommended that at least two biopsies from the antrum and one from the body of the stomach be submitted to the pathologist. The standard hematoxylin and eosin stain is an excellent stain to evaluate gastritis and, if enough organisms are present, to demonstrate *H. pylori*. Special stains can be used if there is a question as to whether the organism is present.

Histology as a method to diagnose *H. pylori* is associated with the disadvantages of the other invasive tests. This test is best employed for patients who are already undergoing endoscopy.

Culture of biopsies

The benefits of culturing gastric mucosal biopsies obtained at endoscopy include accurate identification of the organism (100% specificity) and the opportunity to perform antibiotic sensitivity testing on isolates, in the rare instance that this need arises. The drawbacks of culture are that the organism is difficult to grow, the culture procedure is not reliably reproducible, it requires laboratory expertise, it is not widely available, and it is relatively expensive. Moreover, culture and sensitivity testing delay diagnosis for 3 to 5 days.

H. pylori culture testing is not recommended for most clinical situations. *H. pylori* culture and sensitivity testing are most appropriately used in patients for whom previous courses of *H. pylori* eradication regimens have failed or when there is a question of antibiotic resistance.

Radiologic Studies

There are limited roles for radiologic studies in patients known to have active ulcer disease. When ulcers of the stomach or duodenum are suspected to be secondary to Crohn's disease, a barium enema and a small intestinal barium x-ray study should be performed to evaluate the rest of the small intestine and colon for evidence of disease. Eight weeks after initiation of treatment for active

gastric ulcers, an upper gastrointestinal barium x-ray or endoscopic study should be performed to confirm ulcer healing.

Differential Diagnosis

Differentiating types of ulcers

Clinical manifestations of NSAID-induced ulcers vary from those of *H. pylori*–related ulcers in several ways (Table 2.6). In persons who develop ulcers in association with NSAID use, gastric ulcers are about twice as likely as duodenal ones. With *H. pylori*–induced ulcers, duodenal lesions are much more common. NSAID-induced ulcers are much less frequently associated with chronic active gastritis than are *H. pylori*–related ulcers.

In contrast to *H. pylori*–related ulcers, NSAID ulcers are most commonly asymptomatic. This can be especially problematic because the first manifestation of ulcer disease in asymptomatic patients may be bleeding or perforation. Among patients who present with bleeding ulcers, those who have been using NSAIDs are more than twice as likely to have been asymptomatic before presentation than those with no history of NSAID use (i.e., *H. pylori*–related ulcer patients). In a survey of ulcer patients conducted in 1998, only one in five of those with NSAID-induced ulcer complications had antecedent warning symptoms.

A final difference between NSAID-induced and *H. pylori*–related ulcers is in the nature of their recurrence. When NSAID use is discontinued, NSAID ulcers do not recur. In contrast, *H. pylori*–related ulcers have a recurrence rate of 50% to 80% within 1 year if the organism is not eradicated by antibiotics.

Other diseases

Most patients with PUD present with dyspepsia or other upper gastrointestinal symptoms. The differential diagnosis of these symptoms includes NSAID-induced or *H. pylori*–related PUD, GERD, and nonulcer dyspepsia. Biliary tract disease (in particular, cholelithiasis

Differences between NSAID-Induced and *Helicobacter pylori*–Induced Ulcers		**TABLE 2.6.**
Characteristic	**NSAID-Induced**	***H. pylori*-Induced**
Site of damage	Gastric twice as often as duodenal	Duodenal more often than gastric
Histology	Surrounding mucosa normal (no increase in gastritis)	Surrounding mucosa inflamed (chronic active gastritis and duodenitis)
Symptoms	More often asymptomatic	Usually pain and/or dyspepsia
Pattern of recurrence	Does not recur if NSAID is stopped	Recurs if *H. pylori* is not eradicated

NSAID, nonsteroidal antiinflammatory drug.

and cholecystitis), pancreatitis, and cancer also must be considered (Table 2.7).

GERD is usually suggested by the classic symptoms of substernal heartburn and pyrosis, which are exacerbated postprandially and by recumbency. If these classic GERD symptoms are present and no other concerning symptoms are present (Table 2.4), H2-receptor antagonist therapy should be begun empirically.

Nonulcer dyspepsia

The diagnosis of nonulcer dyspepsia (or functional dyspepsia) usually is made after negative diagnostic evaluations for PUD in patients in whom symptoms persist after empiric therapy. The category comprises various distinct gastric disorders that cause upper gastrointestinal symptoms and includes gastric dysmotility, gastroparesis, and delayed gastric emptying (seen in patients with diabetic mellitus, some rheumatic or connective tissue diseases, or certain neurologic conditions). Signs and symptoms of nonulcer dyspepsia include epigastric fullness and discomfort, belching, bloating, nausea, and food intolerance (Table 2.8).

If the patient's risk factors and clinical presentation suggest a high likelihood of biliary tract or pancreatic disease, the first diagnostic tests should be liver and pancreatic blood tests and abdominal sonography. If the patients' symptoms are not classic for GERD or biliary or pancreatic disease, the possibility of PUD needs to be seriously considered, especially because there is a high degree of overlap in the clinical manifestations of these diseases (Fig. 2.5).

Pregnant patients

GERD is very common during pregnancy, occurring in up to 50% of pregnant patients. The differential diag-

TABLE 2.7.   Differential Diagnosis of Dyspepsia

Peptic ulcer disease
  Related to infection with *Helicobacter pylori*
  Related to use of nonsteroidal antiinflammatory
    drugs
Gastroesophageal reflux disease
Biliary tract disease
  Cholelithiasis
  Cholecystitis
Pancreatitis
Cancer
Nonulcer dyspepsia

TABLE 2.8.   Nonulcer Dyspepsia

Disease associations

Specific diseases
  Gastric dyskinesia
  Diabetes mellitus
  Gastroparesis
  Rheumatic diseases and connective tissue diseases
  Delayed gastric emptying
  Hypothyroidism
  Certain neurologic diseases
Symptoms
  Epigastric fullness and discomfort
  Belching
  Bloating
  Nausea
  Food intolerance

Specific symptom-directed therapy

Dyspepsia: H_2-RA or proton pump inhibitor
Belching and gas: simethicone
Gastroparesis-like symptoms: prokinetic agent
  (cisapride or metoclopramide)

H_2RA, H_2-receptor antagonist (cimetidine, famotidine, nazatidine, or ranitidine); PPI, proton pump inhibitor (lansoprazole or omeprazole).

nosis of upper gastrointestinal symptoms during pregnancy includes PUD, GERD, the nausea and vomiting of pregnancy, hyperemesis gravidarum, pancreatitis, acute cholecystitis, viral hepatitis, appendicitis, and acute fatty liver of pregnancy (in late pregnancy) (Table 2.9).

MANAGEMENT

In the past, the initial treatment of almost all ulcers was similar (i.e., acid-suppressive or-neutralizing therapies). Current therapeutic approaches have been modified. First, the physician should determine the underlying cause of the PUD—*H. pylori*, NSAIDs, or the other, less common associations. Therapy is then specifically directed toward the suspected cause.

Helicobacter pylori–Related Ulcers

Treatment

If *H. pylori* testing (whether serologic or endoscopic biopsy) is positive, antibiotics in combination with acid-suppressive therapy should be administered for 14 days. Cure of the *H. pylori* infection facilitates ulcer healing and decreases the ulcer recurrence rate. Numerous studies

Summary of Diagnosis

- Dyspepsia is the most common presenting symptom of PUD.
- Most PUD is associated with *H. pylori* or use of NSAIDs.
- Very young and elderly patients commonly have asymptomatic PUD or atypical presentations.
- As a first diagnostic step, it is important to determine whether dyspepsia is a consequence of PUD, GERD, or biliary or pancreatic disease.
- If PUD is suspected as a cause for dyspepsia, the patient should be assessed for the presence of alarm features (Table 2.4).
- Patients who either have alarm features or are 50 years of age or older should be referred for endoscopy.
- If the patient has no alarm features and is younger than 50 years of age, use of NSAIDs should be stopped, *H. pylori* should be sought by serology, and, if the result is positive, the infection should be treated.
- All patients with active ulcers or a history of ulcers should be tested for *H. pylori,* including patients with inactive ulcers who are currently asymptomatic.

Differential Diagnosis of Dyspepsia during Pregnancy	TABLE 2.9.

Peptic ulcer disease
Gastroesophageal reflux disease
Nausea and vomiting of pregnancy
Hyperemesis gravidarum
Pancreatitis
Acute cholecystitis
Viral hepatitis
Appendicitis
Acute fatty liver of pregnancy (in late pregnancy)

have confirmed that once *H. pylori* eradication therapy has been successfully completed, reinfection occurs in fewer than 1% of patients per year.

Regimens   Cure of *H. pylori* infection is not easy and requires combinations of one or two antibiotics with one or two nonantibiotic adjunctive agents. Single agents are ineffective. From the various combination therapies have been used in the attempted eradication of *H. pylori,* eight commonly used regimens have been selected for comparison in Table 2.10. There is no "gold standard" regimen. The choice of *H. pylori* treatment should be based on a combination of factors that include reported eradication rate, frequency of dosing, patient compliance with the regimen, previous antibiotic exposure, and *H. pylori* antibiotic resistance.

Selecting an **H. pylori** *eradication regimen*   In selecting an *H. pylori* eradication regimen for a given patient, the following key points should be considered.

Side effects   Side effects are generally mild, and patient withdrawal from therapy because of side effects is uncommon (1% to 4%). Common side effects of the anti–*H. pylori* therapies include nausea (most common), diarrhea (usually mild), diarrhea secondary to pseudomembranous colitis (very rare), skin rash (associated mostly with amoxicillin), taste disturbance (associated mostly with clarithromycin), black stools (commonly seen with bismuth), and monilial vaginitis (commonly seen with tetracycline).

Side effects are more common when metronidazole is given at a dose of more that 1 g per day (nausea) or when clarithromycin is given at a dose of more than 1 g per day (taste disturbance).

Follow-up

Therapy is successful in approximately 80% to 90% of treated patients, and for most patients a follow-up diagnostic test is not required. Because PUD is a recurrent disease, patients in whom *H. pylori* was not successfully eradicated declare themselves by symptomatic recurrences, at which time endoscopy should be performed. Persistent symptoms after treatment should also be evaluated by endoscopy.

Although confirmation of eradication is not needed for most patients, it may be prudent in patients who have had complications of an *H. pylori*–related ulcer. In such patients, however, the effectiveness cannot reliably be determined until at least 4 weeks after therapy is complete. The urea breath test is the most reliable, noninvasive way to assess successful eradication. If urea breath testing is not available, the only reliable alternative follow-up test is an endoscopy to obtain gastric mucosal biopsies. Because antibody serologic tests remain positive for months to years after treatment of *H. pylori* infection, they are not a practical way to determine whether the organism has been successfully eradicated.

KEY POINTS

- Although a cure rate of 80% was once considered acceptable, rates of 90% or higher are now achievable, especially if the organism is susceptible to the antibiotics used.

- Compliance is important for the successful cure of the infection, and regimens with less frequent dosing and fewer side effects may have increased compliance.

- Successful cure of the infection requires at least two agents (dual therapy). If one week of therapy is desired, three or four agents are needed.

- All successful regimens include clarithromycin or metronidazole, or both.

- H. pylori resistance to metronidazole or clarithromycin may lead to reduced efficacy; antibiotic resistance can be assumed if the patient has had previous exposure to metronidazole or clarithromycin.

- In general, if one of the proton pump inhibitors (lansoprazole or omeprazole) is not available in a formulary listing, the other may be substituted without a reduction in efficacy.

Nonsteroidal Antiinflammatory Drug-Induced Ulcers

When an ulcer is thought to have been induced by NSAIDs, a different therapeutic approach is needed. Therapy for NSAID-induced ulcers should be tailored according to whether one is attempting to heal or to prevent NSAID-induced ulcers and whether NSAIDs can be discontinued.

Treatment

Initial treatment of NSAID-induced ulcers is to stop the NSAID use and to search for and treat *H. pylori*, if it

TABLE 2.10.   Selected Regimens for Treatment of *Helicobacter pylori* Infection

Therapy	Drug 1	Drug 2	Drug 3	FDA-approved	Treatment efficacy (%)
Quadruple[a]	Tetracycline, 500 mg q.i.d. for 2 wk	Metronidazole, 250 mg q.i.d. for 2 wk	Bismuth subsalicylate, 2 tablets q.i.d. for 2 wk	Yes	>90[b]
Triple	Clarithromycin, 250 mg b.i.d. for 2 wk[c]	Metronidazole, 500 mg b.i.d. for 2 wk[c]	Omeprazole, 20 mg b.i.d. for 2 wk[c]	No	>90[d,e]
Triple	Clarithomycin, 500 mg b.i.d. for 2 wk	Amoxicillin, 1 g b.i.d. for 2 wk	Lansoprazole, 30 mg b.i.d. for 2 wk	Yes	>90[d]
Triple	Clarithomycin, 500 mg b.i.d. for 2 wk	Amoxicillin, 1 g b.i.d. for 2 wk	Omeprazole, 20 mg b.i.d. for 2 wk	No	80–95[d]
Dual	Clarithromycin, 500 mg t.i.d. for 2 wk	Omeprazole[f], 20 mg b.i.d. for 2 wk	—	Yes	70–85[d]
Dual	Clarithromycin, 500 mg t.i.d. for 2 wk	Ranitidine bismuth citrate, 400 mg b.i.d. for 4 wk	—	Yes	70–80[d]
Dual	Amoxicillin, 1 g t.i.d. for 2 wk	Lansoprazole, 30 mg t.i.d. for 2 wk	—	Yes	70–80
Dual	Amoxicillin, 1 g t.i.d. for 2 wk	Omeprazole, 20 mg b.i.d. for 2 wk	—	No	35–60

[a] Also requires H$_2$-receptor antagonist b.i.d. for 4 wk.
[b] Efficacy is <70% if *H. pylori* is resistant to metronidazole.
[c] Can also be dosed for 1 week.
[d] Efficacy lower if *H. pylori* is resistant to clarithromycin.
[e] Efficacy lower if *H. pylori* is resistant to metronidazole.
[f] 40 mg daily for 2 wk, then 20 mg daily for 2 wk.

is present. Once the NSAID has been stopped, standard healing doses (twice a day) of any of the H2-receptor antagonists (cimetidine, famotidine, nizatidine, ranitidine) should be prescribed.

Complete NSAID withdrawal may not be possible in all patients, but they may tolerate a reduction in NSAID dose. In cases in which NSAIDs must be continued, a proton pump inhibitor (omeprazole 40 mg daily or lansoprazole 30 mg daily) should be prescribed for 8 weeks to allow ulcer healing.

Prevention

The initial approach to prevention of NSAID-induced ulcers involves identifying persons who are at greatest risk for NSAID-related ulceration (Table 2.11). Patients with a previous history of complicated peptic ulcers and those taking corticosteroids or anticoagulants are considered to be at high risk for NSAID-induced ulcers. Some elderly patients and some patients with comorbid diseases such as functionally compromising heart or lung disease may also be in this category. Patients taking high doses of NSAIDs or combinations of more than one NSAID should also be considered to be at high risk.

Alternative analgesia   If only analgesia is desired, it may be prudent to initiate therapy with acetaminophen, another nonnarcotic analgesic, or a nonacetylated salicylate. However, many patients, especially those with inflammatory disease, require potentially ulcerogenic NSAIDs, in which case the lowest therapeutic antiinflammatory dose should be started. If the NSAID-taking patient has significant risk factors for NSAID-induced ulceration, the clinician should consider prophylaxis with a coadministered agent.

Misoprostol   Although misoprostol is the only drug currently approved for the prevention of NSAID-induced ulcers, it is poorly tolerated by many patients. The principal side effect is dose-related diarrhea at the induction of therapy. Patients who are candidates for prophy-

laxis should initially be given a low dose of misoprostol (100 μg four times daily), with incremental increases to 200 μg four times daily as tolerated.

The combination therapy of diclofenac plus misoprostol (Arthrotec)   This is proposed as a means to increase patient compliance with therapy; the prophylactic component is delivered with the NSAID, which the patient is motivated to take to achieve analgesia or to reduce inflammation.

Proton pump inhibitors   These agents have been reported to be as efficacious as misoprostol and more effective than an H2-receptor antagonist for prevention of NSAID-induced ulcers. Certainly, for patients who are unable to tolerate misoprostol or who develop NSAID-induced ulcers while taking misoprostol or an H2-receptor antagonist, proton pump inhibitors are the only alternative. Because the cost of prophylaxis with a proton pump inhibitor may be a factor in the selection of a prophylaxis regimen, it should be kept in mind that NSAID-induced ulcers can effectively be prevented with omeprazole at 20 mg per day (the lowest available daily dose).

COX-2 inhibitors   Two new drugs that selectively inhibit COX-2, celecoxib and rofacoxib, have recently been approved for human use. They appear to be effective antiinflammatory and analgesic agents with few gastrointestinal side effects. These agents may offer another therapeutic alternative to reduce ulcer rates associated with NSAIDs.

Follow-up

Patients who have continuously taken NSAIDs during the period of ulcer healing or those who need to restart previously discontinued NSAID therapy should have follow-up studies to document healing of NSAID-induced gastric ulcers and, in some instances, NSAID-induced duodenal ulcers. Among patients with NSAID-induced duodenal ulcers, those who do not require resumption of their NSAIDs do not require follow-up endoscopy to document ulcer healing.

Asymptomatic Ulcers

One must consider the appropriate course of therapy for a patient with a history of ulcer disease but whose ulcers are currently inactive and asymptomatic. A National Institutes of Health consensus conference in 1994 recommended that all patients with ulcer disease, including those taking NSAIDs and those with a history of ulcer disease, be tested for *H. pylori* infection and be treated if the infection is present.

High-risk Groups for NSAID-Induced Ulcers	TABLE 2.11.

History of peptic ulcer
Age 75 years or older
History of heart disease
High doses of NSAIDs
Combinations of more than 1 NSAID
Concomitant anticoagulant use
Concomitant use of corticosteroids

NSAID, nonsteroidal antiinflammatory drug.

Treatment of Pregnant Patients

The treatment approach to PUD in pregnancy differs from that in nonpregnant patients because of the adverse fetal effects of the medicines used to treat *H. pylori*.

Most pregnant patients with symptoms of PUD can be managed conservatively; symptoms improve or resolve in 90%. Fatty foods, caffeine, alcohol, and nicotine should be avoided because they exacerbate symptoms. Pregnant patients whose suspected PUD does not respond to conservative management with diet and lifestyle modifications should be treated empirically rather than be exposed to the potential risks of diagnostic procedures.

Antacids and sucralfate appear to be safe during pregnancy. These agents should be the initial drugs of choice when more conservative measures have failed. Animal studies show no teratogenic effects from constant ingestion of antacids during pregnancy. Adverse effects of antacids during pregnancy include interference with iron absorption. When sodium bicarbonate is used as an antacid, metabolic alkalosis and fluid overload may occur in both the fetus and the mother. Antacids that contain simethicone should be avoided because use of simethicone during the first trimester in humans has been associated with birth defects. Because sucralfate is not absorbed, it is generally considered to be safe during pregnancy.

For patients who continue to be symptomatic, H2-receptor antagonists may be used in the second or third trimester. Most clinical experience with H2-receptor antagonists during pregnancy has been with ranitidine and cimetidine; ranitidine is preferred because it lacks the antiandrogenic properties of cimetidine. Omeprazole, when given in very high doses to pregnant animals, produces dose-related fetal toxicity. Human data on the fetal safety of omeprazole administration early in pregnancy is not established. Therefore, omeprazole should be considered unsafe for use in pregnancy until information to the contrary is available.

Nonulcer Dyspepsia

After numerous prospective clinical trials, there is no conclusive evidence to suggest that most cases of nonulcer dyspepsia are related to *H. pylori* infection; the frequency of *H. pylori* infection in dyspeptic patients is similar to its frequency in asymptomatic persons. Nevertheless, in addition to specific symptomatic therapies, some propose that patients with nonulcer dyspepsia should also be tested for *H. pylori* and treated if found to be infected. The rationale is that there is no benefit to having an *H. pylori* infection and there are considerable risks associated with long-term infection, even though there is little reason to suspect that eradication of *H. pylori* in most of these patients will result in improvement in symptoms.

Symptomatic treatment is directed toward the principal symptoms that are present. If the principal manifestation is dyspepsia, H2-receptor antagonists or proton pump inhibitors should be given; simethicone should be administered for belching and gas; prokinetic agents (cisapride or metoclopramide) should be prescribed for symptoms of gastroparesis (early satiety, postprandial fullness, nausea, and vomiting).

REFERRAL

Most patients with dyspepsia should be managed initially by a primary care provider. Patients older than 50 years of age who have an ulcer complication or features concerning for malignancy (Table 2.4) should be referred to a gastroenterologist for endoscopy. Patients who remain symptomatic after empiric therapy for dyspepsia or after anti–*H. pylori* therapy also should be referred to a gastroenterologist. If the history and physical examination suggest the possibility of a perforation, a general surgeon should be contacted.

KEY POINTS

- Most PUD is related to *H. pylori* or ingestion of NSAIDs.

- Antibody testing of serum is an accurate, cost-effective test to screen for *H. pylori* infection.

- A 14-day combination regimen containing at least two, but preferably three, drugs is the desirable approach to treat *H. pylori*–related ulcers.

- Most patients do not need a follow-up *H. pylori* test to evaluate the effectiveness of eradication.

- Patients with NSAID-induced ulcers are frequently asymptomatic.

- Dyspepsia in pregnant patients should initially be managed empirically with dietary modifications, antacids, or sucralfate. These patients do not need *H. pylori* testing because they should not receive anti–*H. pylori* therapy until after delivery.

COMMONLY ASKED QUESTIONS

What foods should a patient with peptic ulcer disease avoid?

The older literature suggesting that ulcer risk might be increased (or decreased) by certain foods has not been substantiated. Even though beverages containing alcohol or caffeine stimulate gastric acid secretion, there is no evidence that either substance causes gastric or duodenal ul-

cers. *There is also no evidence that dairy products assist ulcer healing. Many foods, however, cause dyspepsia. The reason patients may be advised to avoid certain foods is to reduce episodes of dyspepsia rather than to reduce the risk of ulcer.*

How is *H. pylori* acquired?

H. pylori *is acquired during childhood from situations in which there is oral-oral, fecal-oral, or gastric-oral contact. Examples include contact between mother and child or between child and child in a day care setting. The association between lower socioeconomic status and higher likelihood of infection most likely reflects less developed sewage and water sanitation systems.*

Once *H. pylori* is treated in an adult, what are the chances of becoming reinfected?

After successful eradication of H. pylori, *rates of reinfection in adults are less than 1% per year. If* H. pylori *infection is found after a course of anti–*H. pylori *therapy, it is most likely to represent a recrudescence of a suppressed but not eradicated infection, rather than reinfection with a new organism. Furthermore, transmission of infection between adults is very rare. Most cases of new* H. pylori *infection in adults have occurred in those who work closely with gastric fluids or in patients in whom the infection was iatrogenically introduced by gastrointestinal instrumentation.*

ACKNOWLEDGMENT

The author would like to acknowledge Cindy Brown for her help in manuscript preparation.

SUGGESTED READINGS

Abramowicz M, ed. Drugs for treatment of peptic ulcers. *Med Lett* 1994;36:65–67.

Cappell MS, Garcia A. Gastric and duodenal ulcers during pregnancy. Gastroenterol Clin North Am 1998;27:169–195.

Cryer B, Feldman M. Strategies for preventing NSAID-induced ulcers. *Drug Therapy* 1994;24:25–32.

Cutler AF, Havstad S, Ma CK, Blaser MJ, Perez-Perez GI, Schubert TT. Accuracy of invasive and noninvasive tests to diagnose *Helicobacter pylori* infection. *Gastroenterology* 1995;109: 136–141.

Fendrick AM, Chernew ME, Hirth RA, Bloom BS. Alternative management strategies for patients with suspected peptic ulcer disease. *Ann Intern Med* 1995;123:260–268.

McColl KE, El-Omar E, Gillen D, Banerjedd S. The role of *Helicobacter pylori* in the pathophysiology of duodenal ulcer disease and gastric cancer. *Semin Gastrointest Dis* 1997;8: 142–155.

National Institutes of Health Consensus Development Panel on *Helicobacter pylori* in Peptic Ulcer Disease. Helicobacter pylori in peptic ulcer disease. *JAMA* 1994;272:65–69.

Silverstein MD, Petterson T, Talley NJ. Initial endoscopy or empirical therapy with or without testing for *Helicobacter pylori* for dyspepsia: a decision analysis. *Gastroenterology* 1996; 110:72–83.

Soll AH, Practice Parameters Committee of the American College of Gastroenterology. Consensus statement: Medical treatment of peptic ulcer disease. *JAMA* 1996;275: 622 629.

3

Gallstones and Their Complications

Lyman E. Bilhartz
University of Texas Southwestern Medical Center, Dallas, Texas 75235

OVERVIEW

Anatomically, the biliary tract in humans consists of the hepatic ducts, the cystic duct leading to the dead-end pouch of the gallbladder, the common bile duct, and the sphincter of Oddi (Fig. 3.1). Physiologically, the biliary tract is a low-pressure, low-flow hydraulic excretory pathway for hydrophobic, water-insoluble waste products. Because of the low-flow nature of the hydraulic system and the tenuous solubility of the bile

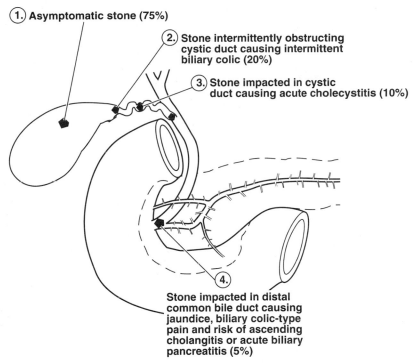

1. Asymptomatic stone (75%)

2. Stone intermittently obstructing cystic duct causing intermittent biliary colic (20%)

3. Stone impacted in cystic duct causing acute cholecystitis (10%)

4. Stone impacted in distal common bile duct causing jaundice, biliary colic-type pain and risk of ascending cholangitis or acute biliary pancreatitis (5%)

FIGURE 3.1.
Schematic representation of the possible clinical sequelae of gallstones. Note that the most common clinical outcome is that the stone remains asymptomatic throughout the patient's life. (Adapted from Bilhartz LF, Horton JD. Gallstone disease and its complications. In: Feldman M, Scharschmidt BF, Sleisenger MH, eds. Sleisenger and Fordtran's Gastrointestinal and Liver Disease, 6th ed. Philadelphia: WB Saunders, 1997:957.)

constituents, bile is vulnerable to precipitation and the formation of concretions. Once formed, the concretions or stones only rarely dissolve spontaneously. Cholelithiasis is the term used to describe the presence of stones in the gallbladder.

TYPES OF GALLSTONES

Based largely on composition, gallstones are categorized as cholesterol stones, black pigment stones, or brown pigment stones. Each category has a unique epidemiology and characteristic risk factors.

Cholesterol Stones

The most common type, accounting for approximately 80% of all gallstones in Western countries, cholesterol stones are composed purely of cholesterol or have cholesterol as the major chemical constituent. Cholesterol gallstones form only in the gallbladder and are strongly associated with age, female gender, and obesity.

Black Pigment Stones

Black pigment stones are composed largely of calcium bilirubinate in a complex with mucin glycoproteins. A regular crystalline structure is absent. Like cholesterol gallstones, black pigment stones form only in the gallbladder, but they are more common in patients with cirrhosis or a chronic hemolytic state.

Brown Pigment Stones

Brown pigment stones are composed of calcium salts of either fatty acids or unconjugated bilirubin, with varying amounts of cholesterol and protein. These stones are usually associated with an infection of the bile ducts. Unlike cholesterol or black pigment stones, brown pigment stones can form *de novo* in the common bile duct.

RISK FACTORS

Irrespective of type, the clinical syndromes produced by all gallstones are identical—only the predisposing risk factors are different.

Ethnic Predisposition

Science is only starting to fully understand the genetic predisposition to gallstone disease. Clearly, certain genetic factors play a key role in the pathogenesis of gallstone disease, but these are likely to be multifactorial and to vary from population to population, because many physiologic factors are also determinants of gallstone formation.

The well-studied Pima Indians in southern Arizona are an example of an extremely high-risk population: 70% of the women older than 25 years of age have gallstones. A second high-risk population is the Scandinavians, 50% of whom develop gallstone disease by age 50. Other high-risk populations include other Amerindian groups in Alaska, Canada, and the continental United States and Mexican-Americans with Amerindian ancestry.

Populations with the lowest rates are from sub-Saharan Africa and Asia. African-Americans have a lower prevalence than Caucasians, and their rate of hospitalization for gallstone-related problems is only 40% of that of whites in the United States.

Within a given population, first-degree relatives of index cases with gallstone disease are 4.5 times more likely to develop gallstones than are matched individuals, which implies a strong genetic influence.

Within a population, gallstones occur sporadically but not randomly. That is, specific risk factors have been identified that predict stone formation. Table 3.1 delineates these risk factors and suggests the physiologic abnormality that accounts for the increased risk.

Age and Gender

Because gallstones rarely dissolve spontaneously, the cumulative prevalence of gallstones, not surprisingly, increases with age. In addition, cholesterol secretion into bile increases with age, whereas bile acid formation may decrease.

Gender is the most prominent risk factor for gallstone formation; most studies report a two- to threefold higher rate in women compared with men. The increased incidence in women is present through the fifth decade, after which the male and female incidences become essentially equal. This may suggest that estrogen has a role in the increased cholesterol secretion into bile that is seen in younger women.

Obesity, Weight Loss, and Total Parenteral Nutrition

Obesity is also a well-known risk factor for cholelithiasis. A large prospective study of obese women found a strong linear association between body mass index (measured in kilograms per square meter) and the incidence of reported cholelithiasis. Those with the highest body mass index (greater than 45 kg/m^2) had a seven-fold increased risk of developing gallstones compared with nonobese controls. This same population had a yearly incidence of gallstone formation of approximately 2%.

Rapid weight loss is a more recently recognized risk factor for the formation of cholesterol gallstones. Approximately 25% of obese patients who undergo strict dietary restriction develop gallstones, and up to 50% of patients who undergo gastric bypass develop gallbladder sludge or gallstones within 6 months after surgery. Up to 40% of these patients become symptomatic from their gallstones in the same 6-month period. Prevention of gallstone formation in this high-risk population may be possible by administration of ursodiol (600 mg daily) prophylactically.

Total parenteral nutrition (TPN) has been associated with the development of acalculous cholecystitis as well as cholelithiasis. Up to 45% of adults and 43% of children develop gallstones after 3 to 4 months of TPN. In general, patients receiving TPN have serious medical problems and are not good candidates for abdominal surgeries. Therefore, prophylactic treatment should be employed if possible. Cholecystokinin-octapeptide has been shown to be effective in preventing gallbladder sludge and gallstone formation and should be used for routine prophylaxis in patients receiving long-term TPN in whom no contraindication exists.

Pregnancy and Parity

Past child-bearing is a frequently touted risk factor for gallstone disease. In reality, the increased risk is small (but probably significant) with increasing parity, especially in younger women. Pregnancy itself is a greater risk factor for the development of biliary sludge and gallstones. During pregnancy, bile becomes more lithogenic owing to increased estrogen levels, which results in increased cholesterol secretion and supersaturated bile. In addition, the volume of the gallbladder doubles and stasis develops; this also promotes sludge and stone formation.

Women who have gallstones before they become pregnant are more likely to develop biliary pain during pregnancy than when in the nonpregnant state. After delivery, gallbladder motility returns to normal, and the bile returns to its prepregnant state. Sludge disappears in 60% to 70% and stones in 20% to 30% of women after delivery.

Drugs

Estrogen is the most extensively studied drug or hormone that is associated with gallstone formation. It is hypothesized to be an important factor in cholesterol

Risk Factors Associated with Cholesterol Gallstone Formation   **TABLE 3.1.**

Risk factor	Proposed metabolic abnormality
Age	Increased cholesterol secretion and decreased bile acid synthesis
Female gender	Increased cholesterol secretion and increased intestinal transit time
Obesity	Cholesterol hypersecretion into bile and increased cholesterol synthesis via increased HMG CoA reductase activity
Weight loss	Cholesterol hypersecretion into bile, reduced bile acid synthesis, and gallbladder hypomotility
Total parenteral nutrition	Gallbladder hypomotility
Pregnancy	Increased cholesterol secretion and gallbladder hypomotility
Drugs	
Clofibrate	Decreased bile acid concentration as a result of suppression of 7a-hyroxylase activity and decreased acyl-CoA:cholesterol acyltransferase (ACAT) activity
Oral contraceptives	Increased cholesterol secretion
Estrogen treatment in women	Cholesterol hypersecretion into bile and reduced bile acid synthesis
Estrogen treatment in men	Cholesterol hypersecretion into bile
Progestogens	Diminished ACAT activity and increased cholesterol secretion
Ceftriaxone	Precipitation of an insoluble calcium-ceftriaxone salt
Octreotide	Decreased gallbladder motility
Genetic Predisposition	
Native Americans	Increased cholesterol synthesis and reduced conversion of cholesterol into bile salts
Scandinavians	Increased cholesterol secretion into bile
Diseases of the terminal ileum	Hyposecretion of bile salts from diminished bile acid pool
Lipid Profile	
Decreased HDL	Increased activity of HMG-CoA reductase
Increased triglycerides	Increased activity of HMG-CoA reductase
APO E-4	Proposed pro-nucleator

APO E-4, apolipoprotein E-4; HDL, high-density lipoproteins; HMG-CoA, 3-hydroxy-3-methylglutaryl coenzyme A. From Bilhartz LE, Horton JD. Gallstone disease and its complications.

In: Feldman M, Scharschmidt BF, Sleisenger MH, eds. Sleisenger and Fordtran's Gastrointestinal and Liver Disease. 6th ed. Philadelphia: WB Saunders, 1997:950.

gallstone formation based on the observation that gallstones occur more frequently in women during their reproductive years.

Lipid-lowering drugs as a whole might be expected to alter the propensity to form gallstones because they alter key pathways in cholesterol and bile acid synthesis and metabolism. The fibric acid derivative clofibrate is the lipid-lowering drug that has the greatest association with increased gallstone formation. Cholestyramine and nicotinic acid have nonstatistical association with gallstone formation. 3-hydroxy-3-methylglutaryl (HMG) coenzyme A–reductase inhibitors reduce the biliary cholesterol saturation index, but their role in prevention or treatment of gallstone disease has not been determined.

Octreotide, the somatostatin analogue, has been shown to increase the incidence of gallstones in patients receiving the drug as treatment for acromegaly. The incidence of newly formed gallstones after initiation of treatment with octreotide may be as high as 30%. Decreased gallbladder motility is the recognized defect associated with octreotide administration.

Diet and Lipid Profile

A high level of serum cholesterol does not seem to be a risk factor for the development of gallstones. However, hypertriglyceridemia is positively associated with an increased incidence of gallstone disease. High-density lipoprotein cholesterol has been shown to be inversely correlated with the presence of gallstones and biliary cholesterol saturation.

Diet would seem to be a logical variable that could explain some of the discrepancies in gallstone prevalence reported from various countries. However, this has not been the case. Studies to date have been conflicting, especially in regard to fat consumption. The studies are too numerous to elaborate on, but even in animal models fat consumption may or may not cause an increase in gallstone formation, depending on which species is used for experimentation. Dietary cholesterol has been shown to increase cholesterol secretion and decrease the bile salt pool, but only in people in whom gallstones already exist.

Systemic Disease

Diabetes is the systemic disease most extensively studied in regard to gallstones, because it is believed that diabetics are more prone to complications associated with cholelithiasis. Given that hypertriglyceridemia and obesity are risk factors for gallstones and that gallbladder motility can be impaired in diabetes, it has long been thought that patients with this disease are at an increased risk for the development of gallstones. However, diabetes as an independent risk factor has been difficult to prove. The data suggest a trend toward an increased prevalence that does not reach statistical significance. If

a real increased risk exists, it may be in those patients with hyperinsulinemia.

Diseases of the ileum are recognized risk factors for gallstones. Crohn's disease is the most common systemic illness that affects the terminal ileum, and it clearly carries an increased risk. The loss of specific bile acid receptors in the terminal ileum results in excessive bile salt excretion and a diminished bile acid pool, which leads to lithogenic bile.

DIAGNOSIS

As shown in Table 3.2, a wide array of imaging technologies is available to evaluate the biliary tract. Each test strengths and limitations, and the tests vary widely in relative cost and risk to the patient. With the possible exception of ultrasound, none of the tests should be ordered "routinely" in the evaluation of the patient with suspected gallstone disease. Rather, the diagnostic evaluation should proceed rationally, based on the individual patient's symptoms, signs, and laboratory studies.

TABLE 3.2.   Imaging Studies of the Biliary Tract

Technique	Condition tested	Findings/comments
Sonography	Cholelithiasis	Stones appear as mobile, dependent echogenic foci within the gallbladder lumen with acoustic shadowing
		Sludge appears as layering echogenic material without shadows
		Sensitivity >95% for stones >2 mm
		Specificity >95% for stones with acoustic shadows
		Best single test for stones in the gallbladder
	Choledocholithiasis	Stones in CBD are seen sonographically in only 50% of cases but can be inferred by the finding of a dilated CBD (>6 mm diameter) in 75%
		Sonography can confirm, but not exclude, CBD stones
	Acute cholecystitis	Sonographic Murphy's sign (focal gallbladder tenderness under the transducer) has a positive predictive value of >90% in detecting acute cholecystitis when stones are seen
		Pericholecystic fluid (in the absence of ascites) and gallbladder wall thickening to >4 mm (in the absence of hypoalbuminemia) are nonspecific findings suggestive of acute cholecystitis
Endoscopic ultrasound (EUS)	Choledocholithiasis	Highly accurate means of excluding or confirming stones in the CBD
		Sensitivity of 93% and specificity of 97%
		Concordance of EUS with ERCP diagnosis is 95%
		With experienced operators, EUS can be used in lieu of ERCP for excluding CBD stones

(continued)

Technique	Condition tested	Findings/comments
Oral cholecystography (OCG)	Cholelithiasis	Stones appear as mobile filling defects in an opacified gallbladder
		Sensitivity and specificity exceed 90% when the gallbladder is opacified, but "nonvisualization" occurs in 25% of tests and can result from multiple causes besides stones
		Opacification of the gallbladder demonstrates patency of the cystic duct, a necessary prerequisite for medical dissolution therapy or lithotripsy
		May be useful in the evaluation of acalculous gallbladder diseases such as cholesterolosis or adenomyomatosis
Cholescintigraphy (hepatobiliary scintigraphy, HIDA, DICIDA scans)	Acute cholecystitis	Assesses patency of the cystic duct—nothing more
		Normal scan shows radioactivity in the gallbladder, CBD, and small bowel within 30–60 min
		Positive scan is defined as nonvisualization of the gallbladder with preserved excretion into the CBD or small bowel
		Sensitivity is 95% and specificity 90% with false-positive results seen in fasted and critically ill patients
		When done with cholecystokinin stimulation, gallbladder "ejection fraction" can be determined and may help in evaluating patients with acalculous biliary pain
		Normal scan virtually excludes acute cholecystitis
Endoscopic retrograde cholangiopancreatography (ERCP)	Cholelithiasis	When contrast flows retrograde into the gallbladder, stones appear as filling defects and can be detected with a sensitivity of 80%, but sonography remains the mainstay of confirming cholelithiasis
	Choledocholithiasis	ERCP is the gold standard test for stones in the CBD, with sensitivity and specificity of 95%
		Ability to extract stones (or at least drain infected bile) is life-saving in severe cholangitis and reduces the need for CBD exploration
Computed tomography (CT), magnetic resonance (MR) imaging	Complications	Although not well suited for detecting uncomplicated stones, a standard CT scan is an excellent test for detecting complications such as abscess formation, perforation of the gallbladder or CBD, or pancreatitis
		Spiral CT and MR cholangiography may prove useful as a noninvasive means of excluding CBD stones

CBD, common bile duct.
From Bilhartz LE, Horton JD. Gallstone disease and its complications. In: Feldman M, Scharschmidt BF, Sleisenger MH, eds.

Sleisenger and Fordtran's Gastrointestinal and Liver Disease, 6th ed. Philadelphia: WB Saunders, 1997:959.

Notably absent from the list of imaging studies of the biliary tract is the plain abdominal radiographic film. Although useful on occasion to evaluate patients with abdominal pain, this method lacks both sensitivity and specificity. Only 50% of pigment stones and 20% of cholesterol stones contain enough calcium to be visible on the plain abdominal film. Because 80% of all gallstones in Western countries are of the cholesterol type, it follows that only one fourth of the stones can be detected by simple radiographs. Plain abdominal films have their greatest utility in the evaluation of patients with some of the unusual complications of

Summary of Diagnosis

- Biliary colic classically causes episodic attacks of epigastric or right upper quadrant pain that last from 1 to 4 hours.
- Neither constant, chronic abdominal pain nor momentary stabbing pain is characteristic of biliary colic, nor are symptoms of gas, flatulence, or dyspepsia.
- Acute cholecystitis usually is preceded by recurrent attacks of biliary colic and manifests with localized right upper quadrant pain and tenderness of more than 6 hours' duration and low-grade fever.
- Ultrasound examination of the gallbladder is a sensitive and specific test for stones in the gallbladder (cholelithiasis).
- Ultrasound may reveal a dilated common bile duct that suggests the presence of a common duct stone (choledocholithiasis), but its sensitivity for this diagnosis is only 75%. If choledocholithiasis is suspected, then a cholangiogram by endoscopic retrograde cholangiopancreatography (ERCP) is usually needed to exclude a common duct stone definitively.
- Abnormal liver function tests suggest bile duct obstruction and generally warrant further investigation of the bile ducts by ERCP.
- The combination of fever, jaundice, and abdominal pain (Charcot's triad) suggests possible cholangitis; urgent administration of antibiotics and evaluation of the bile ducts by ERCP is warranted.

gallstones, such as emphysematous cholecystitis or cholecystenteric fistula, and in the detection of a porcelain gallbladder.

MANAGEMENT OF GALLSTONES

Treatment of Asymptomatic Gallstones

A common situation that all primary care practitioners eventually encounter is the issue of what to recommend to a patient who has been found to have gallstones but who has no symptoms suggesting biliary tract disease. For example, the presence of a calcified gallstone may be noted incidentally on a routine chest film, or the report of an abdominal ultrasound ordered to evaluate symptoms elsewhere in the abdomen (e.g., aorta, pelvis, kidneys) may comment on the incidental finding of cholelithiasis. Is the patient at risk from an incidental gallstone? Would the patient benefit more from having the stones removed before complications arise, or is the cost and risk of prophylactic cholecystectomy not justified?

To answer these questions, some knowledge of the natural history of asymptomatic gallstones is needed. Although precise data on this subject are sparse, enough is known to recommend a conservative, "wait and see" approach in almost all cases. According to the best longitudinal, prospective study, the rate of development of biliary pain was about 2% per year for 5 years, after which it decreased over time. Although these estimates can be criticized on the basis that, because the subjects were mostly male college professors, the results may not accurately reflect the natural history of asymptomatic gallstones in groups at higher risk for this disease (e.g., Mexican-American women), the conclusion that the vast majority of asymptomatic stones remain asymptomatic over time is not questioned.

Prophylactic Cholecystectomy

There may be some subsets of patients in whom the natural history is not so benign and in whom a prophylactic cholecystectomy may be justifiable for the purpose of eliminating future complications. Based on anecdotal cases, inferences on the natural history of asymptomatic stones in specific subsets of patients, and cumulative clinical experience, the following are possible exceptions to the dictum of leaving asymptomatic stones alone.

1. A young patient with sickle cell anemia and incidental cholelithiasis in whom an abdominal pain crisis would be difficult to distinguish from biliary colic or acute cholecystitis
2. A young woman of Amerindian ancestry with incidental cholelithiasis in whom prophylactic cholecystectomy may be warranted to prevent the delayed complication of gallbladder cancer
3. Possibly, a patient with incidental cholelithiasis who is awaiting organ transplantation
4. Any patient with gallbladder wall calcification (porcelain gallbladder) who is an acceptable surgical risk, for the purpose of preventing gallbladder carcinoma as a late complication

5. A patient with incidental cholelithiasis who is planning prolonged space travel or other extremely remote assignments.

Notably absent from this list are diabetic patients with incidental cholelithiasis, who were long considered to have an increased risk of serious complications even though their gallstones were asymptomatic. More recent studies have shown that the natural history of gallstones in diabetics follows the same pattern observed in nondiabetics. Therefore, prophylactic cholecystectomy is generally not recommended in diabetics.

Prevention

For the most part, gallstones cannot be prevented, because the risk factors cannot be easily altered. Exceptions include the prophylactic administration of urso-

diol (600 mg daily) during periods of rapid weight loss and, possibly, the daily administration of cholecystokinin-octapeptide intravenously to patients receiving TPN.

CLINICAL SEQUELAE OF GALLSTONES

As depicted schematically in Figure 3.1, gallstones remain asymptomatic in three out of four cases. When they do cause symptoms, they usually result in one or more of four distinct clinical syndromes: biliary colic, acute cholecystitis, choledocholithiasis, and cholangitis. These four syndromes are discussed separately in the following sections and are compared side by side in Table 3.3.

Four Common Clinical Sequelae of Gallstone Disease   **TABLE 3.3.**

Feature	Biliary colic	Acute cholecystitis	Choledocholithiasis	Cholangitis
Patho-physiology	Intermittent obstruction of the cystic duct / No inflammation of the gallbladder mucosa	Impacted stone in the cystic duct / Acute inflammation of the gallbladder mucosa / Secondary bacterial infection in 50%	Intermittent obstruction of the common bile duct	Impacted stone in the common bile duct causing bile stasis / Bacterial superinfection of stagnant bile / Early bacteremia
Symptoms	Severe, poorly localized epigastric or RUQ visceral pain growing in intensity over 15 min and remaining constant for 1–6 h, often with nausea / Frequency of attacks varies from days to months / Gas, bloating, flatulence, dyspepsia are not related to stones	75% are preceded by attacks of biliary colic / Visceral epigastric pain gives way to moderately severe, localized pain in the RUQ, back, shoulder or rarely chest / Nausea with some emesis is frequent / Pain lasting >6 hr favors cholecystitis over colic	Often asymptomatic / Symptoms (when present) are indistinguishable from biliary colic / Predisposes to cholangitis and acute pancreatitis	Charcot's triad of pain, jaundice and fever is present in 70% / Pain may be mild and transient and is often accompanied by chills / Mental confusion, lethargy and delirium are suggestive of bacteremia
Physical findings	Mild to moderate gallbladder tenderness during an attack with mild residual tenderness lasting days	Febrile, but usually <38.8°C (102°F) unless complicated by gangrene or perforation / Right subcostal tenderness with inspiratory arrest (Murphy's sign)	Often a completely normal examination if the obstruction is intermittent	Fever in 95% / RUQ tenderness in 90% / Jaudice in only 80% / Peritoneal signs in only 15%

(continued)

TABLE 3.3.   *Continued*

Feature	Biliary colic	Acute cholecystitis	Choledocholithiasis	Cholangitis
	Often a completely normal examination	Palpable gallbladder in 33%, especially in patients having their first attack Mild jaundice in 20%	Jaundice with pain suggests stones while painless jaundice with a palpable gallbladder favors malignancy	Hypotension and mental confusion coexist in 15% and suggest gram-negative sepsis
Laboratory findings	Usually normal In patients with findings of only uncomplicated biliary colic, an elevated bilirubin, alkaline phosphatase, or amylase suggests coexisting CBD stones	Leukocytosis of 12,000–15,000 cells/mm^2 with bandemia is common Bilirubin may be 2–4 mg/dL, and transaminase and alkaline phosphatase may be elevated even in absence of CBD stone or hepatic infection Mild amylase elevation is seen even in absence of pancreatitis If bilirubin >4 mg/dL or amylase >1,000 suspect CBD stone	Elevated bilirubin and alkaline phosphatase seen with CBD obstruction Bilirubin >10 mg/dL suggests malignant obstruction or coexisting hemolysis Transient "spike" in transaminases or amylase suggests passage of a stone	Leukocytosis in 80% but remainder may have normal leukocyte count with bandemia as the only hematologic finding Bilirubin >2 mg/dL in 80% but when less the diagnosis may be missed Alkaline phosphatase is usually elevated Blood cultures are usually positive, especially during chills or fever spike, and grows two organisms in 50%
Diagnostic tests	Sonography Oral cholecystography (OCG) Meltzer-Lyon test	Sonography Hepatobiliary scintigraphy (DICIDA, HIDA scans) Abdominal computed tomography	ERCP Transhepatic cholangiogram (THC)	ERCP Transhepatic cholangiogram (THC)
Natural history	After initial attack, 30% have no further symptoms The remainder develop symptoms at rate of 6%/yr and severe complications at 1%/yr	50% resolve spontaneously in 7–10 days without surgery Left untreated, 10% are complicated by a localized perforation and 1% by a free perforation and peritonitis	Natural history is not well defined, but complications are more frequent and severe than for asymptomatic stones in the gallbladder	High mortality rate if unrecognized, with death from septicemia Emergency decompression of the CBD (usually by ERCP) dramatically improves survival
Treatment	Elective laparoscopic cholecystectomy with intraoperative cholangiogram (IOC) ERCP for stone removal if IOC shows stones	Cholecystectomy with IOC If IOC shows stones, then CBD exploration or ERCP for stone removal	Stone removal at time of ERCP and early laparoscopic cholecystectomy	Emergency ERCP with stone removal or at least biliary decompression Antibiotics to cover gram-negative organisms Interval cholecystectomy

CBD, common bile duct; ERCP, endoscopic retrograde cholangiopancreatography; RUQ, right upper quadrant.
(From Bilhartz LE, Horton JD. Gallstone disease and its complications. In: Feldman M, Scharschmidt BF, Sleisenger MH, eds. Sleisenger and Fordtran's Gastrointestinal and Liver Disease, 6th ed. Philadelphia: WB Saunders, 1997:958.)

BILIARY COLIC

Definition

Biliary colic is a syndrome characterized by episodic, self-limited right upper quadrant or epigastric pain arising from a gallbladder that is attempting to contract and secrete bile against an obstructed cystic duct. The pain is visceral in origin and therefore poorly localized, and it is not associated with evidence of inflammation; hence, there is no fever or leukocytosis. Biliary colic by far the most common presenting symptom of cholelithiasis. About 75% of patients with symptomatic gallstone disease seek medical attention because of episodic abdominal pain.

To distinguish this complication from cholelithiasis (the presence of gallstones), the term biliary colic is used to describe the complex of symptoms that occurs when a stone obstructs the cystic duct.

Cause

The syndrome of biliary colic is caused by intermittent obstruction of the cystic duct by one or more gallstones. There is no requirement that inflammation of the gallbladder accompany the obstruction—only that symptoms be caused by it. The term "chronic cholecystitis" should be avoided because it implies the presence of a chronic inflammatory infiltrate that may or may not be present in a given patient. Indeed, there is little correlation between the severity and frequency of colic on the one hand and the pathologic changes in the gallbladder on the other. Bacteria can be cultured from gallbladder bile or from the gallstones themselves in about 10% of patients, but bacterial infection is not thought to contribute to the symptoms.

Patient Presentation

History

The pain of biliary colic is of visceral origin and therefore is poorly localized. In a typical case, the patient experiences episodes of upper abdominal pain, usually in the epigastrium or right upper quadrant but sometimes in other abdominal locations. The pain may be precipitated by eating a meal, but more commonly there is no inciting event, and the pain can even begin at night. The onset of biliary colic is more frequent during periods of weight reduction and marked physical inactivity, such as prolonged bed rest.

The pain of biliary colic is steady rather than intermittent, as would be suggested by the word "colic." The pain gradually increases over a period of 15 to 60 minutes and then remains at a plateau for an hour or longer before slowly ebbing. In one third of the patients, the pain has a more sudden onset, and on rare occasions it may abruptly cease. Pain lasting longer than 6 hours suggests acute cholecystitis rather than simple biliary colic.

In order of decreasing frequency, the pain is felt maximally in the epigastrium, right upper quadrant, left upper quadrant, and various parts of the precordium or lower abdomen. It is therefore incorrect to think that pain located other than in the right upper quadrant is atypical of gallstone disease. Radiation of the pain to the scapula, right shoulder, or lower abdomen occurs in half of the patients. Diaphoresis and nausea with some vomiting are common; however, the emesis is not as protracted as in intestinal obstruction or acute pancreatitis. As with other kinds of visceral pain, the patient with biliary colic is usually restless and active during an attack.

Physical examination

The physical examination is usually normal, with only mild to moderate gallbladder tenderness during an attack and perhaps mild residual tenderness lasting several days afterward.

Complaints of gas, bloating, flatulence, and dyspepsia, although frequently present in patients with gallstones, are probably not related to the stones themselves. Rather, they are nonspecific symptoms that are found with a similar frequency in people without gallstones. Accordingly, patients with gallstones whose only clinical manifestations are dyspepsia and other nonspecific upper gastrointestinal tract symptoms are not appropriate candidates for cholecystectomy.

Diagnosis

Laboratory tests

In a patient with uncomplicated biliary colic, laboratory studies are usually completely normal. Elevations of bilirubin, alkaline phosphatase, or amylase suggest coexisting choledocholithiasis.

Radiologic studies

Ultrasound   In general, the first (and in most cases only) imaging study to be performed for a patient with biliary colic is an ultrasonographic examination of the right upper quadrant. As outlined in Table 3.2, ultrasound is a rapid, noninvasive, highly sensitive, and highly specific means of establishing the presence or absence of stones in the gallbladder. Despite ultrasound's impressive diagnostic accuracy, the sheer number of patients with suspected gallstone disease means that occasionally ultrasound misses a clinically important stone and the correct diagnosis is delayed. Given the relatively benign natural history of biliary colic, it is probably safe to simply monitor the patient for a while and move on to other diagnostic modalities in the event that symptoms recur.

Oral cholecystography   Nowadays, oral cholecystography (OCG) is generally viewed as a secondary imaging study of the gallbladder. It is reserved for patients in whom medical dissolution therapy or lithotripsy of the gallstones is planned. In such cases, it is essential to establish patency of the cystic duct before therapy, and OCG can accomplish this. On rare occasions, OCG may demonstrate a layer of small floating gallstones that were missed by ultrasound.

Differential diagnosis

Reflux esophagitis, peptic ulcer, pancreatitis, renal colic, lesions of the colon such as diverticulitis and carcinoma, radiculopathy, and angina pectoris are the most common diseases to be considered in the differential diagnosis of a patient with recurrent, episodic upper abdominal symptoms. Usually, a careful history goes a long way in sorting out the differential diagnosis of recurrent upper abdominal pain. For example, relief with ingestion of food, antacids, or antisecretory drugs suggests acid peptic disease, whereas a cramping nature to the pain suggests an intestinal problem. Renal stones usually have typical findings on a urinalysis, and the pain of angina pectoris is usually precipitated by exercise and does not last for hours.

The irritable bowel syndrome, like biliary colic, is common in young women, but symptoms should have a distinct relation to bowel movements.

Shingles or a radiculopathy from osteoarthritis may produce symptoms resembling those of biliary colic.

Management

The natural history of biliary colic is cause for concern but not alarm. Approximately 30% of patients having an initial attack of classic biliary colic symptoms will experience no additional attacks over the next 24 months. Therefore, a reasonable approach would be to offer cholecystectomy to the 70% of patients with recurring episodes of biliary colic. In this group, the frequency of recurrent attacks varies widely but the pattern remains relatively similar for an individual patient over time. On average, patients with an initial attack of biliary colic who are observed develop symptoms sufficient to warrant cholecystectomy at a rate of approximately 6% per

year. The probability of development of a severe complication requiring urgent surgical intervention is only approximately 1% per year.

The treatment procedure for recurrent, uncomplicated biliary colic in a patient with documented gallstones is usually an elective laparoscopic cholecystectomy. For patients who have experienced only a single attack of biliary colic, there is one chance in three that they will have no further attacks in the next decade, and a "wait and see" approach is advisable, with referral to a surgeon when a recurrent attack happens.

Cholecystectomy

The decision as to which operation (laparoscopic or open cholecystectomy) to offer a patient is best made by the surgeon and depends on the preoperative concern about common duct stones as well as the experience of the surgeon with laparoscopy. Most patients already know that the laparoscopic approach involves a shorter hospital stay and more rapid convalescence and want to be referred to a surgeon who can offer laparoscopy as an option. However, if the patient or the primary care practitioner has a good, trusting relationship with a general surgeon who does not do laparoscopic surgery, then a traditional open cholecystectomy is a safe and effective means of treating biliary colic.

Medical treatment

Medical treatment of gallstones by dissolution therapy with ursodiol (300 mg twice daily) is effective in only a fraction of patients and is rarely used. The ideal candidate for medical dissolution is a patient with a small number of small (less than 10 mm), noncalcified gallstones and a functioning gallbladder by oral cholecystography. Even in these ideal circumstances, the probability of complete dissolution is only 25% and requires a year or more of treatment.

Referral

When presented with a patient with known gallstones, the primary caregiver has three options: observe the patient, attempt to dissolve the stones, or refer the patient to a surgeon for definitive treatment. Observation is warranted for most asymptomatic patients with gallstones, and perhaps for patients who have experienced only a single attack of colic (a rare situation). Medical dissolution therapy is rarely effective. Therefore, most patients with recurrent biliary colic should be referred to a surgeon. The primary care physician should refer the patient to a surgeon when a recurrent attack happens.

ACUTE CHOLECYSTITIS

Definition

Acute cholecystitis is defined as inflammation of the gallbladder wall associated with a clinical picture involving abdominal pain, right upper quadrant tenderness, fever, and leukocytosis. In approximately 90% of cases of acute cholecystitis, the underlying cause is a gallstone obstructing the cystic duct. In the remaining 10% of cases, cholecystitis occurs in the absence of gallstones and is termed acute acalculous cholecystitis.

Cause

Whereas biliary colic is caused by intermittent obstruction of the cystic duct by a gallstone, acute cholecystitis generally occurs when a stone becomes impacted in the cystic duct, causing chronic obstruction. Stasis of bile within the gallbladder lumen results in damage to the gallbladder mucosa, with consequent release of intracellular enzymes and activation of a cascade of inflammatory mediators.

Enteric bacteria can be cultured from gallbladder bile in approximately half of patients with acute cholecystitis; however, bacteria are not thought to contribute to the actual onset of acute cholecystitis. Antibiotics are used in patients with suspected gallbladder perforation or gangrene or in those patients with particularly toxic presentations, including fever greater than 38.8°C (102°F).

If the gallbladder is examined during the initial few days of an attack of acute cholecystitis, distention and an impacted stone in the cystic duct usually are noted. On opening the gallbladder, bile, stones, inflammatory exudate, and, rarely, pus are present. Later in the attack, the normally present bile pigments are absorbed and replaced with thin mucoid fluid, pus, or blood. If the attack of acute cholecystitis is left untreated for a long period but the cystic duct remains obstructed, the lumen may become distended with clear mucoid fluid—so-called hydrops of the gallbladder.

Patient Presentation

History

Three of every four patients with acute cholecystitis report having had prior attacks of biliary colic. Often, the initial symptom that alerts the patient to the possibility that something more is happening than a simple recurrence of biliary colic is the duration of the pain. The pain of biliary colic usually lasts longer than 1 hour but rarely more than 6 hours. If the pain has been constant for more than 6 hours, it comes increasingly unlikely that the patient has uncomplicated biliary colic.

As inflammation in the gallbladder wall progresses, the poorly localized visceral pain gives way to moderately severe parietal pain that usually becomes localized to the right upper quadrant. Less commonly the back, and rarely even the chest, may be the site of maximal pain.

Nausea with some vomiting is characteristic of acute cholecystitis, but these symptoms almost invariably follow rather than precede the onset of pain. Emesis is not as persistent or as severe as in an intestinal obstruction or acute pancreatitis.

In some cases, the symptoms of acute cholecystitis are nonspecific, with only a mild ache and anorexia, whereas others may present with toxic manifestations including fever, severe right upper quadrant pain with guarding, and localized rebound tenderness.

The natural history of untreated acute cholecystitis is resolution of pain in 7 to 10 days. It is not uncommon for symptoms to remit within 48 hours of hospitalization. Left untreated, approximately 10% of cases become complicated by localized perforation and 1% by free perforation and peritonitis.

Physical examination

Unlike the situation in uncomplicated biliary colic, the physical examination can, in many cases, suggest the diagnosis of acute cholecystitis. Fever is common (due to active inflammation in the gallbladder mucosa), but it is usually less than 38.8°C unless gangrene or perforation of the gallbladder has occurred. The abdominal examination reveals right subcostal tenderness and a palpable gallbladder in 33% of the patients. A palpable gallbladder is more common in patients who are having their first attack of acute cholecystitis, because repeated attacks usually result in a scarred, fibrotic gallbladder that is unable to distend. For unclear reasons, the gallbladder is usually palpable lateral to its normal anatomic location.

A relatively specific finding for acute cholecystitis is Murphy's sign: During palpation in the right subcostal region, pain and inspiratory arrest may occur when the patient takes a deep breath that brings the inflamed gallbladder into contact with the examiner's hand. A positive Murphy's sign in the appropriate clinical setting is a reliable predictor of acute cholecystitis, although confirmation of gallstones by ultrasound is still warranted.

Diagnosis

Laboratory tests

White blood cell count   Leukocytosis with a shift to immature neutrophils is common.

Serum bilirubin   Jaundice is often subtle, with bilirubin concentrations less than 4 mg/dL. A higher bilirubin level suggests the possibility of common duct stones, which are found in one half of jaundiced patients with acute cholecystitis.

Liver function tests   Because common bile duct stones with cholangitis is usually part of the differential diagnosis, attention is directed to the liver function test. Even without any detectable bile duct obstruction, acute cholecystitis often causes mild elevations in the serum concentrations of transaminase and alkaline phosphatase. Even the serum amylase and lipase concentrations may be nonspecifically elevated. An amylase concentration greater than 1,000 U/dL usually indicates coexisting common bile duct obstruction or acute pancreatitis and warrants further evaluation along those lines.

Radiologic studies
Ultrasound   Ultrasound is the single most useful imaging study in acutely ill patients with right upper quadrant pain and tenderness. Not only can it accurately establish the presence or absence of gallstones, but, as discussed previously and as shown in Table 3.2, ultrasound becomes a highly specific extension of the physical examination. A sonographic Murphy's sign is defined as focal gallbladder tenderness under the transducer. With a skillful operator and an alert patient, the positive predictive value of a sonographic Murphy's sign is greater than 90% for the detection of acute cholecystitis if gallstones are also present.

Additionally, ultrasound can detect nonspecific findings of acute cholecystitis, such as pericholecystic fluid and gallbladder wall thickening to greater than 4 mm. Both of these findings lose specificity for acute cholecystitis if hypoalbuminemia (less than 3.2 g/dL) or ascites is present.

Cholescintigraphy   Because gallstones are so prevalent in the background population, many patients with nonbiliary tract diseases (e.g., acute pancreatitis, complications of peptic ulcer disease) who present with acute abdominal pain have only incidental and clinically irrelevant gallstones. The greatest utility of cholescintigraphy is in these patients, because it can exclude acute cholecystitis and allow the clinician to focus on nonbiliary causes of the patient's acute abdominal pain.

As outlined in Table 3.2, a normal cholescintigraphic scan shows radioactivity in the gallbladder, common bile duct, and small bowel within 30 to 60 minutes after injection of the isotope. With only rare exceptions, a normal scan excludes acute cholecystitis due to gallstones, because virtually every patient with that disease has a gallstone obstructing the cystic duct at the time of the attack. If a positive scan is defined as the absence of isotope in the gallbladder, then a falsely negative scan would be one in which the gallbladder filled with dye despite acute cholecystitis—a situation that virtually never occurs. To be sure, a false-positive result, defined as the absence of isotope in the gallbladder in a patient who does not have acute cholecystitis, does occur with regularity, especially in fasted or critically ill patients receiving TPN. Therefore, scintigraphy should not be used as the initial imaging study in a patient with suspected cholecystitis, but rather as a secondary imaging study in patients who are already known to harbor gallstones but whose clinical features hold out the possibility of nonbiliary causes of their acute abdominal pain.

In summary, cholescintigraphy should be thought of as a secondary imaging test aimed at establishing whether the cystic duct is obstructed. As such, cholescintigraphy can exclude acute cholecystitis due to gallstones but cannot confirm it.

Abdominal computed tomography   With respect to acute cholecystitis, abdominal computed tomography (CT) finds its greatest utility not in merely confirming the presence of acute cholecystitis, but rather in detecting complications such as emphysematous cholecystitis or perforation of the gallbladder while excluding other intraabdominal pathologic states that may produce a similar clinical picture. For example, abdominal CT is a highly sensitive means of detecting pneumoperitoneum, acute pancreatitis, pancreatic pseudocyst, hepatic or intraabdominal abscess, appendicitis, or obstruction or perforation of a hollow viscus. In a straightforward case of acute cholecystitis, an abdominal CT scan usually is not warranted; however, if the diagnosis is less certain or the optimal timing of surgery is in doubt, the CT scan can be invaluable.

Differential diagnosis
Given the high incidence of acute cholecystitis, even a weak diagnostician will often be correct in making this diagnosis in patients with right upper quadrant pain, fever, and leukocytosis. However, a surprisingly lengthy list of other conditions can manifest with similar clinical features. The principal conditions to consider in the differential diagnosis are appendicitis, acute pancreatitis, pyelonephritis or renal stone, peptic ulcer disease, acute hepatitis, pneumonia, hepatic abscess or tumor, and gonococcal perihepatitis. To avoid embarrassment or worse, the astute clinician would do well at least to

consider all of these possibilities before recommending a cholecystectomy.

Acute appendicitis   This is the disease most often confused with acute cholecystitis, because the initial diagnostic impression is based largely on localized right abdominal tenderness, which may be lower than expected in cholecystitis or higher than expected in appendicitis. In general, fever, leukocytosis, and tenderness progress more inexorably in appendicitis. A complete abdominal ultrasound examination can usually differentiate between these two entities.

Acute pancreatitis   This disease may also be difficult to distinguish from acute cholecystitis based on the history and physical examination alone. Generally, vomiting is a more prominent feature in acute pancreatitis, and hyperamylasemia is more profound.

Diseases of the right kidney   Kidney disease can produce pain and tenderness similar to that of acute cholecystitis, but urinalysis and ultrasound usually differentiate the two.

Peptic ulcer disease   Whereas the pain of uncomplicated peptic ulcer disease is usually chronic in nature and therefore is seldom confused with acute cholecystitis, a perforated ulcer may, at least initially, mimic severe acute cholecystitis. Signs of generalized peritonitis or a pneumoperitoneum strongly suggest a perforated viscus or at least the need for an emergency laparotomy.

Pneumonia with pleurisy   This disease can cause abdominal pain and tenderness, but the pleuritic nature of the pain and the chest x-ray findings should be helpful in diagnosis.

Acute hepatitis   In some instances, acute hepatitis, especially when it is caused by alcohol consumption, manifests with rather severe right upper quadrant pain and tenderness. Fever and leukocytosis further add to the confusion with acute cholecystitis. In such cases, careful assessment of the liver function test over time, along with ultrasound examination or cholescintigraphy, may serve to exclude acute cholecystitis. Rarely, a liver biopsy is warranted.

Gonococcal perihepatitis   This disease, also known as Fitz-Hugh–Curtis syndrome, produces right upper quadrant pain and tenderness and leukocytosis, which often overshadow any pelvic complaints. Nevertheless, adnexal tenderness is present on physical examination, and a Gram stain of the cervical smear should show gonococci.

Hepatic abscesses and tumors   These lesions can usually be differentiated from acute cholecystitis on the basis of ultrasound findings. Previously undiagnosed gallbladder perforation may manifest with fever from a subhepatic abscess. Finally, pseudolithiasis due to ceftriaxone therapy has caused symptoms resembling acute cholecystitis, although the gallbladder is histologically normal.

Management

The patient with suspected acute cholecystitis should be hospitalized for evaluation and treatment. Volume contraction from vomiting and poor oral intake is common, and intravenous fluid and electrolyte repletion should be given. Oral feeding should be withheld and a nasogastric tube inserted if the patient's abdomen is distended or if there is persistent vomiting.

In straightforward, uncomplicated cases, antibiotics may be withheld. Antibiotics are warranted if the patient appears particularly toxic or a complication is suspected (e.g., perforation of the gallbladder, emphysematous cholecystitis). A variety of antibiotics covering gram-negative enteric bacteria are effective. Coverage with a single agent such as cefoxitin is appropriate for mild cases; more severely ill patients should receive a broader combination, such as ampicillin with an aminoglycoside or a third-generation cephalosporin and metronidazole.

If the degree of leukocytosis exceeds 15,000 cells/mm^3, particularly in the setting of worsening pain, high fever (greater than 38.8°C), suppurative cholecystitis (empyema) or perforation should be suspected and urgent surgical intervention may be required.

Advanced gallbladder disease may be present even if local and systemic manifestations are unimpressive.

Definitive therapy for acute cholecystitis is cholecystectomy; studies have demonstrated the safety and effectiveness of the laparoscopic approach. The morbidity and mortality rates are very low, unless complications such as perforation of the gallbladder or gangrene have already occurred.

Referral

The primary care physician should see to it that the patient with suspected acute cholelithiasis is hospitalized, resuscitated, and given antibiotics if toxic. In most cases, consultation with a general surgeon is appropriate to ensure that timely surgical treatment is accomplished.

CHOLEDOCHOLITHIASIS

Definition

Choledocholithiasis is defined as the occurrence of stones in the common bile duct. Like stones in the gallbladder, choledocholithiasis by itself may remain asymptomatic for years; clinically silent passage of stones from the bile duct into the duodenum is known to occur, perhaps frequently. Unlike stones in the gallbladder, which usually manifest with relatively benign bouts of recurrent biliary colic, stones in the common bile duct, when they do cause symptoms, manifest with life-threatening complications such as cholangitis or acute pancreatitis. Therefore, confirmation of choledocholithiasis generally warrants some type of intervention to remove the stones, whereas the incidental finding of cholelithiasis can be monitored expectantly.

Cause

Gallstones can pass from the gallbladder into the common bile duct, or they can form primarily in the duct. All gallstones from one patient, whether from the gallbladder or the common duct, are of the same type, either cholesterol or pigment. Cholesterol stones form only in the gallbladder, and therefore any cholesterol stones found in the common bile duct must have migrated there from the gallbladder. Likewise, black pigment stones, which are seen with old age, hemolysis, alcoholism, and cirrhosis, also form in the gallbladder and only rarely migrate into the common bile duct. The majority of pigment stones in the common bile duct are the softer brown pigment stones, which form de novo in the common duct as a result of bacterial action on the phospholipid and bilirubin in bile. They are often found proximal to biliary strictures and are frequently associated with cholangitis. Brown pigment stones are associated with recurrent pyogenic cholangitis (oriental cholangiohepatitis).

Fifteen percent of patients with gallbladder stones also have stones in the common duct. Conversely, of patients with ductal stones, 95% also have gallbladder stones. For patients who present with choledocholithiasis months or years after cholecystectomy, it may be impossible to determine whether the stones were overlooked at the earlier operation or have formed since.

Stones in the common bile duct usually come to rest at the lower end of the ampulla of Vater. Obstruction of the bile duct increases bile pressure proximally and causes the duct to dilate. Normal pressure in the duct is 10 to 15 cm of water; it rises to 25 to 40 cm with complete obstruction. When pressure exceeds 15 cm of water bile flow decreases, and at 30 cm it stops.

Patient Presentation

History

Mild jaundice is present in 20% of all patients and reaches 40% in the elderly.

Little information is available on the natural history of asymptomatic common duct stones. Although it is clear that in many patients such stones remain asymptomatic for months or years, the available evidence suggests that the natural history of asymptomatic common duct stones is less benign than that of asymptomatic gallstones.

The morbidity of choledocholithiasis stems principally from biliary obstruction, which increases biliary pressure and diminishes bile flow. The rate of onset of obstruction, its degree, and the amount of bacterial contamination of the bile are the major factors that determine the resulting symptoms. Acute obstruction usually causes biliary colic and jaundice, whereas obstruction that develops gradually over several months may manifest initially with pruritus or jaundice alone. If bacteria proliferate, life-threatening cholangitis may result (see Cholangitis).

Physical examination

The physical examination is usually completely normal if obstruction of the common duct is intermittent. Mild to moderate jaundice may be seen when the obstruction has been present for several days to a few weeks. Deep jaundice, particularly with a palpable gallbladder, suggests a neoplastic obstruction of the common duct, even when the patient has stones in the gallbladder. With longstanding obstruction, secondary biliary cirrhosis may result, with physical findings of chronic liver disease.

Diagnosis

Laboratory tests

As shown in Table 3.3, laboratory studies may be the only hint of the existence of choledocholithiasis.

Bilirubin and alkaline phosphatase   With bile duct obstruction, both bilirubin and alkaline phosphatase concentrations increase. Bilirubin accumulates in serum due to blocked excretion, whereas alkaline phosphatase levels rise because of increased synthesis of the enzyme by the canalicular epithelium. The rise in alkaline phosphatase is more rapid and precedes that of bilirubin. The absolute height of the bilirubin concentration is proportional to the degree of obstruction, but the height of the alkaline phosphatase level bears no relation to either the degree of obstruction or its cause. In cases of choledocholithiasis, the bilirubin value typically falls in the range of 2 to 5 mg/dL and rarely surpasses 12 mg/dL.

Transaminase and amylase　Transient "spikes" in transaminases or amylase concentrations suggest passage of a common duct stone into the duodenum.

Radiologic studies

Standard ultrasound　Ultrasound actually results in visualization of common bile duct stones in only approximately 50% of cases, but dilation of the common bile duct to greater than 6 mm in diameter is seen in approximately 75% of cases. Therefore, ultrasound can confirm or at least suggest the presence of common duct stones but cannot definitively exclude choledocholithiasis. The bile duct dilates to the point that it can be detected either sonographically or by abdominal CT in approximately 75% of cases. In patients who have had recurrent bouts of cholangitis, the bile duct may become fibrotic and unable to dilate. Moreover, dilation is sometimes absent in patients with choledocholithiasis because the obstruction is low grade and intermittent.

Endoscopic ultrasonography　Although it clearly is more invasive than a standard ultrasound examination, endoscopic ultrasonography has the advantage of better visualization of the common bile duct and, in preliminary studies, it can exclude or confirm choledocholithiasis with a sensitivity and specificity of approximately 95%.

Endoscopic retrograde cholangiopancreatography　ERCP is the gold standard for the diagnosis of common bile duct stones, with a sensitivity and specificity of approximately 95%.

Percutaneous transhepatic cholangiography　This study, known as PTC, is also an accurate means of confirming the presence of choledocholithiasis. PTC is most readily accomplished in the setting of dilated intrahepatic bile ducts, and the test is now used primarily when ERCP is unavailable or was unsuccessful.

Laparoscopic ultrasonography　This is a new imaging modality employed in the surgical suite immediately before mobilization of the gallbladder. Preliminary studies suggest that laparoscopic ultrasonography may be as accurate as operative cholangiography in detecting stones in the common bile duct and therefore may obviate the need for the latter.

Spiral computed tomography and magnetic resonance cholangiopancreatography　Rapid CT imaging of the common bile duct after administration of an intravenous contrast agent (spiral CT) and magnetic resonance cholangiopancreatography (MRCP) are promising new techniques of evaluating the common bile duct for stones. The advantage of these techniques over ERCP is the lack of invasiveness (sedation and endoscopy are not needed). The disadvantages of spiral CT or MRCP are the somewhat diminished sensitivity compared with ERCP and the inability to remove the stones if they are found. If the index of suspicion for a stone in the common bile duct is low, then these tests are appropriate; if the suspicion of a stone is high, then an ERCP is a better first test.

Differential diagnosis

Biliary colic　The symptoms caused by obstruction of the common bile duct cannot be distinguished from those caused by obstruction of the cystic duct. Therefore, biliary colic is always part of the differential diagnosis. Of course, the presence of jaundice or abnormal liver function tests strongly points to the bile duct as the source of the problem rather than the gallbladder.

Choledochal cyst or obstruction of the bile duct　In patients presenting with jaundice, malignant obstruction of the bile duct or obstruction from choledochal cyst may be clinically indistinguishable from choledocholithiasis.

Acute congestion of the liver　This condition, associated with cardiac decompensation, can cause intense right upper quadrant pain, tenderness, and even jaundice with bilirubin concentrations as high as 10 mg/dL. However, the temperature remains normal and the white blood cell count is normal or only slightly elevated. The patient typically has other obvious signs of cardiac decompensation. Constrictive pericarditis or cor pulmonale can also cause acute congestion of the liver with only subtle cardiac findings.

Acute viral hepatitis　This disease rarely causes severe right upper quadrant pain with tenderness and fever. The white blood count usually is not elevated, whereas the alanine aminotransferase (ALT) and aspartate transaminase (AST) concentrations are markedly elevated.

AIDS cholangiopathy and papillary stenosis   These entities must be considered in human immunodeficiency virus–infected patients with right upper quadrant pain and abnormal liver function tests.

Management and Referral

Given the high propensity for serious complications such as cholangitis and acute pancreatitis, choledocholithiasis warrants removal of the stones (either culdoscopically or surgically) in almost all cases. The optimal therapy for a given patient depends on the level of symptoms, coexisting medical problems, local expertise, and whether the gallbladder is intact.

Common bile duct stones discovered at the time of a laparoscopic cholecystectomy present somewhat of a dilemma for the surgeon. The operation can be converted to an open cholecystectomy with a common bile duct exploration, but this approach results in greater morbidity and a more prolonged hospital stay. Alternatively, the laparoscopic cholecystectomy can be carried out as planned, and the patient can return for endoscopic removal of the common duct stones by ERCP. Such an approach, if successful, cures the disease but runs the risk of requiring a third procedure, namely a common bile duct exploration if the ERCP was unsuccessful at removing the common duct stones. In general, the greater the level of expertise of the therapeutic endoscopist, the more inclined the surgeon should be to simply complete the laparoscopic cholecystectomy and have the common duct stones removed endoscopically at a later date.

In especially high-risk patients, endoscopic removal of common duct stones may be performed without the need for cholecystectomy at all. This approach is particularly appropriate for elderly patients who have other concurrent, severe illnesses. Studies indicate that subsequent cholecystectomy for symptoms is required in only 10% of patients treated this way.

CHOLANGITIS (BACTERIAL CHOLANGITIS)

Definition

Cholangitis is defined as a bacterial infection within the bile ducts. Synonyms include ascending cholangitis and bacterial cholangitis. Sclerosing cholangitis is a rare, inflammatory lesion of the bile ducts not directly caused by bacterial infection. Of all the complications of gallstones, cholangitis kills most swiftly. Pus under pressure in the bile ducts leads to rapid spread of bacteria, via the liver, into the blood, with septicemia resulting. More-

over, the diagnosis of cholangitis is often problematic (especially in the critical early phase of the disease) due to the absence of clinical features pointing to the biliary tract as the source of sepsis. Table 3.3 delineates the symptoms, signs, and laboratory findings that can aid in an early diagnosis of cholangitis.

Cause

In approximately 85% of cases, cholangitis is caused by an impacted stone in the common bile duct that results in bile stasis. Other causes of bile duct obstruction that may cause cholangitis are neoplasms, biliary strictures, parasitic infections, and congenital abnormalities of the bile ducts.

Bile duct obstruction is necessary, but not sufficient, to cause cholangitis. Cholangitis is relatively common in patients with choledocholithiasis, almost universal in patients with posttraumatic bile duct stricture, but present in only 15% of patients with neoplastic obstruction. It is most likely to result when a bile duct that already contains bacteria becomes obstructed, which is the situation in most patients with choledocholithiasis and stricture but in few patients with neoplastic obstruction. Malignant obstruction, because it is more often complete than is obstruction due to stricture or common duct stones, less commonly permits the reflux of bacteria from duodenal contents into the bile ducts.

The bacterial species most commonly cultured are Escherichia coli, Klebsiella, Pseudomonas, enterococci, and Proteus. Anaerobic species such as Bacteroides fragilis or Clostridium perfringens are seen in about 15% of appropriately cultured bile specimens. Anaerobes usually accompany aerobes, especially E. coli.

The shaking chills and fever of cholangitis are caused by bacteria from bile duct organisms. Regurgitation of bacteria from bile into hepatic venous blood is directly proportional to the biliary pressure and hence to the degree of obstruction. This is the reason that decompression alone often effectively treats the illness so promptly.

Patient Presentation

History

As shown in Table 3.3, Charcot's classic triad of pain, jaundice, and fever is the hallmark of cholangitis. However, the full triad is only present in 70% of cases. The pain of cholangitis can be surprisingly mild and transient, but often it is accompanied by chills and rigors. Particularly in elderly patients, mental confusion, lethargy, and delirium may be the only historical features obtainable.

Physical examination

Physical examination reveals fever to be almost universal (95% of cases). Right upper quadrant tenderness occurs in approximately 90%, but jaundice is clinically detectable in only 80%. Notably, peritoneal signs are found in only 15% of these patients. In severe cases, hypotension and mental confusion may coexist, indicating gram-negative septicemia. Overlooked cases of severe cholangitis may manifest with intrahepatic abscesses as a late complication.

Diagnosis

Laboratory tests

Laboratory studies are often very helpful in pointing to the biliary tract as the source of sepsis.

Bilirubin   In particular, the serum bilirubin concentration exceeds 2 mg/dL in 80% of cases. In cases in which the bilirubin is initially normal, the diagnosis may be overlooked.

White blood cell count   Leukocytosis likewise is present in 80% of patients, but the count is normal in the remainder. However, in many of the patients with a normal leukocyte count, examination of the peripheral blood smear reveals a dramatic shift to immature neutrophil forms.

Alkaline phosphatase and amylase   Alkaline phosphatase is usually elevated, and the serum amylase concentration may also be elevated if pancreatitis is also present.

Blood cultures   Blood cultures are positive for enteric organisms in most cases, especially if the blood is obtained during chills and fever spikes. The organism found in the blood is invariably the same as that in the bile.

Radiologic studies

The principles of radiologic diagnosis are the same as those noted for choledocholithiasis.

Ultrasound   As shown in Table 3.2, stones in the common bile duct are seen sonographically in only about 50% of cases but can be inferred by the finding of a dilated common bile duct in approximately 75%. Because of this lack of sensitivity, a normal ultrasound result does not exclude the possibility of choledocholithiasis in a patient whose clinical presentation suggests cholangitis.

Abdominal computed tomography   Likewise, an abdominal CT scan is an excellent means of excluding complications of gallstones such as acute pancreatitis and abscess formation, but a standard abdominal CT scan is not capable of excluding common bile duct stones.

Spiral computed tomography and magnetic resonance cholangiopancreatography   As noted previously, spiral CT and MRCP may prove useful for excluding stones in the common bile duct.

Endoscopic retrograde cholangiopancreatography   ERCP is the gold standard test for the diagnosis of common bile duct stones. Moreover, the ability of ERCP to simultaneously confirm the presence of common duct stones and establish drainage of infected bile under pressure can be life-saving.

Percutaneous transhepatic cholangiography   If ERCP is unsuccessful, PTC can be employed.

Management and Referral

In cases of suspected bacterial cholangitis, blood cultures should be obtained immediately and therapy with antibiotics effective against the usual causative organisms should be started. For mild cases, it is usually sufficient to initiate therapy with a single drug, such cefoxitin, 2.0 g intravenously every 6 to 8 hours. In severe cases, more intensive therapy (e. g., gentamicin, ampicillin, and metronidazole) is indicated. Early consultation (i.e., within the first few hours after admission) with a gastroenterologist is warranted, because early removal of the common duct stones, or at least decompression of the pus in the bile duct, can be life-saving.

Improvement with antibiotics should be expected within 6 to 12 hours, and in most cases the infection will come under control within 2 to 3 days, with defervescence, relief of discomfort, and a falling leukocyte count. In these cases, definitive therapy can be planned on an elective basis. If, however, after 6 to 12 hours of careful observation, the patient's clinical status declines with worsening fever, pain, mental confusion, or hypotension, then the common bile duct must be decompressed on an emergency basis. If local expertise allows for it, ERCP with stone extraction or at least decompression of the bile duct is the treatment of choice. Controlled studies comparing ERCP with decompression of the bile duct versus emergency surgery with common bile duct exploration have shown dramatically reduced morbidity and mortality rates in those patients treated endoscopically.

KEY POINTS

- Three out of four patients with gallstones never develop symptoms from their stones; accordingly, asymptomatic, incidentally discovered gallstones should generally be left alone.

- Biliary colic from a gallstone manifests with episodic, recurrent attacks of upper abdominal pain lasting 1 to 4 hours. Gas, flatulence, dyspepsia, and constant abdominal pain are not caused by gallstones.

- Ultrasound is an excellent test for the diagnosis of stones in the gallbladder (cholelithiasis), but it is not sensitive enough to definitively exclude stones in the common bile duct (choledocholithiasis).

- Jaundice with abdominal pain and fever suggests ascending cholangitis—a medical emergency requiring urgent administration of antibiotics and decompression of the obstructed bile duct. Early ERCP with stone removal can be life-saving, especially in elderly patients.

COMMONLY ASKED QUESTIONS

During an ultrasound to look at my kidneys, the radiologists mentioned that I have gallstones. I've never had any symptoms caused by the gallstones, but should I have them taken care of now while I'm healthy?

No, the likelihood that the gallstone will ever cause a problem is only one in four, and except in rare circumstances asymptomatic stones should be left alone. Even if the stone should cause problems in the future, there would be time to arrange for elective surgery.

What causes gallstones?

About 80% of gallstones are caused by precipitation of excess cholesterol in bile, and 20% are caused by precipitation of bilirubin, a blood pigment that is secreted into bile. Risk factors for gallstones include advancing age, female gender, obesity, rapid weight loss, pregnancy, sickle cell anemia, and Amerindian ancestry.

Is there a certain diet that prevents gallstones from occurring?

There is no specific diet that reliably prevents stones from forming or that dissolves stones that have already formed. Because obesity is a definite risk factor for cholesterol stones, modest caloric intake that prevents obesity reduces the risk. However, if you are already overweight, then bear in mind that rapid weight loss is actually a strong risk factor for stone formation. There is no correlation between the amount of cholesterol in the diet or blood and the amount of cholesterol in bile.

Why doesn't the surgeon just remove the gallstones rather than removing the entire gallbladder? Don't I need a gallbladder?

If the gallbladder is left in place, then new stones will form over time and the clinical problem will recur. People do fine without a gallbladder—it just means that bile trickles into the intestine all day in-stead of only after meals. Many other mammals, such as horses and rats, do not have gallbladders at all.

Is a laparoscopic cholecystectomy better than an open cholecystectomy?

It depends. The hospital stay and recovery time are shorter when the surgery can be done laparoscopically. In some cases, even if a laparoscopic approach is planned, the surgeon may discover a need to explore the bile ducts or directly manipulate the gallbladder and may therefore switch the operation to an open cholecystectomy.

SUGGESTED READINGS

Bilhartz LE, Horton JD. Gallstone disease and its complications. In: Feldman M, Scharschmidt BF, Sleisenger MH, eds. Sleisenger and Fordtran's Gastrointestinal and Liver Disease, 6th ed. Philadelphia: WB Saunders, 1997: 948–972.

Carey MC. Pathogenesis of gallstones (review). Am J Surg 1993;165:410–419.

Cotton PB. Endoscopic retrograde cholangiopancreatography and laparoscopic cholecystectomy [Review]. Am J Surg 1993;165:474–478.

Egbert AM. Gallstone symptoms: myth and reality. Postgrad Med 1991;90:119–126.

Everson GT, McKinley C, Kern FJ. Mechanisms of gallstone formation in women: effects of exogenous estrogen (Premarin) and dietary cholesterol on hepatic lipid metabolism. J Clin Invest 1991;87:237–246.

Feld R, Kurtz AB, Zeman RK. Imaging the gallbladder: a historical perspective. AJR Am J Roentgenol 1991;156: 737–740.

Fenster LF, Lonborg R, Thirlby RC, Traverso LW. What symptoms does cholecystectomy cure? Insights from an outcomes measurement project and review of the literature [Review]. Am J Surg 1995;169:533–538.

Friedman GD, Raviola CA, Fireman B. Prognosis of gallstones with mild or no symptoms: 25 years of follow-up in a health maintenance organization. J Clin Epidemiol 1989;42:127–136.

Glenn F. Acute cholecystitis. Surg Gynecol Obstet 1976; 143:56–68.

Gracie WA, Ransohoff DF. The natural history of silent gallstones: the innocent gallstone is not a myth. N Engl J Med 1982;307:798–800.

Graham SM, Flowers JL, Schweitzer E, Bartlett ST, Imbembo AL. The utility of prophylactic laparoscopic cholecystectomy in transplant candidates. Am J Surg 1995;169:44–48, 48–49 (discussion).

Leitman IM, Fisher ML, McKinley MJ, et al. The evaluation and management of known or suspected stones of the common bile duct in the era of minimal access surgery. Surg Gynecol Obstet 1993;176:527–533.

Pitt HA, Cameron JL. Acute cholangitis. In: Way LW, Pellegrini CA, eds. Surgery of the gallbladder and bile ducts. Philadelphia: WB Saunders, 1987:295–310.

Polk HC. Carcinoma and the calcified gall bladder. Gastro-enterology 1966;50:582–586.

Ransohoff DF, Gracie WA. Management of patients with symptomatic gallstones: a quantitative analysis. Am J Med 1990;88:154–160.

Shea JA, Berlin JA, Escarce JJ, et al. Revised estimates of diagnostic test sensitivity and specificity in suspected biliary tract disease. Arch Intern Med 1994;154: 2573–2581.

Shiffman ML, Kaplan GD, Brinkman-Kaplan V, Vickers FF. Prophylaxis against gallstone formation with urso-deoxycholic acid in patients participating in a very-low calorie diet program. Ann Intern Med 1995;122: 899–905.

Strasberg SM, Clavien PA. Overview of therapeutic modalities for the treatment of gallstone diseases. Am J Surg 1993;165:420–426.

Thistle JL, Cleary PA, Lachin JM, Tyor MP, Hersh T. The natural history of cholelithiasis: The National Cooperative Gallstone Study. Ann Intern Med 1984;101: 171–175.

Traverso LW. Clinical manifestations and impact of gallstone disease. Am J Surg 1993;165:405–409.

Ware RE, Kinney TR, Casey JR, Pappas TN, Meyers WC. Laparoscopic cholecystectomy in young patients with sickle hemoglobinopathies. J Pediatr 1992;120: 58–61.

Way LW. Retained common duct stones. Surg Clin North Am 1973;53:1139–1147.

Acute and Chronic Viral Hepatitis

Steven L. Leach

University of Texas Southwestern Medical Center, Dallas, Texas 75235

DEFINITION

Viral hepatitis is hepatocellular injury resulting from the direct or indirect effects of viruses that infect the liver. To date, five pathologic hepatotropic viruses have been identified; they have been labeled types A, B, C, D, and E. Another hepatotropic virus, hepatitis G, has been characterized but is probably not pathologic. Other viruses that cause systemic disease, such as Epstein-Barr virus (EBV) and cytomegalovirus (CMV), are known to cause hepatocellular injury and may cause self-limited, acute hepatitis. The spectrum of disease produced by hepatotropic viruses is broad, ranging from asymptomatic, chronic infection with normal transaminases to fulminant hepatitis. Similarly, a variety of extrahepatic manifestations have been documented. Each of the five pathologic hepatotropic viruses causes acute hepatitis. Only types B, C, and D cause chronic hepatitis (infec-

tion lasting longer than 6 months). Viral hepatitis is the most common cause of chronic hepatitis, cirrhosis, hepatocellular carcinoma, and death from liver disease.

In the United States, the Centers for Disease Control and Prevention (CDC) estimate that between 200,000 and 700,000 new cases of viral hepatitis occur each year. Of these, at least 180,000 are attributed to hepatitis A virus (HAV), 128,000 to HBV, and 28,000 to HCV. Although the number of new cases of HBV far exceeds that of HCV each year, HCV is much more likely to result in chronic hepatitis. Consequently, the prevalence of HBV in the United States is estimated at 1 to 1.25 million, whereas that of HCV is estimated at 4 million. Approximately 15,000 deaths per year are attributed to the effects of viral hepatitis. Ten percent of transfusion-related hepatitis and 5% of community-acquired hepatitis cases remain unexplained.

DIAGNOSIS OF ACUTE HEPATITIS

Diagnostic Tests

Abnormal liver tests are some of the most common findings in clinical practice. Consequently, the accurate diagnosis of acute hepatitis depends on recognition of specific patterns of liver injury. Patterns of injury can be broadly classified as infiltrative (e.g., granulomatous hepatitis), obstructive (e.g., cholelithiasis, primary sclerosing cholangitis), or hepatocellular (e.g., autoimmune, drug-induced, or viral types). Biochemically, these are characterized by *predominant* elevations of alkaline phosphatase and gamma-glutamyl transferase in infiltrative/obstructive disease, and transaminases in hepatocellular injury. In addition to the pattern of injury, the degree of abnormality is helpful in classifying the disease process. Transaminase elevations are considered mild if they are less than 2 to 3 times the upper limit of normal, moderate if 3 to 20 times above normal, and marked if more than 20 times greater than normal.

Differential Diagnosis

Hepatitis

The approach to the patient with hepatitis begins with a thorough history and physical examination. Knowledge of risk factors, epidemiologic patterns, and the course of symptoms frequently suggests a specific cause. Acute hepatitis is suspected when symptoms are severe, abrupt in onset, or of short duration. Symptoms of chronic hepatitis are typically mild, insidious in onset, or of prolonged duration.

Laboratory testing allows one to characterize the disease process more precisely. Conditions associated with mild hepatocellular injury include chronic viral hepatitis (HBV or HCV), alcoholic liver disease, hemochromatosis, and nonalcoholic steatohepatitis. Marked transaminase elevations are seen in acute viral hepatitis, drug-induced hepatitis, and ischemic hepatitis. Each of these processes represents a spectrum of disease, and considerable overlaps exist. A broad differential diagnosis is shown in Table 4.1.

Viral hepatitis

Viral hepatitis should be considered in the differential diagnosis of all patients with hepatitis. In patients with history and laboratory findings suggestive of chronic hepatitis, adequate screening for viral causes can be accomplished by checking for hepatitis B surface antigen (HBsAg) and anti-HCV. If these tests are negative, viral hepatitis is very unlikely. HAV and HEV do not cause

---

Summary of Diagnosis

- The spectrum of disease caused by viral hepatitis ranges from asymptomatic with normal transaminase concentrations to fulminant hepatitis. Extrahepatic manifestations are common.
- The symptoms of acute viral hepatitis are similar for all viral types. They include fatigue, malaise, anorexia, nausea, vomiting, headache, myalgias, arthralgias, fever, and right upper quadrant abdominal pain.
- Signs of viral hepatitis may include tender hepatomegaly, splenomegaly, and lymphadenopathy.
- Laboratory tests typically reveal transaminase elevations ranging from 3 to 20 times the upper limit of normal. Bilirubin usually does not exceed 10 mg/dl.

TABLE 4.1.

Differential Diagnosis of Acute Hepatitis

Noninfectious causes
  Alcohol
  Autoimmune hepatitis
  Ischemia
  Drug toxicity
  Drug hypersensitivity
  Biliary obstruction
  Primary biliary cirrhosis
  Wilson's disease
  Alpha$_1$-antitrypsin deficiency
  Hemochromatosis
  Congestive heart failure
Viruses
  Hepatitis viruses A, B, C, D, E
  Epstein-Barr virus
  Cytomegalovirus
  Yellow fever virus
  Herpes simplex virus
  Rubella virus
  Coxsackievirus
Complications of other infections (usually mild)
  Syphilis
  Tuberculosis
  Toxoplasmosis
  Amebiasis

chronic hepatitis; screening for them is unnecessary and not cost-effective. Testing for anti-HDV is indicated only when HBsAg is positive. The approach to acute hepatitis is more complicated. A directed evaluation begins with serologic analyses for hepatitis A, B, and C. A sample of serologic patterns in acute viral hepatitis is presented in Table 4.2.

Acute hepatitis A Acute HAV infection is diagnosed on the basis of the presence of immunoglobulin M (IgM) anti-HAV. These antibodies are present in 90% of infected patients at the time of presentation. Given its high sensitivity and specificity, this test is usually diagnostic and only occasionally needs to be repeated.

Acute hepatitis B Accurate diagnosis of acute HBV infection requires two tests. Although infection with HBV can be diagnosed on the basis of the presence of HBsAg alone, it does not distinguish between acute and chronic hepatitis B. Furthermore, HBsAg may be rapidly cleared and undetectable in the acute phase under various conditions, such as fulminant or subfulminant hepatitis or concomitant infection with HDV. Consequently, IgM antibodies against the core antigen (HBc), the hallmark of acute infection, are essential to secure the diagnosis. Nevertheless, some patients with chronic HBV infection remain positive for IgM anti-HBc indefinitely, so this test is necessary but not sufficient to make the diagnosis. Other causes of acute hepatitis must be ruled out before one can safely conclude that HBV is the causative agent.

Acute hepatitis C Antibodies to HCV are present in only 50% to 70% of patients with acute HCV infection, making this the most difficult type to diagnose. Retesting at 4-week intervals may be necessary. When suspicion is high and the diagnosis is urgent, direct tests for HCV RNA are required. This is rarely necessary, however, because the course is usually mild. IgM and IgG anti-HCV are not effective at distinguishing between acute and chronic infection. As with HBV, the diagnosis of acute HCV infection is depends in part on the exclusion of other causes.

Acute hepatitis D and hepatitis E Additional tests for HDV and HEV infection are obtained depending on the results of tests for types A, B, and C. If evidence of HBV is present, whether acute or chronic, markers for HDV must also be obtained. However, it is not necessary to obtain these in every patient, because coinfection with HBV is mandatory for HDV to be present. HEV infection remains rare in the United States. Nevertheless, it must be considered in the appropriate circumstances (e.g., recent travel to endemic areas). Markers for HEV should be obtained when other causes have been ruled out and the suspicion of viral hepatitis remains high.

This paradigm is effective in most cases. As with all laboratory tests, false-positive and false-negative results do occur. When risk factors or clinical features dictate, alternative tests such as DNA/RNA tests, immunoblot assays, or liver biopsy should be considered. Tests for other causes, including infections, should be obtained on the basis of clinical suspicion. For instance, in India, more

---

TABLE 4.2. Diagnostic Tests in Acute Hepatitis[a]

Type of viral hepatitis	Anti-HAV IgM	HBsAg[b]	Anti-HBc IgM[c]	Anti-HCV[d]	Anti-HDV IgM	Anti-HEV IgM
A	+					
B		+	+			
B + C		+	+	+		
B + D		±	+		+	
C				+		
C + Chronic B		+		+		
D		±			+	
E						+

Anti-HAV, antibody to hepatitis A virus; HBsAg, hepatitis B surface antigen; Anti-HBc, antibody to hepatitis B core antigen; Anti-HCV, antibody to hepatitis C virus; Anti-HDV, antibody to hepatitis D virus; Anti-HEV, antibody to hepatitis E virus
[a] The evaluation of acute hepatitis begins with serologic studies for viral types A, B, and C; Serology results for types D and E are obtained depending on the results of these initial tests.
[b] In severe cases or in HBV/HDV coinfection, HBsAg may be rapidly cleared to undetectable levels; HBsAg does not distinguish between acute and chronic infection.
[c] IgM anti-HBc may be positive in chronic carriers; other causes must be excluded.
[d] Anti-HCV does not distinguish between acute and chronic HCV infection; other causes must be excluded.

than 20% of non-A, non-B viral hepatitis may be attributed to CMV or EBV. Despite careful investigation, some cases of acute hepatitis remain unexplained. Uncharacterized non-ABCDE hepatitis viruses are thought to account for many of these episodes.

CLASSIFICATION

Hepatitis A

Cause

Formerly known as "infectious hepatitis," hepatitis A is the most common form of viral hepatitis worldwide. Several distinct genotypes have been identified, but there is only one serotype. An important characteristic of HAV is its stability, a factor that contributes to its propagation. The virus is stable to temperatures of 60°C and may remain viable in the environment at ambient temperatures for 1 month.

HAV is transmitted by the fecal-oral route, although rare episodes of transfusion-related transmission have been reported. After a brief viremia, replication is limited to the liver. High viral titers are found in the bile and stool of infected persons. Stool viral titers are highest in the late incubation stage or in the prodromal (pre-icteric) stage, when symptoms first become noticeable.

By the time icterus occurs, infectivity is waning. The total duration of viral shedding may be several months, with children harboring the virus longer than adults do.

Figure 4.1 depicts the worldwide distribution of HAV infection. In some countries, seroprevalence rates exceed 90%. Rates of infection are highest in South America, Africa, Southeast Asia, and Greenland. Socioeconomic influences appear to be the most significant factors contributing to this trend. Infection is endemic in developing countries where hygiene and sanitation are inadequate. In these regions, almost all of the population is affected by the end of the first decade of life. Most of these infections go unrecognized because the severity of illness is much less in younger persons. In contrast, seropositivity rates in developed countries are low in childhood but gradually increase with advancing age. Seasonal variations are common, with more frequent infections in fall and winter months. Because there are no chronic carriers of infection, HAV does not have a reservoir. The virus is maintained by serial propagation from an acutely infected person to a susceptible person.

The incidence of HAV infection in the United States has tended to rise and fall in a cyclic pattern lasting approximately 10 years. The current incidence is estimated at 9.1 cases per 100,000 persons per year. The seroprevalence in the United States was determined by the

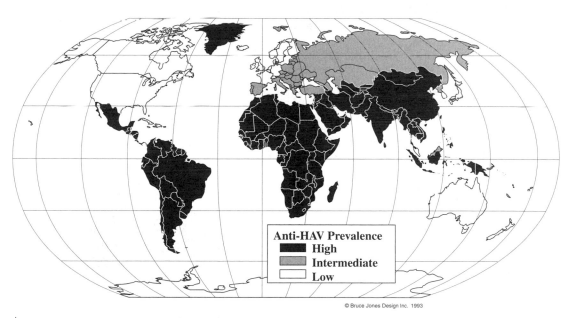

Anti-HAV Prevalence
High
Intermediate
Low

© Bruce Jones Design Inc. 1993

†This map generalized available data. Patterns may vary within countries.

Anti-HAV, antibody to hepatitis A virus

FIGURE 4.1.
Worldwide distribution of hepatitis A virus infection.

Third National Health and Nutrition Examination Survey (NHANES-III), which was conducted from 1988 to 1991. The overall prevalence was 33%. Prevalence was 10% for persons younger than 10 years of age, 18% for those age 20 to 29, 49% for those age 40 to 49, and 75% for those older than 75 years. Prevalence was 67% among Mexican-Americans, 37% among African-Americans, and 29% among whites. Both incidence and prevalence have been declining in the United States.

Figure 4.2 depicts the most frequently reported sources of infection in the United States. Household or sexual contact with an infected person is the most common source, accounting for one fourth of cases. Additional risk factors include employment or attendance in a day care center, recent international travel, and history of injection drug use. Homosexual as well as heterosexual sex has been implicated. Poor sanitation and overcrowding contribute to episodes of infection via water and food, including milk and shellfish. These pathways for infection account for only a very small percentage of infections. Fifty percent of infections have no identifiable source.

Patient presentation

History Hepatitis A is typically a self-limited illness with no long-term sequelae. The incubation period (from the time of infection to the onset of symptoms) ranges from 15 to 50 days, with a mean of 4 weeks. Symptom onset is usually abrupt. The prodromal symptoms (those preceding jaundice) are similar to those of other viral illnesses and include fever, anorexia, malaise, fatigue, headache, myalgias, and arthralgias. Nausea, vomiting, and right upper quadrant abdominal pain may result in weight loss. Pruritus may also be present. Within a week, dark urine and clay-colored stool and/or jaundice appear. With the onset of jaundice, symptoms begin to resolve.

The symptoms of acute HAV usually last 2 to 3 weeks. However, complete recovery maybe delayed for up to 12 weeks. The severity of symptoms depends greatly on age. Seventy percent of infected children younger than than 6 years of age have no symptoms of acute hepatitis. Seventy percent of infected adults have jaundice. Extrahepatic manifestations are unusual, but arthritis, rashes, and leukocytoclastic vasculitis may be seen.

Physical examination The liver is usually slightly enlarged and tender. Splenomegaly and posterior cervical adenopathy are detected in as many as 15% of patients. At the time of presentation, transaminase concentrations usually exceed 1,000 U/L and may be as high as 5,000 U/L. The alanine aminotransferase (ALT) concentration is typically greater than that of aspartate aminotransferase (AST). These elevations are followed by a rise in bilirubin, which rarely exceeds 10 mg/dL. Once they peak, transaminases decline by as much as 75% per week for the first several weeks, then more slowly thereafter. Bilirubin decreases more gradually over a similar period (Fig. 4.3).

Complications Although complete resolution is the norm, fulminant hepatitis may occur. Patients older than 50 years of age and those with chronic liver disease are at greatest risk. The CDC reports approximately 100

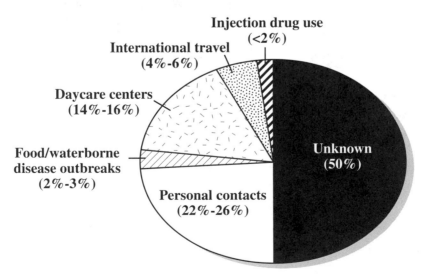

FIGURE 4.2.
Risk factors for hepatitis A virus infection.

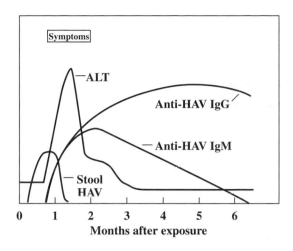

HAV, hepatitis A virus; Anti-HAV, antibody to hepatitis A virus

FIGURE 4.3.

Clinical course and laboratory findings in hepatitis A virus infection.

deaths per year from HAV. The overall case-fatality rate is 0.3%; for those over age 50, it is 1.8%. Fulminant hepatitis resulting from HAV superinfection in chronic HBV has been well documented. Of particular concern is a report of fulminant hepatitis in 7 of 17 patients with chronic HCV who were superinfected with HAV.

Several less common manifestations have been described. Cholestatic hepatitis is a well-documented variant of HAV infection. It is characterized by pruritus, more pronounced elevations in serum bilirubin (more than 10 mg/dL), more prolonged jaundice (duration exceeding 12 weeks), and less dramatic increases in transaminase levels (less than 500 U/L). As a rule, however, these patients also recover completely.

Relapsing hepatitis occurs in 6% to 10% of patients. After a typical case of acute HAV, a second acute hepatitis may ensue 5 to 14 weeks later. Transaminases are again increased to more than 1,000 U/L, IgM anti-HAV remains persistently positive, and virus may be detected in the stool and blood. The relapse usually lasts no longer than 30 days and is followed by complete resolution. Chronic hepatitis does not develop. Rarely more than one relapse may occur. Autoimmune hepatitis triggered by acute hepatitis A is another documented but rare result of infection.

Diagnosis

Although the diagnosis of hepatitis A may be suggested by the history and patterns of liver test abnormalities, definitive diagnosis is confirmed by detection of IgM anti-HAV. No further testing or invasive procedure is neces-

sary. IgM anti-HAV is detectable in virtually all patients at the time of presentation. When suspicion is high and initial tests are negative, repeat testing 3 to 7 days later is occasionally necessary. The serologic tests are highly sensitive and specific. The presence of IgG anti-HAV in the absence of IgM suggests prior exposure and should prompt a search for other causes of acute hepatitis. Vaccination rarely promotes an IgM response; consequently, the development of an IgM response after vaccination is evidence of true infection. In 25% of infected patients, IgM anti-HAV persists for as long as 12 months.

Management

Treatment For information on treating and referring cases of HAV, see the section on Management of Acute Hepatitis.

Prevention There are now two safe, highly effective vaccines for HAV (Havrix and Vaqta), and there is good evidence that vaccination is cost-effective. Recommended dosing schedules for HAV vaccination are listed in Table 4.3.

Despite the availability and efficacy of these vaccines, global vaccination programs are not yet feasible and have not been implemented. Implementation is limited by several factors. Most important is the fact that appropriate dosing and timing of immunizations for children younger than 2 years of age are not known. Infected children in this age group are frequently asymptomatic; this results in a persistent, unrecognized propagation of the virus. A second issue is a lack of public awareness, particularly in countries where endemicity is low, such as the United States. Consequently, prevention is currently accomplished through improvements in sanitation and living conditions in urban centers and in developing countries.

Both vaccines are formalin-inactivated viruses derived from HAV grown in human fibroblast cultures. Purified lysates are adsorbed to an aluminum hydroxide adjuvant. Havrix is preserved in 2-phenoxyethanol; Vaqta is formulated without preservative. Tolerance is excellent. The most common side effects are mild local

Summary of Diagnosis

- The diagnosis of acute HAV infection is based on the detection of anti-HAV IgM.
- Antibody detection is a very sensitive and specific test. These antibodies are present in more than 90% of patients with acute HAV at the time of presentation.

TABLE 4.3.	Recommended Dosing Schedules for Hepatitis A Virus (HAV) Vaccination	
Patient age (yr) or status	Schedule (mo)	Dose
Havirx		
2–18	0, 1, 6–12	360 ELU/0.5 mL
2–18	0, 6–12	720 ELU/0.5 mL
>18	0, 6–12	1,440 ELU/1.0 mL
Vaqta		
2–17	0, 6–18	25 U/0.5 mL
>17	0, 6	50 U/1.0 mL
Immune globulin prophylaxis		
Preexposure		
Short-term (1–2 mo)		0.02 mL/kg
Long-term (3–5 mo)		0.06 mL/kg[b]
Postexposure		0.02 mL/kg

ELU, ELISA units.
[a] 0 represents initial dose.
[b] May repeat every 5 months.

TABLE 4.4.	Centers for Disease Control and Prevention Recommendations for Hepatitis A Virus (HAV) Vaccination

Preexposure

Persons traveling to or working in countries that have high or intermediate endemicity
Children in communities that have high rates of HAV and periodic outbreaks
Men who have sex with men
Illegal drug users
Handlers of HAV-positive primates and those who work with HAV in the laboratory
Persons with chronic liver disease
Persons with clotting factor disorders

Postexposure

Household and sexual contacts of persons confirmed to have HAV
Staff and attendees of day care centers
Food handlers exposed to coworkers with HAV
(Single-case exposures in school or workplace do not require prophylaxis)

Adapted from Centers for Disease Control and Prevention. Prevention of hepatitis A through active and passive immunization: recommendations of the advisory committee on immunization practices (ACIP). MMWR Morb Mortal Wkly Rep 1996;45:1–30.

reactions, headache, and malaise. Vaccination is typically a two-shot series, with the second dose given 6 to 18 months after the first. Injections should be given in the deltoid muscle. The vaccines can be administered simultaneously with other vaccines, including hepatitis B, diphtheria, tetanus, oral typhoid, cholera, Japanese encephalitis, rabies, yellow fever, and HAV immune globulin. However, these injections should be given at separate sites. After vaccination, almost 100% of patients develop protective antibodies in approximately 4 weeks. Concurrent immunization with immune globulin decreases the absolute titers of antibody but does not reduce the proportion of patients developing protective levels. Levels of antibody decline over time, but it is estimated that they remain protective for at least 20 years. Other factors that may lessen immunogenicity of vaccination include age older than 40 years, subcutaneous injection, freezing of the vaccine, and an accelerated dosing schedule. Prevaccination testing is cost-effective in persons who have a high likelihood of prior infection, such as those older than 40 ears of age and those born in areas of high endemicity. Postvaccination testing is not necessary.

The CDC recommendations for immunization are listed in Table 4.4. There is currently no recommendation for routine vaccination of workers in day care cen-

ters, health care institutions, schools, or sewage treatment plants. Nevertheless, vaccination of such persons may be warranted. For travelers, initial vaccination should occur at least 1 month before departure. Contraindications include hypersensitivity to aluminum or 2-phenoxyethanol. Vaccination can be safely performed in immunocompromised patients. Safety has not been established in pregnancy, but the theoretical risk is low. Immune globulin is an effective alternative for persons younger than 2 years of age, those who are allergic to a component of the vaccine, those traveling for only a short period, and those traveling on short notice. Absolute antibody titers are lower than those produced by inactivated virus vaccination, but they remain protective for up to 3 to 5 months. Postexposure prophylaxis is recommended for all household and sexual contacts of infected persons. It is also indicated for staff and attendees of day care centers if one or more children become infected. For food handlers, prophylaxis is recommended only for other food handlers with whom the index case has come in contact. Transmission to consumers may occur, but administration of immune globulin to all patrons is not cost-effective.

Hepatitis B

Cause

Once referred to as "serum hepatitis," HBV is the most common cause of chronic hepatitis worldwide. The World Health Organization estimates that more than 350 million persons are chronically infected, a number that is expected to exceed 400 million by the year 2000. As many as 25% of these persons will die from the direct effects of the virus.

HBV is transmitted via parenteral or mucous membrane exposure to HBV-infected body fluids. HBV has been identified in virtually all body fluids, including saliva, tears, ascites, synovial fluid, breast milk, pleural fluid, gastric fluid, urine, semen, cerebrospinal fluid, and vaginal secretions. HBV replicates primarily in hepatocytes, but there is evidence that it can replicate in some extrahepatic tissues as well. The virus is not directly cytotoxic. Rather, hepatitis is thought to result from the host's immune response to the foreign antigens of HBV presented on the surface of the hepatocyte. HBV is very stable and can remain viable at room temperature for up to 6 months. It is effectively inactivated by heating to 98°C for 1 minute or by exposure to formalin or chloroform.

Hepatitis B is a circular DNA virus that includes four overlapping open reading frames. These reading frames are labeled S (surface or envelope), C (core), P (polymerase), and X (transcriptional activators). The S gene encodes three distinct proteins that together compose the envelope of the virion (HBsAg). The C gene encodes the proteins that make up the nucleo-capsid or core (HBcAg), which directly surrounds the DNA. Hepatitis e antigen (HBeAg) is a modified product of the C gene. Clinically, it serves as a marker for active viral replication.

The life cycle of HBV can be divided into four stages. The typical laboratory findings in each of these stages are summarized in Table 4.5. After the initial infection, replication begins in a state of immune tolerance, characterized by the presence of HBsAg, HbcAg, HBeAg (with the exception of mutants), high titers of HBV DNA, and normal transaminases. In persons with immature or suppressed immune systems, this stage may last indefinitely. The second stage begins when the host mounts an immune response. Reduced levels of HBV DNA occur concomitantly with elevations of transaminases (hepatitis), a result of cell-mediated hepatocellular injury. The severity and duration of this stage depends on the degree of the host response. An incomplete response results in chronic hepatitis. On the other hand, if the host response is adequate to halt viral replication, the virus becomes dormant. In some cases, the virus integrates into the host genome. This marks the third phase of infection. HbeAg becomes negative, and HBV DNA titers drop even further. Nevertheless, in many cases DNA is still detectable by sensitive polymerase chain reaction (PCR) techniques. Transaminases return to normal, and anti-HBe becomes positive. This transition from stage 2 to stage 3 is the goal of treatment for HBV and is associated with improvement in histologic status and long-term survival. HbsAg is still pres-

Stages of Hepatitis B Virus Infection[a]   **TABLE 4.5.**

Disease Marker	Replicative phase		Integrative phase	
	Stage 1	Stage 2	Stage 3	Stage 4
HBsAg	Positive	Positive	Positive	Negative
Antibody to HBsAg	Negative	Negative	Negative	Positive
HBV DNA	Strongly positive	Negative[b]	Negative	Positive
Antibody to HBcAg	Positive	Positive	Positive	Positive
HBeAg	Positive	Positive	Negative	Negative
Antibody to HBeAg	Negative	Negative	Positive	Positive
Aspartate and alanine aminotransferase levels	Normal	Elevated	Normal	Normal

HBV, hepatitis B virus; HBsAg, hepatitis B surface antigen; HBcAg, hepatitis B core antigen; HBeAg, hepatitis B e antigen

[a] Stage 1 is characterized by immune tolerance, with the presence of HBeAg and large quantities of HBV DNA in serum signaling the period of active viral replication. Stage 2 is characterized by active hepatitis with diminished HBV DNA levels. By stage 3, clearance of the bulk of virus-infected cells has occurred, mediated by the host immune response. Replication ceases and HBeAg disappears despite the presence of circulating HBsAg. In stage 4, HBsAg has been cleared and the presence of antibody to HBsAg signals the development of full immunity to the virus.

[b] Although viral DNA is negative by hybridization techniques, it remains detectable by sensitive polymerase chain reaction methods in many patients.

From Lee WM. Hepatitis B virus infection. N Engl J Med 1997; 337:1733–1745.

ent at this point. Relapse to stage 2 is possible but uncommon. Full immunity is not achieved until the fourth stage, when HBsAg finally disappears and antibody to HBsAg (anti-HBs) becomes detectable. At this point, HBV DNA is truly absent.

As with HAV, the incidence and prevalence of HBV vary tremendously, depending on socioeconomic circumstances. The prevalence is highest in developing countries, such as those in Southeast Asia, China, and Africa, where more than half of the population have serologic evidence of prior infection. In these regions, the rate of chronic infection ranges from 8% to 15%. In developed areas such as the United States, Western Europe, Australia, and New Zealand, seroprevalence is less than 20%, and the rate of chronic infection is less than 2%. Intermediate prevalence is seen in Eastern Europe, Southern Europe, Central Asia, Japan, and regions of the former Soviet Union (Fig. 4.4).

The risk factors for HBV infection in the United States are shown in Figure 4.5. The most common risk factors for transmission are sexual activity (homosexual or heterosexual) and injection drug use. The most recent data from the CDC Sentinel Counties study revealed that heterosexual activity now accounts for about one third of infections, a 50% increase since 1988. Infection from homosexual activity has decreased by 60% since

1985 but still accounts for 16% of acute cases. Rates of infection from injection drug use have also decreased 40% since 1988 and now account for 17% of infections.

Although perinatal infection does occur, HBV infection in industrialized countries is much more common in adolescent and adult populations. About 22,000 babies are born to HBsAg-positive mothers in the United States each year. The great majority of these receive immune prophylaxis, and transmission is uncommon. Horizontal transmission in early childhood also occurs, particularly in families that have recently emigrated from areas of high endemicity. Other well-defined risk factors include occupational exposure, blood transfusion (particularly in hemophiliacs receiving clotting factor concentrates), hemodialysis, and organ donation. Transmission from surgeon to patient has also been documented. Overall, it is estimated that the incidence of HBV infection in the United States has decreased 40% since 1985.

The frequency at which chronic hepatitis develops after acute HBV is inversely proportional to the age at infection. When transmission is from infected mother to neonate (vertical transmission), the rate of chronic infection is 70% to 90%. With later infections (horizontal transmission), the rate steadily decreases until it reaches 6% to 10% by the age of 6 years. Aside from

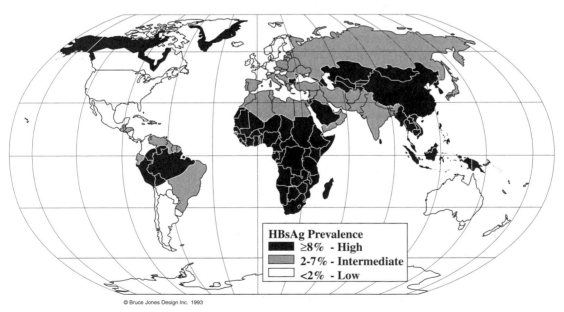

© Bruce Jones Design Inc. 1993

†This map generalized available data. Patterns may vary within countries.

HBsAg, hepatitis B surface antigen

FIGURE 4.4.
Worldwide distribution of hepatitis B virus infection.

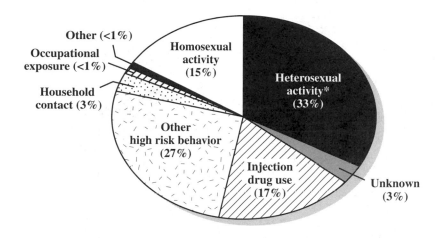

*Includes sexual contact with persons documented to have HBV infection, and the risk of multiple sexual partners.

FIGURE 4.5.
Risk factors for hepatitis B virus infection.

age, immunosuppression from any cause results in a higher likelihood of chronic infection. Consequently, patients infected with the human immunodeficiency virus (HIV), those receiving immunosuppressive agents, those receiving hemodialysis, and those with malignancy are more likely to remain HbsAg positive.

Patient presentation

History   After an incubation period of 30 to 180 days, acute HBV infection follows a course very similar to that of HAV. Prodromal symptoms include malaise, fatigue, arthralgias, myalgias, headache, nausea, and abdominal discomfort. The severity of these symptoms varies with age and comorbid conditions. More severe disease is seen in those with advanced age and an intact immune system. The prodrome is followed by the onset of jaundice, which typically heralds the onset of recovery.

Physical examination   The liver may be slightly enlarged and tender. Adenopathy and splenomegaly are occasionally seen. Fulminant hepatitis occurs in 0.1% to 1.0% of patients with acute HBV.

Course of disease   The pattern of symptoms and laboratory tests seen in acute, self-limited HBV infection is depicted in Figure 4.6. HBsAg is typically detectable in the blood 30 to 60 days after exposure. After a period of asymptomatic antigenemia, the host immune response is heralded by the rise of transaminases and the appearance of IgM anti-HBc. Transaminases rise abruptly and

are associated with the onset of symptoms. The peak in transaminase concentrations, which may be several hundred to several thousand units per liter, roughly correlates with the decline in HBsAg and the rise in bilirubin. As transaminases begin to decline, symptoms also tend to resolve. HBsAg gradually declines over several months. After a period of undetectable surface antigen, the "window period," anti-HBs appears, indicating viral clearance and immunity. IgM anti-HBc is gradually replaced by IgG anti-HBc over 3 to 6 months.

Chronic hepatitis   Persistence of HBsAg for longer than 6 months is the hallmark of chronic hepatitis. Chronic hepatitis can take a variety of forms. In the immune-tolerant patient (stage 1), HBsAg remains present with high levels of HBV DNA but normal transaminases. Progressive liver disease is infrequent in this population. However, after many years of infection, cirrhosis and hepatocellular carcinoma (HCC) can still occur. Furthermore, flares of hepatitis, due to either HBV or superinfection with other viruses, may lead to acute or fulminant disease. In patients with active hepatitis (stage 2 disease), HBeAg is an indicator of high likelihood of disease progression. Fifty percent of HBeAg-positive patients with active hepatitis progress to cirrhosis in 5 years. Approximately 5% of HBeAg-positive patients spontaneously convert to anti-HBe per year; as a result, the severity of hepatitis improves and ALT returns to normal.

Complications   Once cirrhosis is established, the development of complications (e.g., ascites, variceal

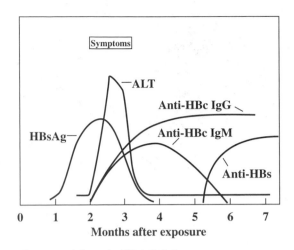

*Represents typical course in self-limited infection.
Patterns vary in persons developing chronic infection.

HBsAg, hepatitis B surface antigen; *ALT*, alanine aminotransferase
Anti-HBc, antibody to hepatitis B core antigen
Anti-HBs, antibody to hepatitis B surface antigen

FIGURE 4.6.
Clinical course and laboratory findings in hepatitis B
virus infection.

bleeding, encephalopathy) is approximately 2% to 5%
per year. Most complications occur after cirrhosis has
been present for at least 2 years. The 5-year mortality
rate is 29%. From the onset of first decompensation,
disease progression is more rapid, resulting in a 5-year
mortality rate of 65%.

HEPATOCELLULAR CARCINOMA   The development of HCC is also of great concern. The incidence
varies widely by geographic region, with HCC being
one of the most common tumors in Southeast Asia and
sub-Saharan Africa. In patients with established cirrhosis, the annual incidence of HCC is estimated to be
1% to 3%. The cumulative probability in one study
was 15% at 10 years. Risk factors for the development
of HCC include advanced age, higher levels of alpha-
fetoprotein, firm liver on examination, and thrombocytopenia. Various forms of treatment for HCC are
now available, including resection, catheter-directed
embolism, cryotherapy, and chemotherapy. Response
to therapy is disappointing, with an overall 1-year mortality rate of about 75%.

EXTRAHEPATIC MANIFESTATIONS   The extrahepatic complications of HBV are well documented
and include polyarteritis nodosum (PAN), glomerulonephritis, and leukocytoclastic vasculitis. PAN is a
multisystem, necrotizing angiitis resulting from the deposition of immune complexes. It is characterized by
weight loss, fever, peripheral neuropathy, renal involve-

ment, gastrointestinal involvement, and heart failure.
The onset of PAN may occur during acute hepatitis,
and it has been documented up to 12 years after infection. The mean time to onset is 12 months, although
most cases occur in the first 6 months.

Glomerulonephritis resulting from HBV infection
may manifest as membranous or membranoproliferative
disease. As with PAN, the cause is thought to be the deposition of immune complexes. The disease is characterized by proteinuria, active urine sediment, and, in some
cases, renal insufficiency.

Diagnosis

The diagnosis of HBV is based on the detection of
serum antigens and antibodies. These tests are highly
sensitive and specific, but their interpretation can be
challenging (Table 4.6).

HBsAg   The presence of HBsAg is diagnostic of
infection. However, it does not distinguish between
acute and chronic infection. Furthermore, in severe hepatitis, HBsAg may be rapidly cleared to undetectable
levels, potentially obscuring the presence of the virus.

Anti-HBc   Serologic proof of acute infection is
more accurately conferred by the presence of IgM anti-
HBc. These antibodies become detectable early in infection and persist for about 6 months. During this time,
they are gradually replaced by IgG anti-HBc, which serve
as a persistent marker of prior infection.

An exception to this pattern is seen in chronic infections, in which IgM anti-HBc may remain positive indefinitely. The persistence of IgM antibodies is typical of
chronic viral hepatitis infections. Consequently, interpretation of the presence of IgM antibodies depends on the
clinical scenario. It is always necessary to rule out the possibility of concurrent infections that could account for
the acute symptoms, particularly if there is a history suggestive of antecedent chronic hepatitis. Nonviral causes
of acute hepatitis, such as drug-induced liver injury or
alcohol-induced hepatitis, must also be considered.

Anti-HBs   The presence of anti-HBs represents
complete recovery from acute infection. It is also the
hallmark of effective immunization and provides immunity to further infection, with rare exceptions. In
some patients, HBsAg and anti-HBs coexist, representing infection with different strains of virus.

HBeAg   Measurement of HBeAg is not necessary
for diagnosis of infection. Its primary value is in identifying patients with active viral replication.

Interpretation of Hepatitis B Serology Results		TABLE 4.6.
Tests	Results	Interpretation
HBsAg	Negative	
Anti-HBc	Negative	Susceptible
Anti-HBs	Negative	
HBsAg	Negative	
Anti-HBc	Negative or positive	Immune
Anti-HBs	Positive	
HBsAg	Positive	
Anti-HBc	Positive	Acutely infected[a]
IgM anti-HBc	Positive	
Anti-HBs	Negative	
HBsAg	Positive	
Anti-HBc	Positive	Chronically infected
IgM anti-HBc	Negative	
Anti-HBs	Negative	
HBsAg	Negative	
Anti-HBc	Positive	Four interpretations
IgM anti-HBc	Negative	Possible[b]
Anti-HBs	Negative	

IgM, immunoglobulin M; HBsAg, hepatitis B surface antigen; anti-HBc, antibody to hepatitis B core antigen; anti-HBs, antibody to hepatitis B surface antigen; HBV, hepatitis B virus

[a] Some patients with chronic HBV infection remain IgM anti-HBc positive indefinitely.

[b] Patient may be in "window period" after acute HBV infection; anti-HBs may be present but below the level of detectability; HBsAg may be below the level of detectability in a chronically infected patient; patient may be susceptible with a false-positive anti-HBc.

Other tests   In addition to serologic studies, direct tests for DNA are available, as are histologic stains for viral elements. These are rarely needed for diagnosis. HBV DNA testing is used primarily in the management of chronic HBV infection.

Management

Treatment   For discussions of the treatment of acute and HBV infections, see the sections on Management of Acute Hepatitis and Management of Chronic Hepatitis.

Prevention   Hepatitis B is a preventable infection. Two recombinant vaccines (Recombivax HB and Engerix-B) and serum immune globulin are available to

Summary of Diagnosis

- IgM anti-HBc is the hallmark of acute HBV infection. However, patients with chronic hepatitis from HBV may remain positive for these antibodies indefinitely. A definitive diagnosis of acute HBV requires the exclusion of other causes.
- Any patient with evidence of HBV infection (acute or chronic) should be tested for HDV.

prevent transmission. In 1991, the Advisory Committee on Immunization Practices at the CDC established a comprehensive plan for eliminating transmission in the United States. This plan is now being implemented. In areas where it has been aggressively employed, there has been a dramatic reduction in the rate of infection. Worldwide, however, the vaccines remain underutilized, largely because of its cost. HBV vaccine alone costs as much as all other immunizations recommended for childhood vaccination combined.

Recombinant vaccines are derived from the expression of HBsAg in yeast. After purification, the antigen is adsorbed onto aluminum hydroxide and preserved in thimerosal. Both vaccines are very safe. Pain at the injection site and low-grade fever are the two most common side effects, although the rates of these symptoms in vaccinated subjects do not exceed those in subjects given a placebo. Hepatitis B immune globulin (HBIg) is derived from plasma known to have high titers of anti-HBs. The process by which it is prepared ensures that HIV cannot be transmitted. Its primary indication for use is postexposure prophylaxis. Recommended schedules for HBV vaccination are listed in Table 4.7.

Vaccination is very effective, with more than 90% of adults and 95% of children developing protective antibodies (anti-HBs, 10 mIU/mL or higher). Several vaccination regimens are possible. In adults, a three-shot regimen is given at 0 (initial dose), 1, and 6 months. If the schedule is interrupted, further doses should be given as soon as possible, but the series does not have to be restarted. The second and third doses must be separated by at least 2 months. For all practical purposes, the two currently available vaccines are interchangeable. Higher doses are required for immunocompromised patients, including those receiving hemodialysis. Injections should be given only in the deltoid muscle of adults and adolescents, or in the thigh of infants and children. Factors that may reduce vaccine immunogenicity include age

TABLE 4.7.	Recommended Dosing Schedules for Hepatitis B Virus (HBV) Vaccination		
Patients	Schedule (mo)[a]	Recombivax HB	Engerix-B
Newborn child of HBsAg+ mother	At birth (≤12hr) with HBIg, 1–2, and 6	5.0 μg/0.5 mL	10 μg/0.5 mL
Newborn child of HBsAg–mother	0–2, 1–4, 6–18	2.5 μg/0.5mL	10 μg/0.5mL
Child (1–10 yr)	0, 1–2, 4–6	2.5 μg/0.5mL	10 μg/0.5 mL
Adolescent (11–19 yr)	0, 1–2, 4–6	5.0 μg/0.5mL	10 μg/0.5 mL
Adult	0, 1–2, 4–6	10 μg/1.0mL	20 μg/1.0 mL
Immunocompromised adult	0, 1, and 6	40 μg/1.0mL	40 μg/2.0 mL

HBsAg, hepatitis B surface antigen; HBIg, hepatitis B immune globulin.
[a] 0 represents initial dose.

older than 40 years, HIV infection, smoking, subcutaneous injection, freezing of the vaccine, and acceleration of the dosing schedule. HBV vaccine may be given with any other vaccines, including HAV vaccine and HBIg, as long as they are given at different sites with separate syringes.

Indications for vaccination are listed in Table 4.8. Contraindications include hypersensitivity to yeast or other components of the vaccine. Immunization is not contraindicated in pregnancy or in HIV infection. Preimmunization testing with anti-HBs or anti-HBc may be cost-effective in persons with significant risk factors. Postvaccination testing is indicated only for those whose further management depends on knowledge of immune status, such as health care workers. Testing should be performed 1 to 2 months after completion of the vaccination series. Approximately half of nonresponders develop antibodies after one to three additional doses. Hemodialysis patients should be evaluated yearly, and booster doses should be given if anti-HBs titers fall to less than 10 mIU/mL. Adequate levels of antibody do not prevent infection in all patients. However, when infection does occur, it is very rarely clinically apparent and does not appear to result in a chronic carrier state. Antibody titers wane over time, but whether additional booster doses of vaccine are necessary will be determined as more long-term data become available.

Current recommendations for postexposure prophylaxis are listed in Table 4.9. Prophylaxis should be provided to anyone with percutaneous, ocular, or mucous membrane exposure to HBV-infected blood or body fluids. Transmission resulting from exposure of intact skin to infected fluids has not been documented. After exposure of a previously unvaccinated person, HBIg should be administered within 24 hours. The

effectiveness of HBIg when administered longer than 7 days after exposure is not known.

Hepatitis C

Cause

With the development of serologic tests for hepatitis B in the early 1970s, it became clear that HAV and HBV could not account for the majority of episodes of posttransfusion hepatitis. Epidemiologic studies indicated that the causative agent in most cases was a transmissible agent, which came to be known as "non-A, non-B hepatitis." It was identified and well characterized as a virus by 1989 and renamed hepatitis C. Since then, six major genotypes and more than 80 subtypes have been identified.

Transmission   Transmission of the virus is primarily by subcutaneous or intravenous inoculation. However, transmission via mucous membrane exposure to HCV-infected fluids also occurs. The primary site of replication the liver, but replicative forms of the virus can also be found in the serum and in peripheral mononuclear cells. The mechanism of liver injury is largely undefined. However, a direct cytopathic effect has not been proven, and injury is thought to be largely immune mediated.

Epidemiology   In 1989, the annual incidence of HCV infection in the United States was estimated at 180,000 new cases per year. The most recent data suggest that this has now been reduced to approximately 28,000 per year. This dramatic decline is a consequence of screening of blood supplies and decreased incidence among injection drug users. Despite this reduction, the overall burden of disease remains enormous, because most infections lead to chronic hepatitis. HCV accounts for about 20%

TABLE 4.8. Centers for Disease Control and Prevention Recommendations for Hepatitis B Virus (HBV) Vaccination

Universal vaccination of all infants and previously unvaccinated children by the age of 11 yr

Health care workers exposed to blood and body fluids

People with multiple sexual partners or sexually transmitted diseases

Sexual partners or household contacts of HbsAg-positive people

Men who have sex with men

Illegal drug users

Patients with chronic renal insufficiency (preferrably before beginning hemodialysis)

Patients receiving clotting-factor concentrates

Travelers to regions of high endemicity

Patients or staff of institutions for the developmentally disabled

Immigrants from areas of high HBV endemicity

Adapted from Centers for Disease Control and Prevention. Hepatitis B virus: a comprehensive strategy for eliminating transmission in the United States through universal childhood vaccination. MMWR Morb Mortal Wkly Rep 1991;40:1–19. HBsAg, hepatitis B surface antigen.

of acute viral hepatitis infections in the United States. However, only 15% of acutely infected patients clear the virus spontaneously. As a result, approximately 3.9 million Americans are chronically infected, with 8,000 to 10,000 deaths per year attributed to the direct effects of the virus. Given the large pool of patients infected, the number of deaths is expected to triple in the next 10 to 20 years. In the United States, HCV accounts for 40% to 60% of all chronic liver disease and is now the leading reason for liver transplantation.

HCV infects people of all ages and ethnicities, but most acute cases are found among young adults between the ages of 20 and 39 years. Minorities are more often infected, including 3.2% of African-Americans, 2.1% of Mexican-Americans, and 1.5% of non-Hispanic whites.

Risk factors The risk factors for HCV are listed in Table 4.10. Identifiable risk factors remain elusive in many cases. Approximately 30% to 40% of patients with acute HCV deny all identifiable risk factors in the 6 months before onset of their illness. Ten to twenty percent of patients with chronic infection deny all well-documented risk factors. Before 1989, most acute infections were attributed to blood transfusions. Serologic testing and other changes in transfusion practices have now almost eliminated the risk of transmission from

Recommendations for Hepatitis B Virus Postexposure Prophylaxis **TABLE 4.9.**

Vaccination and antibody response status of exposed person	Treatment based on virologic status of source		
	HBsAg-positive	HBsAg-negative	Source not tested or status unknown
Unvaccinated	HBIG[a] × 1; initiate HB vaccine series	Initiate HB vaccine series	Initiate HB vaccine series
Previously vaccinated			
Known responder[a]	No treatment	No treatment	No treatment
Known nonresponder[b]	HBIG × 2 or HBIG × 1 and initiate revaccination	No treatment	If known high-risk source, treat as if source were HBsAG positive
Antibody response unknown	Test exposed person for anti-HBs: if adequate, no treatment; if inadequate, HBIG × 1 and vaccine booster	No treatment	Test exposed person for anti-HBs: if adequate, no treatment; if inadequate, initiate revaccination

HB, hepatitis B; HBsAg, hepatitis B surface antigen; HBIG, hepatitis B immune globulin; anti-HBS, antibody to hepatitis b surface antigen

[a] Dose of hepatitis B immune globulin is 0.06 mL/kg intramuscularly.

[b] Responder is defined as a person with adequate levels of serum antibody to HBsAG (i.e., anti-HBs 10 mIU/mL); inadequate response to vaccination is defined as serum anti-HBs <10 mIU/mL). From Centers for Disease Control and Prevention. Immunization of health-care workers. MMWR Morb Mortal Wkly Rep 1997;46:1–42.

TABLE 4.10. Risk factors for Hepatitis C Virus (HCV) Infection

Injection drug use
Blood transfusion before 1990
Hemodialysis
Previous needlestick injury
Multiple sex partners
Sexually transmitted diseases
Known sexual contacts with HCV-infected patients
Intranasal cocaine use
Organ donation recipient
Hepatitis C–positive mother
Tattoos

this source. This risk is currently estimated to be .010% to .001% per unit of transfused blood.

Despite efforts to reduce the number of infections acquired by injection drug use, this remains the most common form of transmission, accounting for half of all new infections. Furthermore, intranasal cocaine use is a documented risk factor. By one estimate, 50% to 80% of new injection drug users will test positive for anti-HCV within 6 to 12 months. The role of sexual transmission remains difficult to delineate. Overall, there is an excess of HCV associated with sexual risk factors (multiple sex partners, sexually transmitted diseases). However, the effectiveness of transmission is thought to be low. It is difficult to provide convincing evidence for increased rates of transmission among monogamous sexual partners. In addition, sharing of toothbrushes and razor blades has been implicated but not proven in household transmission. Overall, household and sexual exposure may account for 10% to 15% of cases. The risk of perinatal infection is about 5%.

The prevalence of infection among hemodialysis patients is estimated at 10% to 20%. Transmission is probably a result of inadequate observation of infection control practices, such as sharing medication vials and hemodialysis equipment. A positive correlation exists between the number of years of hemodialysis treatment and the risk of infection. Occupational exposure among health care workers remains a great concern. Seroprevalence is estimated at 1% among hospital-based health care workers. Accidental needlestick injuries are independently associated with seroconversion. Seroconversion after a needlestick injury averages 3.5%, but in one series in Japan using RNA testing, the incidence was 10%. There has been one reported case of transmission by blood

splash to the conjunctiva. Postexposure prophylaxis with antiviral agents or immune globulin has not been shown to be helpful in reducing the risk of developing hepatitis.

Patient Presentation

The incubation period ranges from 2 to 20 weeks, with an average of 7 weeks. However, HCV RNA is detectable in the blood within 1 to 3 weeks. Transaminase elevations usually begin at 6 to 8 weeks (range, 2 to 26 weeks) after exposure, and typically peak at 10 to 15 times the upper limit of normal. The severity of symptoms associated with these elevations varies. Only one third of patients develop symptoms at all. Clinical jaundice is seen in fewer than one third of symptomatic patients, although more than 70% of symptomatic patients have bilirubin levels higher than 3 mg/dL. Symptoms associated with acute HCV infection are similar to those of other hepatitis viruses and include anorexia, nausea, fatigue, malaise, arthralgias, and myalgias. Signs include low-grade fever, icterus, right upper quadrant abdominal tenderness, and hepatomegaly. The acute illness usually resolves over 2 to 12 weeks. Fulminant hepatitis is rare but has been reported.

As with the acute illness, the symptoms of chronic hepatitis are often intermittent, vague, nonspecific, or absent. The most commonly reported symptom is fatigue. Others include nausea, poor appetite, abdominal pain, myalgias, arthralgias, weakness, and weight loss.

Disease activity in chronic hepatitis varies. The majority of patients have some liver test abnormalities, and fluctuations are common. Approximately one third have normal tests, and only one fourth have transaminase levels more than 2 times normal. Histopathologic activity is determined on the basis of the amount of inflammation/necrosis and fibrosis present. This is expressed as the histologic activity index or Knodell score. It is the best predictor of progression of disease. Correlation between the ALT and histologic activity is inconsistent. Although patients with normal ALT values are generally thought to have a milder form of the disease, they too may have histologic evidence of chronic hepatitis and fibrosis.

Progression to cirrhosis is frequently reported as occurring in 20% of patients after 20 years of infection. Factors influencing disease progression include high viral load, HCV genotype 1b, male sex, age older than 40 years at the time of infection, and concomitant alcohol consumption. Once cirrhosis is established, typical sequelae of advanced liver disease may arise, including liver failure, jaundice, encephalopathy, portal hypertension, ascites, and variceal bleeding. Even after cirrhosis has developed, however, survival rates are high, 91% at 5 years and 79%

at 10 years. Chronic hepatitis is associated with HCC in 1% to 5% of patients after 20 years; it is seen more commonly in certain geographic distributions, in men, and in the elderly.

Extrahepatic manifestations of HCV infection include arthritis, essential mixed cryoglobulinemia, membranoproliferative glomerulonephritis, porphyria cutanea tarda (PCT), lichen planus, and autoimmune diseases. Arthritis is a common manifestation. Antinuclear antibodies (ANA) and rheumatoid factor (RF) may be positive, usually at low titers. High titers suggest that other disease processes are active.

Essential mixed (type II) cryoglobulinemia is a lymphoproliferative disorder characterized by circulating immunoglobulins consisting of polyclonal IgG and monoclonal IgM. These immunoglobulins precipitate at low temperatures in small- to medium-sized blood vessels. Monoclonal IgM possess RF activity. Cryoglobulins are found in as many as one third of patients with HCV, but only 1% to 2% develop clinical features of the disease. More than 80% of patients with type II cryoglobulinemia have detectable HCV RNA. Signs and symptoms include arthralgias, fever, hepatosplenomegaly, neuropathy, vasculitic skin lesions, and purpura. Glomerular disease results from the deposition of polyclonal immunoglobulins in the glomerular capillaries. The nephrotic syndrome or rapidly progressive glomerulonephritis with acute renal failure, or both, may occur. Hypocomplementemia is also common.

A clear relation has been established between HCV infection and membranoproliferative glomerulonephritis and nephrotic syndrome. This process is frequently, but not always, mediated by cryoglobulins. It is the result of deposition of antigen-antibody complexes in the glomerulus. When present, proteinuria frequently improves with interferon therapy.

It is now recognized that HCV is associated with many cases of PCT, the most common of the porphyrias. It is characterized by photosensitivity, with fluid-filled vesicles and bullae developing in sun-exposed areas. Skin is friable, and minor trauma may result in the formation of bullae. Small white plaques called *milia* may also be present. Alcohol consumption, estrogen use, and iron overload are also associated with PCT.

A number of autoimmune processes are seen with increased frequency in HCV infection. Five to twelve percent of infected patients have antithyroid antibodies. Hypothyroidism is present in as many as 5%. There is also an increased incidence of Sjögren's syndrome and idiopathic thrombocytopenic purpura. The pathologic mechanism of this relationship is not well defined.

Diagnosis

As with other forms of viral hepatitis, the diagnosis of HCV infection is usually based on serology. Widespread testing for HCV began in 1989 with the use of enzyme-linked immunoassays (ELISA). Lack of sensitivity led to the development of second-generation tests. These became available in 1992 and have a sensitivity of 92% to 95%. The specificity is not known. A third-generation test with even greater sensitivity and specificity is anticipated. At the onset of symptoms, antibodies are detectable in only 50% to 70% of patients with acute HCV. However, after 3 months of infection, 90% have antibodies. Consequently, repeat serologic testing or testing with supplemental methods may be necessary in acute hepatitis, when anti-HCV is negative and suspicion is high.

Interpretation of test results in asymptomatic persons depends on the prevalence of the disease in the population being tested. In populations with high seroprevalence (e.g., intravenous drug users), the accuracy of this test exceeds 90%. A positive test is diagnostic. However, in low seroprevalence populations (e.g., blood donors with normal ALT concentrations), only about 50% of patients with positive ELISA tests can be demonstrated to have HCV by other supplemental assays. A positive test in this setting necessitates additional testing; a negative test is sufficient to rule out infection.

Confirmatory testing should be performed on asymptomatic patients and those in low-risk groups. Until recently, the most common supplemental test has been the radioimmunoblot assay (RIBA), which detects core and nonstructural gene products. Indeterminate results are possible. The most sensitive tests for HCV are those that directly measure RNA—reverse transcriptase–polymerase chain reaction (RT-PCR) and signal amplification by branched DNA (bDNA). Both qualitative and quantitative tests are available by these methods. Because of their sensitivity and absence of indeterminate results, these methods have become the confirmatory tests of choice. However, these tests are not standardized. Significant variability exists among them, such that comparisons of viral load between tests may be grossly inaccurate. Serial testing is helpful only when evaluating response to treatment; it is otherwise discouraged.

Genotyping and serotyping of HCV are also commercially available. In some studies, types Ia and Ib have been less likely to respond to therapy than types 2 or 3. However, no genotype precludes consideration of treatment. Consequently, genotyping is not a necessary component of the evaluation of these patients.

Summary of Diagnosis

- Clinically significant acute HCV is uncommon.
- Anti-HCV is present in only 50% to 70% of patients with acute infection.
- In the acutely ill patient, direct tests for RNA may be necessary.

Management

Treatment   For discussion of the treatments of acute and chronic HCV infections, see the sections on Management of Acute Hepatitis and Management of Chronic Hepatitis.

Prevention   No vaccine is available for HCV. No postexposure prophylaxis has been shown to be helpful. Consequently, prevention depends on the elimination of risk factors. Increasing public awareness of HCV and its risk for transmission is essential. Advertising campaigns have focused on those at greatest risk, especially intravenous drug users. Emphasis is also placed on physician education to increase early detection of asymptomatic infection. Universal precautions are mandatory. Sexual transmission can be prevented with appropriate safe-sex practices. Barrier protection is recommended for persons with multiple sexual partners or other risk factors for sexually transmitted diseases. So far, there are insufficient data to make this same recommendation for stable monogamous partners. Household exposure can be reduced by avoiding the sharing of razor blades or other objects potentially contaminated with infected blood.

Hepatitis D

Cause

Hepatitis D is a primitive virus that relies on the gene products of HBV for propagation. The only known HDV-related protein is HDAg, which is important in replication of the virus. It forms the core protein, which encapsulates the genome. The mature virus is surrounded in a coat of HBsAg.

Transmission of HDV occurs by the same mechanisms as HBV. These include direct parenteral inoculation via injection drug use, occupational exposure, blood transfusion, or hemodialysis. Sexual transmission is common, as is transmission via household exposure. Perinatal transmission has been documented. In general, patterns of transmission fall into two groups. In areas of endemicity, transmission typically occurs via person-to-person contact. In areas with low rates of infection, transmission occurs by percutaneous exposure, usually via intravenous drug use.

Worldwide, approximately 5% of persons chronically infected with HBV are also coinfected with HDV. Because of its dependence on HBV for propagation, the epidemiologies of the two viruses parallel one another, though there are some significant differences. As a general rule, areas that are endemic for HDV are regions with a high prevalence of HBV infection. However, the corollary is not necessarily true; high prevalence of HBV does not predict a high rate of infection with HDV.

In the United States, rates of HDV infection in HBsAg-positive persons vary from as low as 1.4% in the southeast to 12.0% in southern California. Infection is most common in persons with a history of injection drug use or hemophilia. Public health measures to reduce injection drug use and improve the quality of donated blood have substantially reduced the incidence of infection.

Patient presentation

Hepatitis D infection occurs in one of two ways—either as simultaneous coinfection with HBV, or as superinfection in a chronic carrier of HBV. Simultaneous infection has an incubation period ranging from 5 weeks to 6 months. The acute viral illness is indistinguishable from other forms of viral hepatitis. Infected persons may be entirely asymptomatic, or they may have self-limited disease with typical symptoms of malaise, fatigue, arthralgias, myalgias, headache, low-grade fever, nausea, vomiting, or abdominal pain. A biphasic course is not uncommon, with a recurrence of typical hepatitis symptoms and elevation of bilirubin and transaminase concentrations 2 to 5 weeks after resolution of the first episode. Serologically, this correlates with the variable appearance of products of the two viruses. Simultaneous infection results in chronic disease in only about 3% of patients. However, when it does occur, chronic coinfection appears to lead to a more rapid disease progression. There is an excess incidence of fulminant hepatitis in patients with simultaneous infections.

Serologic markers of simultaneous infection follow a variable pattern. HDAg may appear before, after, or concurrently with HBcAg. Detectability of HDAg in the blood ranges from 1 to 21 days after the onset of symptoms. It is rapidly cleared and is typically undetectable by 3 weeks. IgM antibodies are detectable within 2 to 3 weeks after onset of symptoms and remain present for 2 to 3 months. Only 50% of patients develop long-lasting IgG antibodies. Simultaneous infections have been associated with decreased HBV replication and early clearance of HBsAg.

Superinfection in chronic carriers of HBsAg follows a slightly different course. After a much shorter incubation period of 2 to 8 weeks, typical symptoms of acute hepatitis occur in most patients. The course of the acute disease does not differ significantly from that seen in simultaneous infection, except that biphasic disease is uncommon. However, chronic coinfection occurs at a significant rate. This has been associated with progression to cirrhosis in 20% to 60% of patients in 2 to 6 years, although the direct effect of HDV in this process is debated. As with simultaneous infection, fulminant hepatitis occurs at higher than expected rates. Fourteen percent of cases of fulminant hepatitis worldwide are caused by HDV superinfection.

No extrahepatic diseases have been independently attribute to HDV. Likewise, no association with the development of HCC has been clearly identified.

Diagnosis

The diagnosis of HDV should be considered in all patients with evidence of HBV infection and in all patients with fulminant hepatitis. The only commercial assay available currently is a blocking radioimmunoassay for total anti-HDV. However, the development of anti-HDV is delayed in some patients, necessitating the testing of convalescent titers or a more definitive test such as HDV RNA, HDAg immunoblot assay, or tissue staining of hepatocytes for HDAg. Simultaneous infection is characterized by the presence of HBsAg, IgM anti-HBc, and anti-HDV. However, simultaneous infection may result in rapid clearance of HBsAg. Consequently, acute HBV may be missed if one screens for acute hepatitis with HBsAg alone. In either case, an appreciation for the limits of serologic testing is necessary. In patients with chronic HBV, HDV superinfection is characterized by the presence of HBsAg and anti-HDV and the absence of IgM anti-HBc. In fulminant hepatitis, markers for HDV infection may be absent in the serum and detectable only by biopsy.

Management

Treatment   For discussion of the treatment of acute and chronic HDV infections, see the sections on Management of Acute Hepatitis Management of Chronic Hepatitis.

Prevention   There is no effective vaccine for HDV. The prevention of HDV infection depends on the concerted effort to prevent the spread of HBV. A national program of HBV vaccination is now in place in the United States. However, because vaccination on a global scale remains unfeasible, public health measures to reduce transmission via injection drug use, sexual transmission, occupational exposure, and household contact remain the cornerstone. In patients with preexisting HBV infection, this is the only means of prevention.

Hepatitis E

Cause

Previously known as "enterically transmitted non-A, non-B hepatitis," hepatitis E virus has now been well studied and characterized. Although HEV is generally unrelated to HAV, in many ways the viruses behave similarly.

Transmission of HEV is by the fecal-oral route. A brief period of viremia does occur, and transfusion-related transmission has been postulated but not proven. Viremia typically clears within 10 days of icterus. Chronic viremia does not occur. High titers of the virus are found in the stool and bile of infected persons. Viral shedding in the stool has been documented for up to 52 days.

Hepatitis E is typically found in endemic areas of Asia, Africa, and South America. Worldwide incidence and prevalence are not known, but some estimates are as high as 2 million cases a year in India alone. Mortality rates are estimated at 0.4% to 3.8%, accounting for a substantial proportion of cases of fulminant hepatitis. It is most common in developing countries where contamination of drinking water is common. Epidemics frequently occur in the rainy season as a result of flooding. Common-source infection is the rule. Secondary infection (e.g., from household exposure) is rare, occurring in only 2% of cases, in contrast to 15% in HAV. There is no known chronic carrier state, although prolonged viremia in some patients has been documented. The role of zoonotic reservoirs has not been defined.

Hepatitis E occurs in both epidemic and sporadic forms. In countries where the disease is endemic, the estimated seroprevalence of IgG anti-HEV ranges from 5% to 30%. Based on serologic studies of healthy blood donors, the incidence in the United States and other Western countries has ranged from 0.4% to 2.0%. It has been presumed that essentially all of these infections have been the result of exposure during travel to endemic areas.

Summary of Diagnosis

- HDV infection occurs only in conjunction with HBV. All patients with HBV should be tested for HDV. Severe infections may result in early clearance of HBV markers.

At least one infection has been documented to have originated in the United States.

Clinically apparent disease is most common in young adults from 15 to 40 years of age. However, children as young as 2 months of age have been documented to have acute disease. A particularly important characteristic is the high fatality rate among pregnant women, especially in the third trimester. Intrauterine infection can occur. In one cohort of eight pregnant women with overt acute HEV, six of the babies had evidence of acute HEV, two of whom died. Infection during pregnancy results in an abortion rate of 12% and a mortality rate as high as 20%.

Patient presentation

The natural history of acute HEV infection is similar to that of HAV. After infection, the incubation period of HEV ranges from 2 to 9 weeks, with the average being 40 days. The virus appears in the stool before the development of transaminase elevations. The symptoms are those of other forms of acute hepatitis and include fatigue, malaise, nausea, decreased appetite, and right upper quadrant pain. In the presence of cholestasis, pruritus and clay-colored stool may be present. On physical examination, tender hepatomegaly, splenomegaly, and occasionally lymphadenopathy may be noted. Rashes and arthritis are uncommon. The pattern of liver injury is typically "hepatitic," but cholestasis may be present in 25% of patients. Transaminase elevations are typically several hundred to several thousand units per liter, and bilirubin is usually only mildly elevated (average, 5 mg/dL).

Diagnosis

IgM and, frequently, IgG anti-HEV antibodies are present in almost all patients at the time of presentation. Consequently, the diagnosis of HEV is usually based on serology. The sensitivity of current ELISA tests may be as high as 97%. The specificity is not known. In areas where incidence is high and IgM is not detected, a comparison of acute and convalescent titers of IgG may be necessary to secure the diagnosis. Supplemental tests for HEV include immune electron microscopy of stool samples, RT-PCR, fluorescent antibody-blocking assay, Western blot, and direct staining of liver tissue for HEAg. These are primarily research tools and are rarely needed in clinical practice.

Management

Treatment   For discussion of the treatment of acute HEV infection, see the section on Management of Acute Hepatitis.

Summary of Diagnosis

- HEV infection is rare in the United States.
- Serologic testing is indicated in patients with an appropriate travel history when other causes have been ruled out.

Prevention
Given the significant incidence and mortality of HEV worldwide, particularly in pregnant women, there is a great deal of interest in developing effective vaccines. No vaccine is currently available for the prevention of HEV, but clinical trials of combinant vaccine are underway. Because transmission in the United States is extremely rare, the risk of infection is of concern primarily for travelers. Immune globulin derived from U.S. populations is not protective because the rate of infection here is too low to produce adequate protective levels of antibodies. Serum derived from populations where infection is common is an attractive possibility but is currently not available. Consequently, prevention of HEV depends on the application of public health measures aimed at providing safe sources of drinking water. For travelers, strict avoidance of food or water potentially contaminated by human feces is essential.

Table 4.11 summarizes the hepatotropic viruses.

MANAGEMENT OF ACUTE VIRAL HEPATITIS

Treatment

The management of acute viral hepatitis is similar for all viral types. Most patients have mild, self-limited disease with no long-term sequelae and can be managed without hospital admission. In most cases, symptoms are improving at the time of presentation. The most important task initially is to secure the diagnosis and rule out other possible causes or comorbid conditions. Once the diagnosis is clear, treatment is typically supportive. No medication has been shown to improve outcome. Adequate rest, volume repletion, abstinence from alcohol, and avoidance of hepatotoxins are recommended. In the event of cholestasis, replacement of fat-soluble vitamins may be necessary. Monitoring for the development of extrahepatic manifestations of disease, such as glomerulonephritis or PAN, is also essential.

The decision to admit a patient to the hospital is often subjective. No clearcut criteria have been established to

Summary of Hepatotropic Viruses **TABLE 4.11.**

Classification	A Heparnavirus	B Hepadnavirus	C Flavivirus–like	D Plant viroid–like	E Calicivirus–like
Type of virus	Nonenveloped Single- stranded RNA	Enveloped Partially double- stranded RNA	Enveloped Single- stranded RNA	Enveloped Single- stranded RNA	Nonenveloped Single- stranded RNA
Transmission	Fecal-oral	Percutaneous Sexual Perinatal	Percutaneous Sexual Perineatal	Percutaneous Sexual Perinatal	Fecal-oral
Incubation	2–7 wk	4–6 wk	2–20 wk	4 wk–6 mo	2–9 wk
Clinical characteristics					
Fulminant hepatitis	.1–3%	0.1–1%	<0.1%	5–20%[a]	1 2%
Chronic infection	No	Yes	Yes	Yes	No
Treatment	Supportive	Interferon Lamivudine	Interferon Ribavirin	Interferon	Supportive
Prophylaxis	Immune globulin Inactivated virus vaccine	HBIG Recombinant vaccine	None	HBV vaccinations	None[b]

HBIG, hepatitis B immune globulin; HBV, hepatitis B virus; HDV, hepatitis D virus.
[a] Fulminant hepatitis is much more common in HDV superinfecting chronic HBV than in simultaneous infection.
[b] Vaccine is in development.

determine who should or should not be admitted. Consequently, clinical judgment is essential. Table 4.12 lists a number of factors that may prompt consideration of admission. It is of paramount importance to identify those patients at greatest risk for fulminant hepatitis. Individuals with underlying chronic liver disease (e.g., HBV, HCV), HBV/HDV coinfection, significant systemic illnesses, age greater than 50 years, or symptoms that do not begin to resolve with the onset of jaundice are at high risk. Hypoalbuminemia, increased prothrombin time greater than 3 seconds, ascites, volume depletion, and increasing total bilirubin in the setting of rapidly improving transaminases are all concerning signs. These patients should be considered for hospitalization and referred to an experienced hepatologist for further evaluation. When the course of the infection is severe or unpredictable, monitoring of disease progression with transaminases, total bilirubin, and prothrombin time measurements every 24 to 48 hours may be necessary. Worsening coagulopathy is particularly concerning for fulminant hepatic failure, and the onset of encephalopathy is diagnostic. Death from fulminant hepatic failure is usually the result of progressive cerebral edema, high-output heart failure, or in-

fection. Renal failure and hypoglycemia may also complicate this development.

Liver transplantation is a consideration for all patients with fulminant viral hepatitis. The importance of early referral to a transplantation center cannot be overemphasized. The issues surrounding funding and preoperative evaluation are complicated and time-consuming. Consequently, in order to facilitate appropriate care, evidence of fulminant hepatitis must be anticipated and responded to quickly.

Referral

Although many cases of acute hepatitis can be managed safely by primary care physicians, a low threshold for referral is warranted. Referral is indicated when the diagnosis is unclear, complications occur, risk for fulminant hepatitis is present, liver function tests are worsening, or infection with multiple viruses is suspected. Although nospecific treatment has been shown to improve recovery in acute hepatitis, treatment early after infection with HCV is associated with improved response to therapy. Consequently, delayed referral in this case could be detrimental, even in mild disease.

TABLE 4.12.	Factors Influencing the Decision to Admit Patients with Acute Hepatitis

Age older than 50 yr
Pregnancy
Underlying systemic disease
Underlying chronic hepatitis (viral or non-viral)
Volume depletion
Encephalopathy
Ascites
Prothrombin time >15 sec
Total bilirubin >15 mg/dl
Albumin <3 mg/dl
Hypoglycemia
Worsening protime or bilirubin with improving
   transaminases
Social issues including access to follow-up

MANAGEMENT OF CHRONIC HEPATITIS

Hepatitis B

Interferon

The only treatment of proven long-term efficacy for chronic HBV infection is interferon (IFN). IFNs are a group of proteins that function as cytokines in the regulation of immune function. IFNs presumably work by upregulating the immune response to the virus, but they may also be capable of intracellular viral inactivation without hepatocyte destruction. IFNs available for clinical use are produced by recombinant technology.

Treatment goals   The goal of therapy is termination of viral replication, which is manifested by clearance of HBeAg from the serum and reduction of HBV DNA titers to undetectable levels. This correlates with histologic resolution of active hepatitis. Responders remain HBsAg positive in an inactive carrier state, and many subsequently become HBsAg negative. A patient is considered to have a complete response if HBeAg disappears from the serum by the end of therapy and a sustained response if HBeAg persists for at least 6 months after completion of therapy.

Treatment recommendations   Treatment is recommended for patients with ALT at least 1.5 to 2 times the upper limit of normal, detectable levels of HbsAg and HBV DNA in the serum, active hepatitis on liver biopsy, and compensated liver disease. Therapy is con-

traindicated in those with decompensated liver disease, in persons with serious infections or other serious systemic illnesses, and those with contraindications to IFN. Response to therapy is affected by a number of additional factors. The best predictors of response are high transaminase levels (ALT greater than 100 U/L), presence of HbeAg, low HBV DNA levels (less than 200 pg/mL), shorter duration of disease, and fibrosis with active inflammation on liver biopsy. Treatment is rarely helpful and is not costeffective in patients with normal or near-normal transaminase levels or with compromised immune status. In the past, treatment of HIV-infected patients was discouraged. With improved mortality rates from effective HIV therapy, treatment of HIV patients, particularly early in their infection, is appropriate.

The standard therapy includes subcutaneous or intramuscular injection of IFN, 5 million units daily or 10 million units three times per week for 16 weeks. With this regimen, long-term remissions can be expected in 25% to 40% of patients.

IFN is associated with a number of troubling side effects, which usually begin 6 to 8 hours after injection (Table 4.13). These consist of an influenza-like reaction with headache, fatigue, myalgias, fever, and chills. Symptoms typically lessen with time and can be reduced by pretreatment with antiinflammatory agents. Additionally, laboratory abnormalities such as thrombocytopenia and leukopenia are common. Less often, more severe reactions occur, such as severe depression, seizures, induction of autoimmune processes (e.g., idiopathic thrombocytopenic purpura, thyroiditis), bacterial infection, or acute cardiopulmonary or renal disease. Ten to forty percent of patients require dose reductions or termination of therapy because of side effects. During therapy, patients are regularly monitored for the development of laboratory abnormalities and response to treatment. Transient rises in transaminase concentrations are common with the initiation of therapy. This should not prompt discontinuation of treatment unless the elevations are severe or are associated with jaundice or synthetic dysfunction.

Other treatments

Treatment with many other agents has been studied, including lamivudine, famciclovir, prednisone, acyclovir, foscarnet, zidovudine, ribavirin, and others. To date, lamivudine and famciclovir appear most promising.

Oral lamivudine   This agent rapidly reduces HBV DNA levels, resulting in histologic improvement and normalization of transaminases. However, on with-

Side Effects of Interferon Therapy   **TABLE 4.13.**

Category	Examples
Systemic effects	Fatigue, fever, headache, myalgia, arthralgia, backache anorexia, weight loss, nausea, vomiting, diarrhea, abdominal cramps, hair loss, and sensitivity reactions
Neurologic effects	Difficulty concentrating, lack of motivation, sleep disturbance, delirium, disorientation, coma, seizures, electroencephalographic changes, decrease in hearing, tinnitus, dizziness, vertigo, decrease in vision, retinal hemorrhages, cotton-wool spots
Psychological effects	Anxiety, irritability, depression, social withdrawal, decreased libido, paranoid or suicidal ideation, return of craving for alcohol or drugs
Hematologic effects	Decrease in platelet count, leukocyte count, and hematocrit
Immunologic effects	Increased susceptibility to bacterial infections, especially bronchitis, sinusitis, furuncles, urinary tract infections; in rare instances, pneumonia, lung abscess, brain abscess, septicemia, bacterial peritonitis
Autoimmune effects	Development of autoantibodies and anti-interferon antibodies, hyperthyroidsim, hypothyroidism, lichen planus, diabetes, hemolytic anemia, thrombocytopenic purpura, lupus-like syndromes
Other effects	In rare instances, pneumonitis, proteinuria, interstitial nephritis, nephrotic syndrome, cardiac arrhythmia, congestive heart failure, acute exacerbation of liver disease

From Hoofnagle JH, Di Bisceglie AM. The treatment of chronic viral hepatitis. N Engl J Med 1997;336:347–356.

drawal of therapy, transaminases return to pretreatment levels in 80% of patients after 1 year. Furthermore, induction of viral mutations has been noted in about 19% of patients over a similar period, resulting in resistance to antiviral therapy. Trials are ongoing with monotherapy and combination therapy in conjunction with IFN and other agents.

Advanced disease   Patients with advanced disease frequently are not candidates for IFN therapy. The management of chronic HBV infection in these patients consists of monitoring for the development of extrahepatic disease (e.g., PAN, glomerulonephritis) and the development of portal hypertension, varices, and HCC. Alpha-fetoprotein determinations every 6 to 12 months and periodic sonograms are recommended.

Orthotopic liver transplantation   Transplantation is a viable treatment for complications of chronic HBV. However, transplantation has been plagued by high re-infection and limited survival rates, factors that made the procedure undesirable for some time. Advances have been made with the use of HBIg for prophylaxis against re-infection. Although appropriate dosing is still being evaluated, preliminary results are encouraging. A disadvantage is high cost. Lamivudine is also being investigated, alone and in combination with HBIg, for this purpose.

Hepatitis C

Interferon

All treatment for HCV is based on IFN. To date, three forms of IFN have been approved by the U.S. Food and Drug Administration (FDA) for the treatment of HCV: interferon alfa-2b (Intron A), interferon alfa-2a (Roferon-A), and interferon alfacon-1 (Infergen), a synthetic consensus interferon. Clinical efficacy appears to be similar for all three. The mechanism of action and the side effects of IFN treatment are the same as those delineated for HBV (Table 4.13).

Response   Response to therapy is determined biochemically by the normalization of ALT or virologically by reduction of viral load to below detectable levels. These reductions begin within the first few weeks of therapy and are maximal by 12 weeks. If a complete response has not occurred by this point, treatment is terminated. A patient is said to have an end-of-treatment response (ETR) if biochemical or virologic tests are normal at the end of treatment, and to have a sustained response if normalization persists for longer than 6 months after completion of the therapy.

Standard therapy   Standard therapy for chronic HCV consists of IFN, 3 million units three times a week for 12 to 18 months. With this regimen, approximately 50% of patients have a biochemical ETR (normalization of ALT) and 30% have a sustained response. This correlates with a viral ETR (undetectable RNA) in 30% to 40% and a sustained response in 10% to 20%.

The FDA has approved ribavarin for the treatment of chronic HCV. It is used in conjunction with IFN and results in significantly improved sustained response rates. When used alone, it is not effective.

Timing   There is good evidence that treatment early after infection leads to higher rates of viral clearance than does later treatment. After acute infection, standard doses of IFN result in rates of viral clearance that exceed 40%. The best time to begin therapy in acute disease is unknown. However, in most instances, IFN is not introduced until the transaminase levels are improving and symptoms have resolved.

Whom to treat   Factors that have been associated with improved response rates include low serum HCV levels (less than 1,000,000 copies/mL), absence of cirrhosis, and HCV genotype 2 or 3. Patients with persistently increased transaminase levels, portal or bridging fibrosis, and at least moderate inflammation on liver biopsy have the highest risk for progression to cirrhosis. Treatment is particularly encouraged for this population. Treatment is not recommended for patients with normal or near-normal ALT, because therapy may precipitate transaminase elevations. It is also not recommended for patients with decompensated cirrhosis.

Interferon treatment in other groups of HCV patients

Treatment recommendations for other groups are less certain and must be individualized. In patients with increased transaminase levels but with histologically little or no evidence of disease, progression to cirrhosis is likely to be slow, if it occurs at all. Consequently, observation with close attention to biochemical evidence of change in disease activity is an acceptable alternative. Periodic liver biopsy every 3 to 5 years is also advisable. In patients with compensated cirrhosis, there is no definitive evidence that treatment prolongs survival or prevents the development of HCC. On the other hand, because of their advanced disease and the risk of disease progression, patients in this group may have the most to gain. These patients frequently have low platelet and leukocyte counts, both of which may be worsened by IFN. Strict caution must be used if treatment is pursued. Data remain incomplete regarding patients younger than 18 or older than 60 years of age.

Failure of therapy   has been associated with the development of anti-IFN antibodies and the development of quasispecies. Retreatment with standard therapy rarely produces a sustained response but may improve the histology. Higher doses of IFN have been shown to increase the rate of ETR, but the data on long-term, virologic sustained response are so far inconclusive.

Orthotopic liver transplantation   Transplantation is an effective and acceptable treatment for the complications of advanced liver disease caused by HCV. HCV infection now accounts for 20% to 25% of all liver transplantations in the United States. Reinfection of the graft is common, but the course of disease is usually mild, making long-term survival favorable.

Hepatitis D

The management of HDV infection is the same as that for HBV. The treatment of HDV infection has been disappointing. So far, IFN is the only therapy shown to be of any benefit. Nevertheless, response to IFN remains poor. Histologic improvement is seen with treatment, and complete responses do occur. However, relapse is common. The current approach is to treat patients with the same doses of IFN used to treat HBV infection. If complete response is not seen in 3 months, the therapy is stopped. In the absence of an alternative therapy, patients must be monitored frequently because of the aggressive course of HBV-HDV coinfection. Liver transplantation may be an alternative for some patients.

Referral

All patients with chronic hepatitis are candidates for referral to a hepatologist or gastroenterologist experienced in the treatment of viral hepatitis. These patients should be evaluated for the appropriateness of IFN therapy. In addition, assessment of disease status and prognosis may be attained. Patients with advanced disease require evaluation and management of portal hypertension, varices, or other sequelae of cirrhosis. Furthermore, these patients need to be observed for the development of extrahepatic manifestations of disease and the development of HCC.

KEY POINTS

- Viral hepatitis is the most common cause of chronic hepatitis and death from liver disease.

- Most cases of viral hepatitis are preventable with appropriate vaccinations and public health measures.

- All patients with laboratory evidence of hepatitis should be tested for viral hepatitis.

- Patients with chronic viral hepatitis should be referred to a gastroenterologist or hepatologist for consideration of treatment with IFN and management of sequelae of chronic liver disease.

- HAV infection is the most common cause of acute viral hepatitis. It is an enterically transmitted virus that typically cause mild, self-limited disease.

- HBV infection is the most common cause of chronic viral hepatitis worldwide. Many patients with hepatitis B subsequently develop cirrhosis and HCC. Sexual transmission is common.

- Most acute HCV infections go unrecognized and result in chronic hepatitis. Hepatitis C is the most prevalent form of viral hepatitis and the most common reason for liver transplantation in the United States.

- HDV is a primitive virus that causes acute and chronic infection only in conjunction with HBV. It results in a substantial number of cases of fulminant hepatitis.

- HEV is an enterically transmitted (usually waterborne) virus similar to HAV that causes both endemic and epidemic disease in regions of Asia, Africa, and South America.

COMMONLY ASKED QUESTIONS

Can HCV be transmitted sexually?
Yes. Sexual transmission accounts for about 15% of infections. The risk of infection increases with multiple partners and the presence of sexually transmitted disease. However, in most cases, the effectiveness of transmission is thought to be low. In some studies of monogamous partners, no transmission was documented over more than 20 years. Consequently, there is currently no formal recommendation for barrier protection for monogamous partners. Otherwise, safe-sex practices are strongly recommended.

If a patient begins a vaccination series but does not complete it on schedule, is it necessary to restart the series?
No. HAV vaccine is highly immunogenic. If the patient has an intact immune system, memory cells should be adequate to respond well to another dose of vaccine, even when it is given later than recommended. Likewise, HBV immunization does not have to be restarted. Simply give the second dose, followed by the third one 2 to 6 months later.

Who requires postvaccination testing after immunization for HBV? What do I do if the antibody levels are not protective?
Postvaccination testing is indicated for anyone at high risk for HBV exposure, including health care workers. Persons receiving routine immunization do not need to be tested. Postvaccination testing should be performed 1 to 2 months after completion of the series. If anti-HBs titers are less than 10 mIU/mL, a second series should be adminis-

tered. If antibodies remain low, the patient is considered a nonresponder and is susceptible to infection. Once responder status is determined, no further testing is required. Only immunocompromised patients (e.g., HIV-positive patients) and hemodialysis patients require repeat testing to maintain anti-HBs levels at 10 mIU/mL or higher.

SUGGESTED READINGS

General

Centers for Disease Control and Prevention. Immunization of health-care workers. *MMWR Morb Mortal Wkly Rep* 1997; 46:1–42.

Hoofnagle JH, Di Bisceglie AM. The treatment of chronic viral hepatitis. *N Engl J Med* 1997;336:347–355.

Lemon SM, Thomas DL. Vaccines to prevent viral hepatitis. *N Engl J Med* 1997;336:196–204.

Hepatitis A

Glikson M, Galun E, Oren R, Tur-Kaspa R, Shouval D. Relapsing hepatitis A: review of 14 cases and literature survey. *Medicine (Baltimore)* 1992;71:14–23.

Gordan SC, Reddy KR, Schiff L, Schiff ER. Prolonged intrahepatic cholestasis secondary to acute hepatitis A. *Ann Intern Med* 1984;101:635–637.

Vento S, Garofano T, Di Perri G, Dolci L, Concia E, Bassetti D. Identification of hepatitis A virus as a trigger for autoimmune chronic hepatitis type I in susceptible individuals. *Lancet* 1991;337:1183–1187.

Vento S, Garofano T, Renzini C, et al. Fulminant hepatitis associated with hepatitis A virus superinfection in patients with chronic hepatitis C. *N Engl J Med* 1998;338:286–290.

Hepatitis B

Lee WM. Hepatitis B virus infection. *N Engl J Med* 1997; 337:1733–1745.

Margolis HS, Alter MJ, Hadler SC. Hepatitis B: evolving epidemiology and implications for control. *Semin Liver Dis* 1991;11:84–91.

McMahon BJ, Alward WLM, Hall DB, et al. Acute hepatitis B virus infection: relation of age to the clinical expression of disease and subsequent development of the carrier state. *J Infec Dis* 1985;151:599–603.

Wong KH, Cheung AM, O'Rourke K, Naylor CD, Detsky AS, Heathcote J. Effect of alpha-interferon treatment in patients with hepatitis B eantigen-positive chronic hepatitis B. *Ann Intern Med* 1993;119:312–333.

Hepatitis C

Cuthbert JA. Hepatitis C: progress and problems. *Clin Microbiol Rev* 1994;4:505–532.

National Institutes of Health. National Institutes of Health Consensus Development Conference Panel Statement: management of hepatitis C. *Hepatology* 1997;26 (Suppl 1): 2S–10S.

Poynard T, Leroy V, Cohard M, et al. Meta-analysis of inter-
    feron randomized trials in the treatment of viral hepatitis C:
    effects of dose and duration. *Hepatology* 1996;4:778–789.

Hepatitis D
Govindarajan S, Chin KP, Redeker AG, Peters RL. Fulminant
    B viral hepatitis: role of delta agent. *Gastroenterology* 1984;
    86:1417–1420.

Polish LB, Gallagher M, Fields H, Hadler SC. Delta hepati-
    tis: molecular biology and clinical and epidemiological fea-
    tures. *Clin Microbiol Rev* 1993;6:211–229.

Hepatitis E
Khuroo MS, Kamili S, Jameel S. Vertical transmission of
    hepatitis E virus. *Lancet* 1995;345:1025–1026.
Krawczynski K. Hepatitis E. *Hepatology* 1993;17:932–941.

CHAPTER 5

Acute and Chronic Pancreatitis

David Magee
University of Texas Southwestern Medical Center, Dallas, Texas 75235

DEFINITION

The definition and classification of pancreatitis have been confusing. Unlike other inflammatory diseases of the gastrointestinal tract (e.g., esophagitis, gastritis, hepatitis, colitis) in which the organ in question can be directly visualized or biopsied, the diagnosis of pancreatitis is almost never confirmed histologically. Without a histologic "gold standard," the diagnosis has depended on evolving clinical criteria. Variation in the definitions, severity, and complications of pancreatitis led to an international symposia in 1992, which created a consistent, clinically based classification of pancreatitis and its complications (1):

Acute pancreatitis   This acute inflammatory process of the pancreas has variable involvement of other regional tissues or remote organ systems.

Severe acute pancreatitis   This is acute pancreatitis associated with organ failure and/or local complications (e.g., necrosis, abscess, pseudocyst). Organ failure is defined as shock (systolic blood pressure lower than 90 mm Hg), pulmonary insufficiency (oxygen partial pressure of 60 mm Hg or less), renal failure (creatinine concentration greater than 177 mol/L [2 mg/dL] after rehydration), or gastrointestinal bleeding (more than 500 mL in 24 hours). Severe acute pancreatitis is further characterized by three or more Ranson criteria (2) or an Acute Physiology and Chronic Health Evaluation (APACHE II) score of 8 or more (3).

Mild acute pancreatitis   This type of acute pancreatitis is associated with minimal organ dysfunction and an uneventful recovery. No complications or organ failures are involved, in contrast to severe acute pancreatitis.

Acute fluid collections   These occur early in the course of acute pancreatitis, are located in or near the pancreas, and always lack a wall of granulation or fibrous tissue.

Pancreatic necrosis   This term refers to one or more diffuse or focal areas of nonviable pancreatic parenchyma that are typically associated with peripancreatic fat necrosis.

Acute pseudocyst   This is a collection of pancreatic juice enclosed by a wall of fibrous or granulation tissue. It can arise as a consequence of acute pancreatitis, trauma, or chronic pancreatitis. Its formation requires 4 weeks or longer from the onset of acute pancreatitis. When pus is present, the lesion is termed a *pancreatic abscess.*

Pancreatic abscess   This circumscribed intra-abdominal collection of pus, usually in proximity to the pancreas, contains little or no pancreatic necrosis and arises as a consequence of acute pancreatitis or trauma. Abscesses occur late in the course of acute pancreatitis, often 4 weeks or longer after onset.

Infected pancreatic necrosis   This is a pancreatic necrosis that has become secondarily infected with bacteria. It is diagnosed by a transcutaneous needle aspiration with Gram's stain and culture.

Chronic pancreatitis   In this inflammatory disease of the pancreas, progressive and irreversible structural and functional changes to the pancreas occur. These changes result in permanent impairment of pancreatic exocrine and endocrine functions.

ACUTE PANCREATITIS

CAUSE

The causes of acute pancreatitis vary from one country to another and within different populations from the same country. Overall, gallstones are the most common cause, accounting for about 45% of cases; alcohol is a

close second, accounting for approximately 35%. After gallstones and alcohol, a number of miscellaneous causes account for another 10% of cases (Table 5.1), and 10% remain idiopathic. Obesity is also a risk factor for severe acute pancreatitis.

Patients thought to have idiopathic pancreatitis can often be found on further evaluation to have a presumed cause. For example, if bile is examined microscopically, cholesterol or bilirubinate crystals may be found in up to 75% of patients with idiopathic pancreatitis (4,5); one study revealed a hypertensive sphincter of Oddi on manometry in 15% of cases of idiopathic pancreatitis (6).

PATIENT PRESENTATION

History

Acute pancreatitis usually has a rapid onset. It is accompanied by upper abdominal pain and is associated with variable abdominal findings that range from mild tenderness to rebound. Abdominal pain is usually constant and boring and often is severe. Generally in the epigastric or periumbilical region, the pain may radiate to the midback. Because of its retroperitoneal nature, the pain may be lessened when the patient sits upright and leans forward, compared with lying flat. Nausea and vomiting are common and may occur without an ileus or gastric outlet obstruction. Vomiting, however, typically does not relieve the pain.

Physical Examination

Low-grade fever is present in more than half of the patients. High-grade fever may indicate cholangitis or sepsis. Tachycardia is common, and hypotension is present in up to 40% of patients. Abdominal tenderness and guarding are typical, and rebound tenderness may be present. Bowel sounds are generally diminished or absent. Pleural effusions, if present, are usually left-sided but may be bilateral. Mild jaundice is not uncommon and may indicate extrahepatic biliary obstruction or underlying liver dysfunction. Blue or dark discoloration of the flanks (Grey Turner's sign) or periumbilical region (Cullen's sign) may arise in the setting of retroperitoneal hemorrhage.

DIAGNOSIS

Because acute pancreatitis varies from mild, self-limited symptoms to fatal illness, combinations of clinical and laboratory data criteria have been formulated to predict its severity. The most widely used are the Ranson and the modified Glasgow criteria (Table 5.2), in which the severity of pancreatitis increases with the number of positive criteria (7,8). Patients with fewer than three risk factors have very low mortality rates.

TABLE 5.1. Causes of Acute Pancreatitis

Structural causes
  Gallstones or microlithiasis
  Hypertensive sphincter of Oddi
  Pancreas divisum
  Choledochocele
  Ampullary or pancreatic tumors
  Iatrogenic—post-ERCP
  Trauma
Toxins
  Ehyl or methyl alcohol
  Scorpion venom
Drugs[a]
  Definite association—azathioprine and 6-mercap-
    topurine, didanosine, pentamidine, tetracycline,
    metronidazole, sulfonamides, furosemide, val-
    proic acid, sulindac, estrogen
  Probable or possible association—thiazides, cime-
    tidine, ranitidine, salicylates, acetaminophen,
    methyldopa, erythromycin, nitrofurantoin,
    ampicillin, isoniazid, dexamethasone, cortico-
    steroids, bumetanide, octreotide, enalapril,
    cyclosporine, cisplatin, amiodarone, tryptophan
Metabolic causes
  Hypertriglyceridemia
  Hypercalcemia
Infections
  Viral—cytomegalovirus, varicella, hepatitis A,
    hepatitis B, non-A, non-B hepatitis, Epstein-Barr
    virus, mumps, rubella, coxsackie virus B, human
    immunodeficiency virus, adenovirus
  Parasitic—ascariasis, clonorchiasis
  Bacterial—mycoplasma, *Mycobacterium avium*
    complex, *Mycobacterium tuberculosis, Legionella,*
    leptospirosis, *Campylobacter jejuni*
Vascular causes
  Ischemia—postcardiac and abdominal surgery
  Vasculitis—systemic lupus erythematosus, poly-
    arteritis nodosa
  Atherosclerotic emboli
Miscellaneous causes
  Familial
  Penetrating peptic ulcer
  Hypothermia
  Tropical causes
  Inflammatory bowel disease
  Idiopathy

ERCP, endoscopic retrograde cholangiopancreatography.
[a] Data from McArthur KE. Review article: drug-induced pancreatitis. Alimentary Pharmacology and Therapeutics 1996;
10:23–38; and Underwood TW, Frye CB. Drug-induced pancreatitis. Clinical Pharmacy 1993;12:440–448.

TABLE 5.2. Adverse Prognostic Factors in Pancreatitis.

Criterion	Gallstone	Nongallstone
Ranson Criteria		
On admission		
Age (yr)	>55	>70
WBC (cells/mm³)	>16,000	>18,000
Glucose (mg/dL)	>200	>220
LDH (U/L)	>350	>400
AST (U/L)	>250	>250
At 48 hours		
Fall in HCT (points)	>10	>10
Rise in BUN (mg/dL)	>5	>2
Calcium (mg/dL)	<8	<8
Arterial P_{O_2} (mm/Hg)	<60	—
Base deficit (mmol/L)	>4	>5
Fluid deficit (L)	>6	>4
Modified Glasgow criteria - within 48 hours		
Age (yr)	>55	>55
WBC (cells/mm³)	>15,000	>15,000
Glucose (mg/dL)	>180	>180
BUN (mg/dL)	>45	>45
LDH (U/L)	>600	>600
Albumin (mg/dL)	<3.3	<3.3
Calcium (mg/dL)	<8	<8
Arterial P_{O_2} (mm Hg)	<60	<60

AST, aspartate aminotransferase; BUN, blood urea nitrogen; HCT,
hematocrit; LDH, lactate dehydrogenase; P_{O_2}, partial pressure of
oxygen; WBC, white blood cell count.

The APACHE II system has been used to assess acute pancreatitis (9). It can be used daily; however, a disadvantage for routine use is its complexity.

Laboratory Tests

Serum amylase

Despite its limitations, the serum amylase level remains central to the diagnosis of acute pancreatitis because of its availability, simplicity, and low cost. Although many tissues synthesize amylase, most of the serum activity originates from the pancreas and the salivary glands. The increased serum amylase concentration during pancreatitis results from enhanced release and decreased renal clearance. Serum levels increase in the first hours after the onset of pancreatitis and parallel the rise in lipase levels. Amylase falls more rapidly than lipase. Amylase levels tend to be higher with gallstone disease (10). Hyperamylasemia an occur in many other conditions (Table 5.3).

TABLE 5.3.	Causes of Hyperamylasemia

Pancreatic isoamylase
    Pancreatitis
    Pancreatic cancer
    Choledocholithiasis
    Penetrating duodenal ulcer
    Intestinal perforation
    Intestinal ischemia
    Intestinal obstruction
    Ruptured abdominal aortic aneurysm
    Renal failure
Salivary isoamylase
    Salivary problems—tumor, infection, alcohol
    Neoplasm—ovarian, lung, breast, prostate,
        myeloma
    Ovarian cyst, ruptured ectopic pregnancy
    Esophageal perforation
    Diabetic ketoacidosis
    Lactic acidosis
    Renal failure
Macroamylase
    Macroamylasemia

Serum lipase

The serum lipase level is more specific and approximately as sensitive as amylase for acute pancreatitis (10). It is a useful early marker. In addition, because the lipase concentration remains elevated longer than the amylase does, serum lipase may help to diagnose pancreatitis after an attack has subsided. However, hyperlipasemia is not specific to pancreatic disease; it can be seen in renal failure, intestinal perforation, ischemia, or obstruction.

Laboratory testing can aid the differentiation between gallstone-induced pancreatitis and nonbiliary forms, which has important therapeutic implications. Emergency therapeutic endoscopic retrograde cholangiopancreatography (ERCP) with stone removal is indicated in severe gallstone-induced pancreatitis (11,12). A common bile duct stone (choledocholithiasis) is often accompanied by elevations of bilirubin, alkaline phosphatase, and alanine aminotransferase (ALT) or aspartate aminotransferase (AST). Marked elevation of amylase also favors a biliary source. An increase of ALT to 3 or more times the baseline is highly specific, but not sensitive, for gallstone-induced pancreatitis (5).

Radiologic Studies

Imaging techniques are an important adjuvant in confirming the diagnosis of gallstone-induced pancreatitis.

Abdominal radiographs

A variety of abdominal radiographic findings have been associated with acute pancreatitis; none, however, is specific. Pleural effusions may be seen, and intestinal gas may demonstrate an ileus or an isolated dilated loop of small bowel overlying the pancreas (sentinel loop). Loss of the psoas margins and increased separation between the stomach and colon suggest pancreatic inflammation. Pancreatic calcification or calcified gallstones may be seen.

Ultrasound

In the evaluation of acute pancreatitis, visualization of the entire pancreas by ultrasound is often limited by intestinal gas and adipose tissue. The greatest value of ultrasound is in evaluating the biliary tract for duct dilation and detecting cholelithiasis in patients with suspected gallstone-induced pancreatitis. Ultrasound is unreliable for the detection of choledocholithiasis.

Computed tomography

A computed tomographic (CT) scan is a valuable tool in acute pancreatitis, but usually it is not needed to make the diagnosis. Its routine immediate use in acute pancreatitis cannot be recommended. Intravenous contrast agents can worsen renal function, and there is concern that if intravenous contrast studies are done early, it may worsen the course of pancreatitis, although prospective studies are needed to confirm this (13).

A dynamic CT scan can provide valuable information on the degree of pancreatic necrosis by assessing areas of the pancreas that do not enhance. This is reserved for the patient with suspected severe disease and clinical deterioration. Patients with more than 50% necrosis have a poor prognosis. A CT severity index has been developed that can assess severity, similar to clinical criteria systems (14). This system grades pancreatic enlargement, inflammation, number of fluid collections, and degree of necrosis.

The main role of the CT scan in acute pancreatitis is to evaluate for early and late complications. A CT scan early (1 to 3 weeks) can give information on necrosis. If the clinical picture indicates possible infection, a guided needle aspirate can be safely obtained for Gram's stain and culture to assess for infected necrosis. If infected necrosis is found, surgery should be performed. Later deterioration (after 4 weeks) can be assessed by CT scan to evaluate for pseudocyst, abscess, perforation or obstruction of the colon, or formation of a pseudoaneurysm.

Endoscopic cholangiopancreatography

ERCP can diagnose gallstone pancreatitis. However, the primary value of ERCP in acute pancreatitis is to remove gallstones quickly in cases of severe acute biliary pancreatitis; it generally should not be used early in less severe cases. When mild to moderate acute pancreatitis begins to resolve, ERCP can be employed to clear the common bile duct if no other cause of pancreatitis has been found.

Differential Diagnosis

In the differential diagnosis of acute pancreatitis, one must be aware of the numerous acute abdominal conditions that can present with similar pain and elevation of enzymes. These include perforated peptic ulcer, intestinal ischemia, perforation or obstruction of the bowel, choledocholithiasis, pancreatic cancer, ruptured abdominal aortic aneurysm, ruptured ectopic pregnancy, and past ERCP manipulation. If concern for any of these conditions exists, an abdominal CT scan is the best test to perform. Enzyme elevation may also be present in renal failure. Possible causes that ERCP can establish include microlithiasis, choledochocele, ampullary or pancreatic tumor, pancreas divisum, hypertensive sphincter of Oddi, and periampullary diverticulum.

Summary of Diagnosis

- Pancreatic enzymes can be nonspecific.
- Liver function tests may help identify gallstone-induced pancreatitis.
- Prognostic indicators are useful but must be individualized to each patient.
- Radiographic studies are of diagnostic, prognostic, and therapeutic value in managing pancreatitis.

MANAGEMENT

Treatment

Seventy-five to eighty percent of all attacks of acute pancreatitis are mild, and treatment is mainly supportive. Conversely, up to 25% of attacks are severe, leading to complications with a mortality rate approaching 9% (15). Pancreatic infection is the leading cause of death. The treatment of acute pancreatitis involves removal of precipitating factors, close monitoring, supportive care, and recognition and treatment of complications.

Mild acute pancreatitis

The diagnosis of pancreatitis requires hospitalization, because severity may not be evident for 24 to 48 hours.

Treatment is supportive. Monitoring of renal function, electrolytes, and oxygenation for evidence of organ failure is essential. Intravenous hydration, analgesia, and elimination of oral intake are mainstays of therapy. Nasogastric suction is necessary only in patients with ileus or severe vomiting.

A search for and removal of factors that may have precipitated the attack is appropriate. Suspected severe gallstone-induced pancreatitis may require emergency ERCP to remove a bile duct stone. Pancreatitis caused by passage of gallstones requires cholecystectomy. The timing of cholecystectomy must be individualized and determined by specialists. Potential offending medications should be discontinued. Serum triglyceride and calcium levels need to be checked on admission and appropriately lowered if elevated. Triglycerides should be maintained below 500 mg/dL.

Early complications

Early complications can occur within the first to third week of hospitalization and are best managed in the intensive care unit. Early pancreatic complications involve sterile and infected necrosis. Suspected infected necrosis should be confirmed by guided needle aspiration with Gram's stain and culture. Infected necrosis requires surgical intervention. Early systemic complications can lead to multisystem organ failure, most commonly involving the cardiovascular, pulmonary, and renal systems. The presence of multiorgan-system failure classifies acute pancreatitis as severe.

Late complications

Late complications occur after 4 weeks and include pseudocyst or abscess formation. Symptomatic pseudocysts can be drained percutaneously, surgically, or endoscopically. An abscess can be drained percutaneously or surgically. Other unusual complications include gastric varices from splenic-vein thrombosis, stress ulceration, rupture of pancreatic pseudoaneurysm, obstruction or fistulization of the colon, and hydronephrosis of the right kidney.

Severe acute pancreatitis

Severe acute pancreatitis requires management in the intensive care unit. Specific interventions to reduce morbidity and mortality have generally been unhelpful. Nutritional support with total parenteral nutrition has not shown benefit. Jejunal enteral feeding has been shown to be successful at least in mild pancreatitis (16); its use in severe pancreatitis needs to be evaluated. Antibiotics have not been shown to decrease mortality; however, the use of imipenem in severe necrotizing pancreatitis reduced the risk of pancreatic sepsis in one study (17). The role of surgery is confined to infected pancreatic necrosis and late complications.

Prevention

Prevention of acute pancreatitis is aimed at removing presumed etiologic factors. Often these are unknown before the first attack. Because gallstones and alcohol are the most common causes, these factors must be addressed. Strict alcohol abstinence should ensue. Cholecystectomy is the primary treatment for gallstone-induced pancreatitis. ERCP may be indicated if choledocholithiasis is suspected or for diagnosis in idiopathic pancreatitis. Potentially causative medications should be discontinued, and triglyceride levels should be controlled.

Follow-up

In mild cases of acute pancreatitis that resolve, when the causative agent has been found and removed (e.g., cholecystectomy in the case of gallstone removal), no specific follow-up is indicated. If no specific cause can be identified, a follow-up evaluation by a gastroenterologist is indicated.

In severe pancreatitis, the patient should be monitored for the next 6 months with attention to the possible development of late complications.

REFERRAL

If it is suspected that a case of mild acute pancreatitis is gallstone-induced, then referral for a cholecystectomy is appropriate. If no identifiable cause is found, then referral to a gastroenterologist for evaluation is appropriate.

For severe acute pancreatitis and late complications, immediate referral to a gastroenterologist and surgeon is appropriate. Severe pancreatitis is defined by evidence of end-organ dysfunction and is suggested by a score of 3 or higher on the Ranson or Glasgow criteria.

CHRONIC PANCREATITIS

CAUSE

Worldwide, malnutrition is the leading cause of chronic pancreatitis, but in Western societies, alcoholism accounts for about 70% of cases. Idiopathic chronic pancreatitis has been reported in up to 30% to 40% of patients with chronic pancreatitis (18,19). In addition, metabolic and mechanical disturbances as well as a genetic predisposition have been implicated (Table 5.4).

The risk of alcohol-induced chronic pancreatitis increases with the duration and amount of alcohol con-

TABLE 5.4.   Causes of Chronic Pancreatitis

Alcohol
Idiopathy
Tropical causes
Miscellaneous causes—obstruction, hereditary, cystic fibrosis, hypertriglyceridemia, hyperparathyroidism

sumed (20); however, there is a wide variation in individual sensitivity to alcohol, and only 5% to 10% of heavy drinkers develop pancreatitis (21). Chronic pancreatitis can progress even after cessation of alcohol. The genetic and nutritional factors in the development of alcoholic pancreatitis are unknown.

Any disease process that causes obstruction of the pancreatic duct can lead to chronic pancreatitis. Strictures caused by pancreas divisum, pseudocysts, traumatic injury, and periampullary tumors account for a small subset of cases of chronic pancreatitis. In general, these conditions are characterized by a dilated pancreatic duct and exocrine insufficiency.

PATIENT PRESENTATION

History

The presenting symptom for most patients with chronic pancreatitis is abdominal pain. The pain is epigastric, dull, and usually constant. Radiation, if present, is through to the back. Pain may be intermittent, with attacks lasting several days and intervening pain-free intervals, or it may be almost constant. The pain is often quickly aggravated by food ingestion. In about 15% of patients, chronic pancreatitis is painless or relatively painless (22).

Nausea, vomiting, anorexia, and weight loss are common. Weight loss is primarily a result of decreased caloric intake, although malabsorption or uncontrolled diabetes may also play a role. Diarrhea and steatorrhea occur when the exocrine secretion of pancreatic enzymes is insufficient for normal digestion. Malabsorption does not occur until enzyme secretion is reduced to less than 10% of normal (23). In addition to malabsorption, clinically evident diabetes occurs relatively late in the course of chronic pancreatitis. Other clinical presentations of chronic pancreatitis may include jaundice secondary to common bile duct stricturing and ascites or pleural effusions due to pancreatic duct leakage or a ruptured pseudocyst.

Physical Examination

The physical examination is usually of limited assistance in the diagnosis of chronic pancreatitis. There is epigastric tenderness during painful episodes; the physical findings, however, are generally not as great as the patient's complaints. Complications of chronic pancreatitis, such as pseudocysts or ascites, may be detected on physical examination.

DIAGNOSIS

Laboratory Tests

Serum pancreatic enzyme levels
Concentrations of serum pancreatic enzymes (amylase and lipase) in chronic pancreatitis may be elevated, normal, or low. Advanced chronic pancreatitis characteristically has low serum levels; however, the diagnosis is usually obvious on clinical grounds.

Cholestatic liver function tests
An elevated alkaline phosphatase or bilirubin concentration may develop if bile duct stricturing occurs.

Glucose
Glucose intolerance occurs typically as the disease progresses (i.e., diabetes).

Exocrine pancreatic function tests
Exocrine pancreatic function can be assessed directly or indirectly.

Direct measurement Duodenal juice is collected and assayed for its volume and bicarbonate and protein concentrations after either the ingestion of a standard meal or intravenous administration of secretin. Direct measurements of pancreatic function have the disadvantages of the inherent invasiveness of the duodenal juice collection and a lack of standardized assays; accordingly, they are rarely used in clinical practice. Easier but less sensitive and less specific techniques involve the oral administration of substrates for pancreatic digestive enzymes, followed by the measurement of their products of digestion. These include the bentiromide and the pancreolauryl tests. They are not readily available in most institutions and are rarely used.

Indirect tests These include measurement of chymotrypsin activity in the stool and the dual-labeled Shilling's test looking for exocrine pancreatic insufficiency, although both lack specificity.

Fecal fat levels Fecal fat levels may be elevated as a result of pancreatic exocrine insufficiency; this can be confirmed by a 72-hour stool collection for fecal fat. While ingesting a high-fat diet (100 g fat per day), a normal individual excretes only about 7 g of fat in the stool per day. Patients with exocrine pancreatic insufficiency often excrete more than 20 g of fat per day. Correction of steatorrhea with pancreatic enzyme replacement therapy (pancrelipase) confirms the diagnosis of exocrine pancreatic insufficiency. Needless to say, the 72-hour stool collection is cumbersome and unpopular with patients and health care providers.

Pancreatic function tests
In general, exocrine pancreatic-function tests are relatively insensitive, especially in early disease, and they should be viewed as complementary diagnostic tests in chronic pancreatitis.

Radiologic Studies

Abdominal radiographs
The demonstration of diffuse, speckled calcification of the pancreas on a plain film of the abdomen is diagnostic of chronic pancreatitis. Although insensitive, an abdominal radiograph is an easy first diagnostic test when attempting to establish this diagnosis.

Ultrasound
Ultrasound, although less sensitive than a CT scan, ultrasound can be useful in the evaluation of chronic pancreatitis. Findings on ultrasound that correlate with chronic pancreatitis include pancreatic duct dilation, cavities, and calcifications.

Computed tomography
A CT scan is more sensitive than ultrasound for the diagnosis of chronic pancreatitis. The most common diagnostic findings are calcifications, duct dilation, and cyst formation. CT may be helpful in the differentiation of chronic pancreatitis from pancreatic cancer. Three-dimensional magnetic resonance pancreatography allows evaluation of pancreatic duct anatomy and needs to be further studied.

Endoscopic cholangiopancreatography
ERCP is considered to be the most sensitive and specific test available for the diagnosis of chronic pancreatitis. Minimal changes are limited to the side branches and fine ducts. Moderate changes include pancreatic duct dilation, tortuosity, or stenosis. Advanced changes include cyst or stone formation and contraction of the

pancreas. It can be difficult to differentiate a pancreatic duct stricture of chronic pancreatitis from pancreatic cancer, and obtaining samples for cytologic analysis by endoscopic techniques may be of benefit.

Differential Diagnosis

The differential diagnosis of chronic pancreatitis can be a dual challenge. The first challenge is the patient with suspected chronic pancreatitis in whom no morphologic changes can be demonstrated. Pancreatic-function tests may be of value in this setting. The second challenge is differentiating chronic pancreatitis from pancreatic cancer. There may be an increased risk of pancreatic cancer in patients with chronic pancreatitis (24). ERCP with cytology may be of value in these cases.

Summary of Diagnosis

- Pancreatic enzymes can be nonspecific.
- Pancreatic function tests for chronic pancreatitis are relatively insensitive and are at best a complementary tool in diagnosis.
- Radiographic studies are of diagnostic, prognostic, and therapeutic value.

MANAGEMENT

Treatment

Treatment for chronic pancreatitis involves primarily the management of pain and secondary complications such as malabsorption, diabetes, pseudocysts, and biliary obstruction. Chronic pancreatitis is generally incurable, with the possible rare exception of chronic pancreatitis induced by hyperparathyroidism, which may be cured by surgical removal of the parathyroid glands.

Treatment of pain

Pain in chronic pancreatitis is the symptom that most often requires treatment. Noninvasive therapies include alcohol abstinence, analgesic medications, celiac nerve blocks, and pancreatic enzyme replacement. Persistent pain should be evaluated by ultrasound or CT to assess for pseudocyst, pancreatic stones, or tumor. ERCP evaluation is also reasonable in cases of persistent pain to define the morphology of the pancreatic duct. Dilated ducts, frequently with areas of strictures, can be found in up to half of the patients (25). Dilated pancreatic ducts may be surgically decompressed by an internal surgical drainage procedure such as a longitudinal pan-

creatic jejunostomy. Smaller ducts are not amenable to internal surgical drainage. Surgical drainage procedures are effective in the short term but become less effective after 5 years.

An alternative to surgery involves the selective use of stents that are endoscopically placed into the pancreatic duct. Short-term results are encouraging; however, long-term benefits have yet to be proven. Endoscopic biliary stent placement has also been effective in the treatment of biliary strictures caused by chronic pancreatitis, particularly in patients who are not considered good candidates for surgery.

Treatment of secondary complications

Malabsorption occurs when more than 90% of exocrine function is lost. Steatorrhea (loss of dietary fat into the stool) is more problematic than azotorrhea (loss of dietary protein). The initial treatment is a low-fat diet. For persistent symptoms, pancreatic enzyme replacement should be given before meals. Gastric acid may need to be neutralized to prevent degradation of these products in the stomach.

Prevention

Prevention of chronic pancreatitis involves alcohol abstinence and improved nutrition. Once the diagnosis is established, the disease is usually incurable.

Follow-up

Chronic pancreatitis is a lifelong process and probably will require serial follow-up with a team approach, including a primary care provider and consultation with specialists in pain management, gastroenterology, and surgery.

REFERRAL

If the pain from chronic pancreatitis is not responsive to noninvasive techniques, then referral to a gastroenterologist and surgeon is appropriate.

KEY POINTS

- Most cases of acute pancreatitis are mild.
- Alcohol and gallstones are the most common causes of acute pancreatitis.
- Etiologic factors of acute pancreatitis should be sought and addressed.
- Specialists should manage severe acute pancreatitis in the intensive care unit.
- Chronic pancreatitis is a progressive, incurable disease.

■ It can be difficult to differentiate chronic pancreatitis from pancreatic cancer.

COMMONLY ASKED QUESTIONS

What caused my pancreatitis?
Alcohol and gallstones are the most common causes. There are other, miscellaneous causes, which are outlined in Table 5.1.

Does pancreatitis recur?
In acute pancreatitis, unless an etiologic factor is found and removed, the chances are good that it will recur. ERCP can often find presumptive causes in cases previously thought to be idiopathic.

Does acute pancreatitis lead to chronic pancreatitis?
Except in the case of continued alcohol abuse, acute pancreatitis usually does not lead to chronic pancreatitis. A rare exception may be seen in complicated disease with stricture of the pancreatic duct.

If I stop drinking, will my chronic pancreatitis disappear?
Unfortunately, while the pain and rate of attacks may diminish, chronic pancreatitis is an incurable disease.

Does surgery relieve the pain of chronic pancreatitis?
Although short-term results of pain relief are promising for selected patients (e.g., those with dilated pancreatic ducts), long-term pain relief is achieved in only 50% to 60% of cases.

SUGGESTED READINGS

Acute Pancreatitis

Agarwal N, Pitchumoni CS, Sivaprasad AV. Evaluating tests for acute pancreatitis. *Am J Gastroenterol* 1990;85:356–366.

Balthazar EJ, Robinson DL, Megibow AJ, Ransom JH. Acute pancreatitis: value of CT in establishing prognosis. *Radiology* 1990;174:331–336.

Bradley EL. A clinically based classification system for acute pancreatitis. *Arch Surg* 1991;128:586–590.

Ranson JHC, Rifkind RM, Roses DF. Prognostic signs and the role of operative management in acute pancreatitis. *Surg Gynecol Obstet* 1975;139:69–80.

Steinberg W, Tenner S. Acute pancreatitis. *N Engl J Med* 1994; 330:1198–1210.

Chronic Pancreatitis

DiMagno EP, Go VLW, Summerskill WHJ. Relations between pancreatic enzyme outputs and malabsorption in severe pancreatic insufficiency. *N Engl J Med* 1973;288:813–815.

Kalthoff L, Layer P, Clain JE. The course of alcoholic and nonalcoholic chronic pancreatitis. *Dig Dis Sci* 1984;29:953.

Lowenfels AB, Maisonneuve P, Cavallini G. Pancreatitis and at the risk of pancreatic cancer. *N Engl J Med* 1993;328: 1433–1437.

Mergener K, Baillie J. Chronic pancreatitis. *Lancet* 1997; 350:1379–1385.

Steer ML, Waxman I, Freedman S. Chronic pancreatitis. *N Engl J Med* 1995;332:1482–1490.

REFERENCES

1. Bradley EL. A clinically based classification system for acute pancreatitis. *Arch Surg* 1993;128:586–590.
2. Ranson JHC, Rifkind RM, Roses DF. Prognostic signs and the role of operative management in acute pancreatitis. *Surg Gynecol Obstet* 1975;139:69–80.
3. Larvin M, McMahon MJ. APACHE-II score for assessment and monitoring of acute pancreatitis. *Lancet* 1989;2: 201–205.
4. Lee SP, Nicholls JF, Park HZ. Biliary sludge as a cause of acute pancreatitis. *N Engl J Med* 1992;326:589–593.
5. Ros E, Navarro S, Bru C, Garcia-Puges A, Valderramer R. Occult microlithiasis in idiopathic acute pancreatitis: prevention of relapses by cholecystectomy or ursodeoxycholic acid therapy. *Gastroenterology* 1991;101:1701–1709.
6. Venu RP, Geenen JE, Hogan W, Stone J, Johnson GK, Soergel K. Idiopathic recurrent pancreatitis: an approach to diagnosis and treatment. *Dig Dis Sci* 1989;34:56–60.
7. Ranson JHC. Etiological and prognostic factors in human acute pancreatitis: a review. *Am J Gastroenterol* 1982; 77:633–638.
8. Blamey SL, Imrie CW, O'Neil J, Gilmour WH, Carter DC. Prognostic factors in acute pancreatitis. *Gut* 1984; 25:1350–1356.
9. Larvin M, McMahon MJ. Apache-II score for assessment and monitoring of acute pancreatitis. *Lancet* 1989;2: 201–205.
10. Agarwal N, Pitchumoni CS, Sivaprasad AV. Evaluating tests for acute pancreatitis. *Am J Gastroenterol* 1990;85: 356–366.
11. Neoptolemos JP, Carr-Locke DL, London DL, Bailey IA, James D, Fossard DP. Controlled trial of urgent endoscopic retrograde cholangiopancreatography and endoscopic sphincterotomy versus conservative treatment for acute pancreatitis due to gallstones. *Lancet* 1988; 2:979–983.
12. Fan ST, Lai ECS, Mok FPT, Lo CM, Zheng SS, Wong J. Early treatment of acute biliary pancreatitis by endoscopic papillotomy. *N Engl J Med* 1993;328:228–232.
13. McMenamin DA, Gates LK Jr. A retrospective analysis of the effect of contrast-enhanced CT on the outcome of acute pancreatitis. *Am J Gastroenterol* 1996;91:1384–1387.
14. Balthazar EJ, Robinson DL, Megibow AJ, Ranson JH. Acute pancreatitis: value of CT in establishing prognosis. *Radiology* 1990;174:331–336.
15. Steinberg W, Tenner S. Acute pancreatitis. *N Engl J Med* 1994;330:1198–1210.
16. McClave SA, Snider H, Owens N, Sexton LK. Clinical nutrition in pancreatitis. *Dig Dis Sci* 1997;42:2035–2044.
17. Barie PS. A critical review of antibiotic prophylaxis in severe acute pancreatitis. *Am J Surg* 1996;172s:38s–43s.
18. Owyang C, Levitt MO. Chronic pancreatitis. In: Yamada T, ed. *Textbook of gastroenterology*, 2nd ed. Philadelphia: JB Lippincott, 1995:2092.
19. Steer ML, Waxman I, Freedman S. Chronic pancreatitis. *N Engl J Med* 1995;332:1482–1490.

20. Mergener K, Baillie J. Chronic pancreatitis. *Lancet* 1997; 350:1379–1384.
21. Bisceglie AM, Segal I. Cirrhosis and chronic pancreatitis in alcoholics. *J Clin Gastroenterol* 1984;6:199–200.
22. Kalthoff L, Layer P, Clain JE. The course of alcoholic and nonalcoholic chronic pancreatitis. *Dig Dis Sci* 1984;29:953.
23. DiMagno EP, Go VLW, Summerskill WHJ. Relations between pancreatic enzyme outputs and malabsorption in severe pancreatic insufficiency. *N Engl J Med* 1973;288: 813–815.
24. Lowenfels AB, Maisoneuve P, Cavillini G. Pancreatitis and the risk of pancreatic cancer. *N Engl J Med* 1993;329: 1433–1437.
25. Nagata A, Homma T, Tamai K. A study of chronic pancreatitis by serial endoscopic pancreatography. *Gastroenterology* 1981;81:884–891.

Infectious Diarrhea

Naiel N. Nassar,* M. Shahbaz Hasan,** and Clark R. Gregg†
*Center for AIDS Research, Education, and Services, Sacramento, California 95814
**Veterans Administration Medical Center, Dallas, Texas 75216
†University of Texas Southwestern Medical Center and Veterans Administration Medical Center, Dallas, Texas 75216

DEFINITION

Diarrhea is one of the most frequently encountered syndromes in general medical practice. Worldwide, infectious diarrhea is the second leading cause of death overall, and among children younger than 5 years of age it is the leading cause, with 4 to 6 million children dying annually from diarrhea-related illnesses. The preponderance of fatal diarrhea occurs in the developing world. Gastroenteritis and acute diarrhea account for 1.5% of hospitalizations of adults in the United States, but fatalities are rare.

Diarrhea is commonly defined as the passage of three or more unformed stools per day. Most infectious causes of diarrhea are mild and self-limited, lasting 3 to 5 days. Diarrhea that subsides within 14 days can be termed *acute;* if it lasts longer than 4 weeks it is called *chronic.* Diarrhea is termed *persistent* if it lasts for an intermediate duration (i.e., 2 to 4 weeks).

This chapter reviews the epidemiology, pathogenic mechanisms, and directed approaches to the diagnosis and treatment of infectious diarrhea. The special situation of travelers' diarrhea (TD) is also covered. Diarrhea complicating the acquired immunodeficiency syndrome (AIDS) is discussed in Chapter 10.

CAUSE

Pathogenesis

Transmission

Microbial pathogens that cause diarrhea are predominantly acquired through the fecal-oral route. This transmission may occur by direct contact with feces or indirectly through consumption of inadequately prepared food substances that have been contaminated by fecal microorganisms during growth, harvesting, or handling. Contamination may be conveyed by an infected person, an insect vector such as a fly, or fomites including fertilizers and processing equipment. A small proportion of cases result from direct inoculation, which can occur during oral-anal sexual intercourse or possibly via inhalation of airborne droplets (e.g., rotavirus, Norwalk-like viruses).

Predisposing factors

Acquisition and establishment of gastrointestinal infection and subsequent development of diarrheal disease occur as a result of the interplay of three principal factors: conditions leading to exposure, predisposing host factors, and microbial virulence factors.

Hygiene Laxity or breakdown in personal or community hygiene practices almost always precedes the acquisition of enteric infection. At the community level, such breakdown or unsanitary practice may involve an institutional failure to treat raw sewage or water supplies adequately. Poor sanitary conditions are the major reason that infectious gastroenteritis is endemic in developing nations, where overcrowding, environmental contamination, and illiteracy coexist. Epidemics of cholera and other enteric infections frequently occur in refugee camps, and outbreaks of gastrointestinal infections occur after natural disasters. Failure to purify water supplies adequately is occasionally responsible for community outbreaks of diarrhea even in developed nations.

Another common breakdown in public health practice involves inadequate food processing and preparation, which can be responsible for significant outbreaks of foodborne gastroenteritis, including salmonellosis, campylobacteriosis, enterohemorrhagic *Escherichia coli* (EHEC) infections, listeriosis, and many others. The conditions for spreading infection are amplified by today's global economy, in which foods can be rapidly transported from the developing world to be distributed and consumed in faraway industrialized nations.

Host factors The human gastrointestinal tract possesses some native resistance to infection. Gastric acidity provides a chemical barrier to survival of ingested microorganisms; achlorhydric patients are susceptible to infection by enteropathogens at inocula that are much smaller than usual. Intestinal motility helps flush out microorganisms as well as their toxins. The normal enteric flora help prevent the replication and establishment of virulent microorganisms by a competitive process known as colonization resistance. This protection is absent in newborn infants and may be breached in persons receiving anti-

microbial drugs. Finally, local immunity may be compromised in neutropenic patients and in patients with AIDS or immunoglobulin A (IgA) deficiency.

Microbial virulence factors Microbes may produce diarrhea by toxin production, adherence to intestinal mucosa, invasion of the gut wall, or disruption of mucosal villous cells.

TOXIN PRODUCTION A number of microorganisms produce one or more enterotoxins that act locally on the mucosa or are absorbed systemically to produce pathologic effects. Locally acting toxins are of two forms: those that alter the secretory function of mucosal cells without physically damaging them (e.g., cholera toxin, heat-labile toxin of enterotoxigenic *E. coli* [ETEC]) and those that are cytotoxins and cause mucosal destruction and inflammation (e.g., *Shigella* spp., *Clostridium difficile*, EHEC, *Entamoeba histolytica*). Examples of absorbed toxins include those associated with staphylococcal and *Bacillus cereus* food poisoning.

ADHERENCE Some organisms, such as ETEC, enteropathogenic *E. coli* (EPEC), and enteroaggregative *E. coli* (EAEC), adhere to and colonize the intestinal mucosa. They do not invade the mucosa, and EPEC and EAEC do not seem to elaborate toxins. The exact mechanisms by which adherence of these bacteria results in diarrhea are unclear.

INVASIVENESS Some microorganisms directly invade the intestinal mucosa to cause an inflammatory gastroenteritis and may cause regional or disseminated extraintestinal infection; examples include *Salmonella* spp., *Shigella* spp., *Yersinia enterocolitica*, *Campylobacter jejuni* and *E. histolytica*. These infections may manifest primarily as a systemic illness or enteric fever with associated diarrhea or other intestinal symptoms.

DISRUPTION OF THE MUCOSAL VILLOUS CELLS By selectively disrupting the function of small intestinal microvilli, certain viruses (e.g., rotaviruses, Norwalk-like viruses) and protozoan parasites can cause malabsorption.

Specific Causes
Bacteria

Bacterial pathogens are responsible for about one third of all cases of diarrhea in the developed world. In developing countries, where ETEC is an important cause of diarrhea, bacteria are responsible for more than 50% of all diarrheal illnesses. *Shigella*, *Salmonella*, and *Campylobacter* species together cause approximately 15% of diarrhea cases. *Aeromonas* spp., *Plesiomonas*, *Vibrio cholerae*, noncholera vibrios, and *Listeria monocytogenes* are important pathogens in certain settings and seasons. EHEC (e.g., O157:H7) causes diarrhea associated with dysentery and hemolytic uremic syndrome in certain parts of the world. *C. difficile* is the principal bacterial cause of nosocomial diarrhea.

Shigella   Shigellosis is caused by one of four species, each with a corresponding serogroup: *Shigella dysenteriae* (serogroup A), *Shigella flexneri* (serogroup B), *Shigella boydii* (serogroup C), and *Shigella sonnei* (serogroup D). Shigellosis is most common in children and is spread by the fecal-oral route. Outbreaks have been associated with contaminated water or food, swimming pool exposures, household contact, and day care centers. Enteric disease is produced by direct invasion of the intestinal epithelium by the organism, which leads to inflammation, mucosal and submucosal ulcerations, and formation of microabscesses. Other virulence factors with *Shigella* infections include the production of cytotoxins that mediate systemic effects, including neurotoxicity and seizures as well as hemolytic uremic syndrome.

Salmonella   Salmonellosis is the most frequently reported foodborne disease in many parts of the world, including some developed countries. Fecal-oral transmission is typical, with outbreaks commonly associated with contaminated eggs, dairy products, and meats. Modern food processing and distribution methods can amplify outbreaks of salmonellosis. Nonhuman reservoirs, including poultry, pigs, cattle, and household pets (especially reptiles), also play an important role in disease transmission. Children younger than 1 year of age have the highest attack rate, but there is also a high attack rate and increased mortality in the elderly and in patients with sickle cell disease, immunosuppression, malaria, achlorhydria, or human immunodeficiency virus (HIV) infection.

Campylobacter   *Campylobacter* species, predominantly *C. jejuni*, represent the most common foodborne bacterial pathogen in many developed countries. Transmission again is fecal-oral, and undercooked chicken is the most frequent vehicle of infection. Outbreaks have also been associated with consumption of unpasteurized dairy products and with animal contact, especially contact with young dogs or cats.

Yersinia enterocolitica   This bacterium causes a spectrum of illness that ranges from simple gastroenteritis to invasive colitis and ileitis. Swine are the major natural reservoir, but transmission is usually via ingestion of milk or meat from contaminated cows. Person-to-person spread is rare, but infection has occurred as a consequence of blood transfusion from asymptomatic but nonetheless bacteremic donors.

Vibrio cholerae   This agent is spread mainly by contaminated water, and cholera is responsible for about 150,000 deaths per year around the world. Of the 139 serogroups, only groups O1 and O139 are associated with epidemics. The seventh pandemic, caused by *V. cholerae* O1 El Tor biotype, began in Southeast Asia in 1961 and reached the Americas in 1991. Disease from the first non-O1 strain (O139 Bengal) was reported from the Indian subcontinent in 1992. Although serogroup O139 strains are genetically related to the O1 strains, they have a greater capacity to produce toxin. There is no cross-immunity among strains of *V. cholerae*, which raises the possibility of yet another pandemic.

Noncholera vibrios   *Vibrio parahaemolyticus* is acquired through exposure to seawater or consumption of raw seafood, especially mollusks.

Clostridium difficile   This bacterium was first proven to be a pathogen in the late 1970s and is now the leading single cause of nosocomial diarrhea. *C. difficile* is part of the normal colonic microflora in the majority of infants and in up to 3% of healthy adults, but *C. difficile* disease is associated with new acquisition of the pathogen. Environmental contamination by *C. difficile* in health care facilities is common. Person-to-person spread also probably occurs. The use of antibiotics, perhaps in combination with conditions that affect gut motility (e.g., abdominal surgery, stool softeners, enemas, tube feedings), facilitates colonization and overgrowth of *C. difficile* by altering the normal colonic microflora. Pathogenic strains of *C. difficile* elaborate two toxins: toxin A, an enterotoxin that is responsible for the colitis, and toxin B, a cytotoxin.

Enterohemorrhagic Escherichia coli   EHEC was first recognized as a pathogen in 1982. Since then the incidence of hemorrhagic colitis caused by this bacterium has been rising, so that the annual incidence in the United States is now estimated at 3 cases per 100,000 population. EHEC is responsible for 15% to 36% of all cases of bloody diarrhea in the developed countries, especially in higher latitudes, where most cases occur between June and September. Of the more than 30 serotypes of *E. coli* that have been associated with hemorrhagic colitis, the most common single type is O157:H7. These bacteria share the ability to produce one of two cytotoxins, known as Shiga-like toxins (SLT-I and SLT-II), which bear chemical and biological similarity to the verotoxin produced by *S. dysenteriae*. Cattle are the main reservoir, and infection occurs after consumption of contaminated ground beef (e.g., hamburgers, beef patties) or other meats, unpasteurized dairy products or apple juice, fruits, vegetables, or water. Children may excrete the organisms for prolonged periods (longer than 3 weeks), and person-to-person transmission has also been observed in high-risk environments such as day care centers.

Aeromonas   Species of this bacterium can be isolated from fresh water and from a variety of animals, including fish, shellfish, farm animals, and reptiles. Aeromonas-associated diarrhea has a seasonal peak in the warmer months of summer and early autumn.

Plesiomonas   These species rarely cause enteric infections; they are associated with travel to the Far East or Mexico or with the consumption of raw oysters. Little is known about the pathogenic mechanisms, spectrum of clinical disease, diagnostic methods, or efficacy of antimicrobial treatment for *Plesiomonas*-associated diarrhea.

Viruses

Viruses are responsible for most of the diarrheal disease in infants. Rotavirus is the most important viral agent, but adenoviruses, Norwalk-like viruses, astroviruses, and caliciviruses also account for much of nonbacterial diarrhea.

Rotaviruses are medium-sized, RNA viruses whose wheel-shaped appearance on electron microscopy gives them their name. The virus penetrates mature small-bowel enterocytes, and the resulting cell death causes villus atrophy and a sprue-like small-bowel malabsorption syndrome.

Rotaviruses are the most common cause of dehydrating acute watery diarrhea in children. In tropical countries infection occurs throughout the year, but in temperate climates a seasonal trend is typical, with most cases occurring in colder months. The route of transmission is fecal-oral; however, there is speculation that airborne transmission is also possible. The infective dose is very small (100 to 1,000 organisms), whereas symptomatic patients excrete massive amounts of viruses (more than 10^{12} organisms per milliliter of stool). Rotaviruses are classified into groups A through G based on the antigenic characteristics of an inner capsid protein known as VP6, but only groups A through C have thus far been associated with human illness.

Parasites

Giardia lamblia, *E. histolytica*, and *Cryptosporidium parvum* are the three major parasitic agents in diarrheal disease; *Cyclospora cayetanensis*, however, may be a more common cause than was previously thought. Microsporidia and *Isospora* are considered causes of watery diarrhea in patients with AIDS and are discussed in Chapter 10.

Giardia   is transmitted via the fecal-oral route and is the most common cause of parasitic diarrhea in the developed world. In many cases, consumption of untreated alpine surface water is implicated in transmission. Nonhuman reservoirs of the parasite include dogs, cats, sheep, and beavers. Outbreaks have been reported among children in day care centers, homosexual men, wilderness hikers, institutionalized persons, travelers to Russia, and even visitors to upscale ski resorts.

Entamoeba histolytica   Eight species of amebas parasitize the human gastrointestinal tract: *E. histolytica*, *Entamoeba dispar*, *Entamoeba coli*, *Entamoeba hartmanni*, *Entamoeba gingivalis*, *Dientamoeba fragilis*, *Endolimax nana*, and *Iodamoeba buetschlii*. Only *E. histolytica* is a pathogen. The highest prevalence of amebiasis is in developing countries, but the overall prevalence of intestinal carriage in the United States is 4%. Transmission may be fecal-oral or person-to-person, especially within institutionalized populations, among sexually active male homosexuals, and among recent immigrants from and travelers to endemic countries.

Cryptosporidium parvum   This parasite has been prominent as a cause of watery diarrhea in AIDS patients (see Chapter 10), but it can also cause diarrhea in nonimmunocompromised hosts. These cases have been related to exposure to animals, day care settings, contaminated water, and travel to the developing world. An epidemic of 400,000 cases of cryptosporidiosis in Milwaukee, Wisconsin, in 1993 resulted from contamination of the municipal water system.

Cyclospora cayetanensis   This is a coccidian protozoan pathogen that causes waterborne or possibly foodborne diarrhea in children, immunocompetent adults, and AIDS patients. It is also occasionally implicated in TD.

Toxigenic bacterial food poisoning

Staphylococcus aureus, *B. cereus*, and *Clostridium perfringens* are the most common causes of acute toxigenic bacterial food poisoning in the United States. Disease caused by each of these is mediated by bacterial exotoxins, through either ingestion of preformed toxin or, in the case of *C. perfringens* and some *B. cereus* syndromes, production of toxin in the intestinal tract after ingestion of large numbers of the viable microorganisms.

Inadequately refrigerated macaroni salad, cream-filled pastries, and ham are the foods most commonly implicated in *S. aureus* food poisoning. Attack rates for groups of people eating these foods can be high.

Travelers' Diarrhea

TD is a common medical complaint among persons who go from developed to developing areas of the world. It occurs in approximately 11 million travelers annually, 30% of whom are confined to bed and an additional 40% required to severely limit their activities.

Risk associated with destination

Destination of travel is probably the most important factor that determines risk for TD. North America, northern Europe, Australia, and New Zealand are characterized by a low (4% to 8%) incidence of diarrhea in travelers from other industrialized countries during short-term travel (2 weeks), whereas travelers to tropical or underdeveloped areas usually experience much higher incidence rates (20% to 55%). Intermediate-risk destinations for travelers include southern Europe, Caribbean countries, Israel, Japan, and South Africa.

Host factors

Certain background medical conditions are associated with especially high risk of TD. In achlorhydric persons, including those who have undergone gastrectomy or are receiving antacid therapies, even a small ingested inoculum might lead to diarrhea, whereas a host with normal protective gastric acidity might remain well after similar exposure. AIDS and secretory IgA deficiency probably are also risk factors. Persons with chronic gastrointestinal disorders, diabetes, or renal or cardiac failure and those taking diuretics may suffer greater morbidity and more complications if they develop diarrhea and should be counseled about this risk before they travel.

Other risk factors

The cause of TD varies significantly with the season in any given area. For instance, *Campylobacter* and rotaviruses are isolated most frequently in the winter, whereas ETEC is the most common pathogen for summer and fall travelers. Affluent travelers from countries with high standards of hygiene seem to be at increased risk of TD, presumably because they have not previously encountered the many enteric pathogens in the developing world. No mode of travel or standard of accommodation exempts travelers from the syndrome, but trekking, camping, and adventure tourism are typified by higher attack rates. There is no gender preference, but younger travelers are more frequently affected, perhaps because of their more adventurous behavior, poorer accommodations, lack of previous tropical experience, lower compliance with dietary restrictions, or larger appetites. The circumstance in which food is consumed can also be a risk factor for di-

arrhea: those who eat in public places have attack rates as high as 45%, whereas apartment dwellers who cook for themselves are at very low risk. The duration of a stay abroad is also an important factor, with the attack rate varying from 22% for stays shorter than 1 week to 45% for stays longer than 3 weeks.

Infectious causes

TD is caused by any of an array of foodborne or waterborne pathogens that are transmitted via the fecal-oral route. Bacteria are the presumed or proven cause in 80% of cases, most commonly *E. coli* (particularly ETEC) and *Shigella* species. Other occasional bacterial causes of TD include EAEC, *Campylobacter* spp., salmonellae, vibrios, *Aeromonas,* and *Plesiomonas. Salmonella* is an uncommon cause of TD. *V. cholerae* is a very rare cause of TD, but noncholera vibrios, especially *V. parahaemolyticus,* account for up to 70% of TD in Japan and have also been found in several Asian countries and locales bordering the Gulf of Mexico.

The most common protozoan cause of TD is *G. lamblia.* Although *Cryptosporidium* and *Cyclospora* infections sometimes occur, *E. histolytica* is rare as a cause of TD. Norwalk-like agents and rotaviruses are the most notable viral agents of TD.

PATIENT PRESENTATION

Clinical Stratification

The workup of a patient with infectious diarrhea should focus initially on differentiating those patients who have severe illness. This first evaluation consists of a focused history to determine the type, severity, and duration of the diarrhea and other features that may suggest complicated or serious acute diarrhea (Table 6.1).

Diarrhea can be categorized as mild (one to two unformed stools per day without abdominal pain or cramps), moderate (three to three unformed stools per day or any number of unformed stools with abdominal pain or cramps), or severe (more than six unformed stools per day, disabling associated symptoms, or any number of unformed stools associated with fever and dysentery). Distressing symptoms are those that force a change in activities, such as missed school or work, change in travel plans, or confinement to bed. Other key features include the duration of symptoms, occurrence of fever or dysentery, whether the illness is worsening, and whether there are symptoms of volume depletion.

Patients with mild disease may be treated symptomatically or simply observed until their symptoms resolve

TABLE 6.1.	Clinical Features Suggesting Serious Diarrhea

Age >70 yr
Immunocompromise
Frequency of stools >6 per day
Duration of diarrhea >48 hr
Abdominal cramps
Tenesmus
Fever
Dysentery
Gastrointestinal hemorrhage
Hypotension, tachycardia
Dry mucous membranes, poor skin turgor
Oliguria

spontaneously, whereas those with more threatening illness should be subjected to a more extensive and timely workup.

History

The physician should attempt to recognize the epidemiologic circumstances that may have contributed to acquisition of the infection. Such a history may suggest a microbial cause, information that may be crucial in deciding on empiric antimicrobial therapy.

Exposure history

The patient should be questioned about any recent travel or recent exposure to antibiotics, which may indicate infection with imported pathogens, resistant bacteria, or *C. difficile.* Persons who practice oral-anal sexual intercourse are predisposed to acquire not only enteropathogens but also a number of sexually transmitted infections. In addition, a history of such behavior should raise the possibility of an HIV-related diarrhea. Persons exposed to day care centers are also at a high risk for infection by *Giardia, Shigella,* EHEC, or *Cryptosporidium.*

Food history

When a single case of diarrhea is encountered, it is difficult to incriminate a specific food or beverage vehicle. Identification of a common food source may be possible, however, when diarrhea in one patient is associated with an outbreak among others who consumed the same product.

Incubation period

Nausea and vomiting may be prominent with food poisoning or viral gastroenteritis. During an outbreak, the incubation period of the illness may suggest a specific pathogen (Table 6.2). When diarrhea and vomiting occur within 6 hours after eating a food item in question, enterotoxin-producing bacteria such as *S. aureus* or *B. cereus* should be suspected. The incubation period for toxigenic *C. perfringens* diarrhea is usually 8 to 14 hours. If vomiting is a prominent feature of the diarrheal disease and the incubation period exceeds 14 hours, a Norwalk-like agent should be suspected, especially in the winter. EHEC disease may begin with watery diarrhea days after exposure, but this is usually followed by hemorrhagic stools.

Physical Examination

The history is followed by a directed physical examination seeking evidence of serious illness, such as volume depletion or extraintestinal dissemination.

Diarrheal stools may be watery or bloody and perhaps mucoid. Most viruses, parasites, and enterotoxigenic bacteria cause a watery diarrhea. Microscopically, this watery stool tends to be noninflammatory, in contrast to the inflammatory diarrhea seen with infections by organisms that invade the gastrointestinal mucosa or elaborate cytotoxins. An inflammatory or invasive process is usually present when fever and/or bloody stools are documented.

Fever is classically present in infections caused by *Shigella* spp., *Salmonella* spp., and *C. jejuni.* In addition, *C. difficile, Aeromonas* spp., invasive *E. coli,* noncholera vibrios, and viruses may also produce febrile illness. Patients with hemorrhagic colitis caused by EHEC typically have minimal fever.

Diarrhea results in the loss of both fluid and electrolytes. Clinical features of volume depletion range from mild dehydration, such as increased thirst, lassitude, dry mucosa, and decreased skin turgor, to severe manifestations including postural hypotension, mental obtundation, oliguria, and finally shock.

Specific Infections

Shigella

Initial presentation   Patients with shigellosis often present with lower abdominal pain, fever (40%), and bloody mucoid stools (30%). However, the disease can be biphasic, with initial symptoms of high fever, abdominal pain, and voluminous watery diarrhea followed in 3 to 5 days by tenesmus, decreasing stool volume, and increasing mucus and blood in the stool. The duration of diarrhea, even when untreated, is usually 4 to 5 days, although symptoms may persist for 3 to 4 weeks in severe cases.

TABLE 6.2.	Typical Incubation Periods of Common Gastrointestinal Infections
Time since exposure	Likely cause
6 hr	Preformed toxins: *Staphylococcus aureus, Bacillus cereus*
8–14 hr	*Clostridium perfringens* toxin
≥48 hr + vomiting	Viral gastroenteritis
>12 hrs + fever/ dysentery	Invasive bacteria: *Salmonella, Shigella, Campylobacter, Yersinia*
≥24 hr + hemorrhagic colitis	Enterohemorrhagic *Escherichia coli*

Complications   Complications of *Shigella* infection include neurotoxicity with seizures in 10% to 40% of infected children, hemolytic uremic syndrome, intestinal perforation, urinary tract infection, and chronic carriage with relapsing or persistent diarrhea. However, bacteremia is unusual. A syndrome of asymmetric reactive oligoarthritis, conjunctivitis, and keratitis, usually associated with histocompatibility type HLA-B27, may develop 2 to 3 weeks after the onset of diarrhea.

Salmonella

Several major clinical syndromes have been described with *Salmonella* infections. *Gastroenteritis* is the most common; it occurs after a short incubation period of 6 to 48 hours with nausea, vomiting, and abdominal cramps progressing to diarrhea and fever (50%) that usually last 3 to 4 days. *Bacteremia and dissemination* are unusual in older children and adults but may complicate 5% to 40% of *Salmonella* gastroenteritis in infants. *Localized infections* occur in 10% of those with bacteremia and include meningitis, endocarditis, arthritis, osteomyelitis, and focal abscesses.

Typhoid or enteric fever is classically caused by *S. typhi* and is characterized by insidious onset of malaise, progressive high-grade fever with abdominal pain or constipation, and relative bradycardia, followed by the development of diarrhea and a "rose spots" rash. If not treated, typhoid fever may progress during the third week to cause hepatitis, myocarditis, cholecystitis, gastrointestinal bleeding or perforation, and manifestations of the systemic inflammatory response syndrome.

A chronic asymptomatic biliary or enteric carrier state occurs in 14% of patients and is encountered with higher frequency in women, infants, and persons with preexisting biliary tract disease.

Campylobacter

Initial presentation   The clinical syndrome is similar to that of shigellosis, with slightly longer incubation period of 2 to 4 days, followed by fever, abdominal pain, and diarrhea.

Complications   Complications are uncommon and include gastrointestinal hemorrhage, toxic megacolon, pancreatitis, cholecystitis, bacteremia, meningitis, and septic arthritis. Postinfectious complications including hemolytic uremic syndrome, reactive arthritis, and Guillain-Barré syndrome have also been reported.

Yersinia

Enterocolitis is the most commonly reported syndrome caused by *Y. enterocolitica*; it is a nonspecific illness of fever, abdominal cramps, and diarrhea lasting about 2 weeks. In older children and young adults, the clinical presentation may mimic that of acute appendicitis when the mesenteric and iliac lymph nodes are involved. Systemic infection with hepatic or splenic abscesses, osteomyelitis, meningitis, or endocarditis has been documented in immunosuppressed patients, diabetics, and those with conditions associated with iron overload, such as thalassemia or hemochromatosis. Postinfectious reactive arthritis and erythema nodosum have also occurred.

Vibrio cholerae

Pathogenic *V. cholerae* produces an enterotoxin that results in intestinal secretion of sodium and chloride and voluminous diarrhea. Incubation periods vary from a few hours to 4 days. The disease is characterized by the acute onset of copious watery ("rice water") diarrhea that can be severe enough to cause prostration, hypovolemic shock, and acute renal failure. About one third of patients also have a low-grade fever and vomiting. The illness lasts for 2 to 7 days and is shortened by antibiotic therapy given early in the course. Asymptomatic infection is not uncommon in endemic areas.

Noncholera vibrios

V. parahaemolyticus is capable of producing both an enterotoxin and a cytotoxin. After a short incubation period (12 to 24 hours), *V. parahaemolyticus* infection typically causes explosive watery diarrhea that is self-limited (median, 3 days). Almost 25% of patients develop an inflammatory diarrhea, and rarely a dysenteric syndrome occurs. Other marine vibrios, including *Vibrio vulnificus*, cause systemic infections and do not usually cause gastroenteritis.

Enterohemorrhagic Escherichia coli

Initial presentation   Hemorrhagic colitis caused by EHEC has an incubation period of 1 to 14 days (median, 3 to 4 days) and usually begins with watery, nonbloody diarrhea with abdominal cramps. There may be nausea and vomiting but only mild fever. The colitis progresses to a bloody diarrhea that lasts 3 to 8 days and is self-limited.

Complications   Hemolytic uremic syndrome and thrombotic thrombocytopenic purpura are variants of a diffuse thrombotic microangiopathy that is suspected in persons who exhibit a microangiopathic hemolysis, thrombocytopenia, and, usually, renal insufficiency days to weeks after the bloody diarrhea. This syndrome occurs in 2% to 7% of patients, usually children and the elderly, and is associated with a 5% to 10% mortality rate.

Aeromonas

Aeromonas infections usually occur in children younger than 2 years of age, but they may occur in adults, particularly those with liver disease or malignancy. Diarrhea is usually mild and of brief duration. However, chronic diarrhea and extraintestinal disease, including meningitis, bacteremia, endocarditis, septic arthritis, and urinary tract infection, have been documented.

Clostridium difficile

Initial presentation   The spectrum of diseases caused by *C. difficile* ranges from an asymptomatic carrier state to life-threatening toxic megacolon. Diarrhea begins a few days to several weeks after the provocative event (e.g., antibiotic exposure, surgery). In most there is a mild to moderate watery diarrhea.

Complications   In severe cases, a dysenteric syndrome may occur that includes bloody diarrhea, fever, abdominal cramps, distention, and dramatic leukocytosis. Such cases may progress to toxic megacolon, colonic perforation, and peritonitis necessitating surgery.

Rotavirus

Initial presentation   After an incubation period of 1 to 3 days, there is an acute onset of watery diarrhea, often with vomiting. The illness usually lasts 5 to 7 days. Rotavirus infections may occur again throughout life, but the primary episode tends to be the most severe.

Complications   Rarely, extraintestinal manifestations such as encephalitis, hemorrhagic shock, hepatitis, or febrile convulsions may occur.

Giardia

Onset of symptoms is generally days to weeks after exposure to *Giardia*. Intestinal malabsorption and chronic intermittent diarrhea are the typical syndromes associated with this infection. Patients often complain of flatulence, bloating, nausea, anorexia, foul-smelling stools, and weight loss.

Entamoeba histolytica

Initial presentation   Most amebic infections are asymptomatic; however, clinical disease may occur, and it is usually characterized by subacute, intermittent, watery, foul-smelling diarrhea with mucus, blood, flatulence, and crampy abdominal pain. More severe illness may occur in persons who are predisposed because of malnutrition, malignancy, glucocorticoid use, pregnancy, or young age.

Complications   Complications are somewhat unusual and include amebic liver abscess, intestinal perforation, and toxic megacolon. About 5% of patients with symptomatic amebic dysentery simultaneously are found to have a single liver abscess that usually involves the upper outer quadrant of the right lobe. Onset of fever and tender hepatic enlargement from amebic liver abscess is usually insidious but may be acute and is sometimes complicated by contiguous extension to the right pleural space or through the left lobe of the liver into the pericardium.

Cyclospora

Diarrhea with cyclosporiasis is not generally severe but is often associated with anorexia, weight loss, and fatigue that may last for 1 to 15 weeks. In immunosuppressed hosts, diarrhea caused by *C. cayetanensis* can be chronic and unremitting.

Toxigenic bacterial food poisoning

Persons with food poisoning syndromes should be questioned thoroughly about what foods were consumed at what time and by which companions early in the course of disease, while memories may be more reliable. Prompt reporting of outbreaks of food poisoning will assist in investigation by public health authorities.

Staphylococcus aureus   Nausea, vomiting, and abdominal pain, sometimes followed by watery diarrhea, develop within 1 to 6 hours after food ingestion, and symptoms usually last less than 12 hours. Rarely, the absorbed staphylococcal toxin acts as a superantigen and provokes a systemic inflammatory response that can be severe.

Bacillus cereus   This organism causes two distinct forms of gastroenteritis. The emesis syndrome is similar to that associated with *S. aureus*. It typically occurs 1 to 6 hours after ingestion of cooked fried rice that has been held at room temperature, which has allowed the spores of *B. cereus* to germinate and produce its heat-stable toxin. The other form of *B. cereus* food poisoning is the diarrheal variant. In this form, *B. cereus* diarrhea is mediated by a second heat-labile enterotoxin produced in vivo by the bacterium after ingestion. Abdominal cramps and watery diarrhea occur 6 to 24 hours later and resolve in approximately 1 day.

Clostridium perfringens   This bacterium is also associated with two distinct syndromes. The more common in the developed world is a self-limited food poisoning mediated by a heat-labile enterotoxin produced by the clostridia in the stomach and small bowel as the ingested bacteria begin to sporulate. The foods implicated most often are undercooked or inadequately reheated meat with gravy or vegetables. Crampy abdominal pain and watery diarrhea develop 6 to 24 hours after ingestion and last several hours to 1 day. The other enteric syndrome caused by *C. perfringens* is called enteritis necroticans; although rare, it is life-threatening. This disease is associated with ingestion of undercooked pork and has been described mostly from the developing world.

Travelers' diarrhea

TD is generally defined as the passage of three or more loose stools in a 24-hour period coincident with foreign travel and in association with at least one other symptom of enteric disease, such as nausea, vomiting, abdominal cramps, fever, fecal urgency, tenesmus, or bloody, mucoid stools.

Typically there is an abrupt onset of watery or loose stools that may be accompanied by cramps, nausea, vomiting (15%), fever, and/or blood in the stools (22%). In young children, TD tends to follow a more prolonged and severe course. The clinical signs and symptoms of the syndrome are remarkably similar regardless of where in the world it occurs. TD usually resolves without treatment in 3 to 4 days, although the duration may be as long as 1 week or even longer than 3 months, depending on the causative organism and other conditions. However, a syndrome lasting longer than 14 days is referred to as persistent diarrhea and is often not caused by infection.

DIAGNOSIS

Laboratory Tests

Diagnostic testing in infectious diarrhea should be focused rather than all-inclusive, aiming to detect specific microbial pathogens as suggested by the patient's history and physical examination. Furthermore, laboratory evaluation of diarrheal disease should be reserved for patients with moderate-to-severe or persistent illness.

Fecal screening tests

A methylene blue or Wright's stain of a fresh fecal smear for polymorphonuclear leukocytes (WBC smear) is used commonly as a screening test to distinguish inflammatory (positive) from noninflammatory (negative) diarrhea. A reliable surrogate test for leukocytes is the stool lactoferrin assay. Detection of fecal leukocytes indicates diffuse colonic inflammation.

The most commonly identified pathogens in patients with a positive fecal leukocyte test result are *Shigella*, *Campylobacter*, *Aeromonas*, *Yersinia*, noncholera vibrios, and *C. difficile*. Small numbers of fecal leukocytes may be found in patients with salmonellosis or intestinal amebiasis. Fecal leukocyte testing detects a pathologic rather than an etiologic process, and, even with a positive smear, stool cultures often yield no pathogens.

Stool cultures

Stool cultures are among the most expensive yet least informative tests performed to evaluate patients with acute diarrhea. Routine stool cultures cost $950 to $1,200 per positive result. This expense can be substantially reduced by limiting the use of stool cultures to patients who meet one or more of the following clinical criteria: severe diarrhea, febrile or dysenteric disease, persistent diarrhea (longer than 14 days), hemorrhagic (possibly EHEC) diarrhea, and fecal leukocyte–positive diarrhea.

Cultures must be performed with care in order to obtain the highest possible yield. Stool should be collected during the acute phase of disease, preferably before the initiation of antibacterial therapy. It is submitted in a clean, nonabsorbent plastic container and processed as soon as possible. Rectal swabs are generally less satisfactory, although *Shigella* are sometimes isolated more readily by this method. Specimens not inoculated within 2 hours after collection should be refrigerated at 4°C or placed in a suitable transport medium for subsequent processing. In most laboratories, routine stool specimens are cultured only for *Salmonella*, *Shigella*, and *Campylobacter*. Other enteric pathogens (e.g., *Yersinia*, *Vibrio*, *E. coli*) may not be detected by routine surveyed culture. If one of these unusual pathogens is suspected, the laboratory should be alerted so that the appropriate diagnostic measures may be used. All patients with hemorrhagic colitis should have stool samples cultured for *E. coli* O157:H7.

Examination for ova and parasites

Routine stool examination for ova and parasites (O&P) in cases of acute diarrhea is even less rewarding than stool culture. An O&P examination is indicated in the setting of persistent diarrhea, diarrhea in a homosexual man, travel to Russia or to a mountainous region of North America, or regular contact with a day care center. There are few data on the optimal number of stool specimens that should be submitted for O&P testing. Although these tests are sensitive, three sequential fresh specimens should be adequate.

G. lamblia, the most common parasite identified in clinical laboratories, can be detected by routine O&P examination or by a specific fluorescent antibody stain or enzyme immunoassay (EIA). Most laboratories do not routinely examine for *Cryptosporidium, Cyclospora,* or *Isospora belli,* so if these protozoa are suspected, specific testing for them must be requested. In amebic dysentery, direct microscopy of a fresh fecal sample at 37°C may reveal motile trophozoites and a cellular exudate. Stool O&P testing is almost never useful in the evaluation of nosocomial diarrhea.

Viral testing

During winter months, watery diarrheal stools, especially those from children, should be screened for rotavirus by EIA before an extensive workup for other enteric pathogens is undertaken. Enteric adenovirus type 40/41, which causes diarrheal disease similar to rotavirus but without the seasonal variation, also may be detected by EIA. Diagnosis of Norwalk-like virus and other small round structured enteric viruses requires electron microscopy or immune electron microscopy, which are not practical in most cases.

Endoscopy

Flexible sigmoidoscopy or other endoscopic procedures may be useful in evaluating homosexual men with acute or persistent diarrhea, other patients with signs and symptoms of proctitis, patients in whom inflammatory or ischemic bowel disease cannot be excluded, and patients with suspected *C. difficile* colitis.

Other Tests for Specific Infections

Salmonella

A diagnosis of salmonellosis is usually made by stool cultures or, in cases of typhoid fever, by bone marrow

or blood cultures. Localized infections such as abscesses yield positive cultures by direct sampling of infected tissue. Serology for *Salmonella* infection is imprecise and often nonspecific, but it is occasionally used as an adjunct in diagnosis.

Yersinia

The diagnosis of yersiniosis is established by culture of stool, blood, peritoneal fluid, or mesenteric lymph nodes. Stool culture requires selective media to inhibit other, more rapidly growing organisms and may require cold enrichment techniques for primary isolation in the laboratory.

Enterohemorrhagic Escherichia coli

Stool screening studies show erythrocytes and leukocytes. The O157:H7 strain can usually be detected in stool with the use of sorbitol-MacConkey agar, on which their morphology is distinctive. Identity of the organism is confirmed by serotyping or toxin testing.

Clostridium difficile

C. difficile colitis is usually a nosocomial diarrhea. Stool assays for *C. difficile* toxin should be obtained for a patient with diarrhea who is currently receiving or has recently (within 6 weeks) received antimicrobial therapy. This test may remain positive for weeks after clinical resolution of *C. difficile* colitis and therefore should not be requested as a test of cure. Stool WBC smears are negative in approximately one half of cases of *C. difficile* diarrhea. Stool culture for *C. difficile* is an epidemiologic and research test and in general should not be ordered for diagnosis in individual patients.

With *C. difficile*–associated diarrhea, the colon is exclusively involved, but lesions may be inapparent or patchy on endoscopic examination. The fully developed "volcano lesions" of pseudomembranous colitis are familiar to experienced endoscopists and are virtually pathognomonic of *C. difficile* colitis.

Entamoeba histolytica

Diagnosis of amebic dysentery is confirmed by identification of mature trophozoites or characteristic quadrinucleate cysts on O&P examination of fresh stool or on biopsy specimens obtained by sigmoidoscopy. Trophozoites of *E. histolytica* often exhibit active directional motility and erythrophagocytosis, findings that are useful in distinguishing them from nonpathogenic amebas, but a specific polymerase chain reaction–based assay is currently the most reliable way to differentiate *E. histolytica* from *E. dispar.*

Serologic tests for *E. histolytica* are positive only with tissue invasion syndromes, not with uncomplicated dysentery, and are considered diagnostic when a high titer is found in a patient with hepatic abscess. If the patient has an amebic liver abscess, needle aspiration of the abscess reveals anchovy paste–like, odorless fluid that on microscopic examination is free of leukocytes and yields negative bacterial cultures.

Blastocystis

B. hominis is a relatively common microscopical finding on routine O&P examination of stool. No toxigenicity has been identified and no anatomic site of invasion or other pathogenic mechanism has been found that would explain the occurrence of diarrhea sometimes associated with this microorganism. However, it has been hypothesized that some pathogenic variants occur.

Differential Diagnosis

Most cases of acute diarrhea resolve within 1 to 2 weeks with observation or specific therapy. Diarrhea lasting 2 weeks or longer should suggest a number of possible diagnoses, including parasitic infection or a noninfectious process. Important considerations in persistent and chronic diarrhea are irritable bowel syndrome, inflammatory bowel disease, ischemic bowel disease, partial bowel obstruction, and pelvic abscess contiguous with the rectosigmoid colon. Lactase deficiency, small-bowel bacterial overgrowth, pernicious anemia, pellagra, malaria, Whipple's disease, diabetic autonomic neuropathy, small-bowel scleroderma, small-bowel diverticulosis, and various malabsorption syndromes are unusual causes of acute or persistent diarrhea that resemble more common infections.

MANAGEMENT

Two basic concepts are important in the management of diarrhea. First, most diarrheas are self-limited and can be managed with hydration and antimotility drugs. Second, despite the variety of microorganisms that can cause infectious diarrhea, specific antimicrobial therapy has proved beneficial with only a few.

Treatment

Fluid replacement

Diarrheal fluid is isotonic with and similar in electrolyte composition to serum. For most patients, rehydration can be accomplished with the use of oral supplements. Intravenous therapy is reserved for the most severely volume-depleted patients and those whose oral intake is limited by vomiting. In the developing world, reusable and poorly

Summary of Diagnosis

- Most cases of diarrhea do not mandate laboratory evaluation.
- Fecal screening tests (WBC smear, lactoferrin assay) help distinguish inflammatory from noninflammatory diarrhea.
- A stool culture is indicated only in selected cases of infectious diarrhea. The laboratory must be notified if cultures for uncommon bacterial pathogens are needed.
- The diagnostic test of choice for antibiotic-associated diarrhea is a stool assay for *C. difficile* toxin.
- O&P examination is appropriate for certain epidemiologic histories, but not for nosocomial diarrhea.

sterilized equipment and supplies are sometimes used for intravenous therapy, and there may be an associated risk of transmission of bloodborne pathogens. There are several commercially formulated oral rehydration solutions (ORS) available that provide 60 to 90 mEq/L of sodium, 20 mEq/L of potassium, 80 mEq/L chloride, 30 mEq/L of citrate or bicarbonate, and 20 g/L of glucose. Because of the risk of hypernatremia in treating young children, pediatric ORS are made with lower concentrations of sodium.

For patients with moderate diarrhea, a rough guide for rehydration is to supplement the ordinary daily fluid requirements with additional doses of ORS to equal the stool volume losses. For adults, this amount is approximately 2 to 3 L per day, with an additional 200 mL after each loose stool. Intravenous therapy should consist of normal saline with potassium supplements or lactated Ringer's solution. Sodium bicarbonate may be added for patients who are in shock or who are acidotic.

Nutritional support

To provide nutritional support during the diarrhea, the general rule is to match the food to the form of the stool being passed. For example, when the stools are unformed, clear soups, broths, juices, jellies, and yogurt are well tolerated along with crackers. Milk products, fatty foods, spices, and other irritant substances may aggravate the diarrhea and are best avoided until the patient has fully recovered.

Antidiarrheal medications

Various pharmaceutical agents are useful in the treatment of moderate to severe diarrhea. By decreasing the number and volume of stools, they provide symptomatic relief and may allow the patient to return to regular activities or travel sooner. There are three classes of such agents: adsorbents, antisecretory agents, and antimotility drugs.

Adsorbents (kaolin-pectin, kaolin) By adsorbing water, these compounds provide some form to the stool, thereby decreasing its frequency, and they may even have a role in adsorbing some bacterial enterotoxins in the gut. Although not particularly palatable, they have no systemic side effects. The recommended dose is 2 tablespoons (1.2 g) repeated after each loose stool, not to exceed 14 tablespoons (8.4 g) per day.

Antisecretory agents (bismuth subsalicylate) The salicylate component of bismuth subsalicylate (Pepto-Bismol) blocks to some degree the effect of enterotoxins on the intestinal mucosa and may reduce the number of stools in some cases by 50%. The bismuth component possesses modest antibacterial activity, which makes it a useful prophylactic agent for TD. The dose is 30 mL or 2 tablets as often as every 30 minutes, up to a maximum of 8 daily doses for up to 2 days. Adverse effects include a disconcerting dark-gray coloration of the tongue and stool and, occasionally, tinnitus due to mild salicylism. This agent should be used cautiously with aspirin or warfarin and is not recommended for pregnant women. Overuse can result in bismuth encephalopathy. It should not be taken within 2 hours of administration of quinolones or tetracyclines because it blocks their absorption from the gut.

Antimotility drugs (loperamide, diphenoxylate, opiates) These drugs act by slowing intestinal motility, which allows time for the absorption of fluid. Loperamide, the preferred antimotility drug, can reduce the number of stools and the duration of diarrhea by 80%, compared with placebo. It is given as 2 mg four times a day, or as 4 mg initially followed by 2 mg after each loose stool, not to exceed 8 tablets per day for up to 2 days.

Diphenoxylate with atropine (Lomotil) is cheaper than loperamide, but it has the disadvantage of potentially causing anticholinergic and central opiate toxicity, which are manifested by dry mouth, blurred vision, possibly urinary retention, and altered mental function. Lomotil is administered as 4 mg four times a day for up to 2 days.

True opiates, such as tincture of opium, paregoric, and codeine, are sometimes used in patients with re-fractory noninflammatory diarrheas, especially in HIV patients.

Antimotility agents are best avoided in patients with from inflammatory diarrhea, such as dysentery, pseudomembranous colitis, or diarrhea due to EHEC. It is believed, although not well substantiated, that these drugs may prolong or aggravate these conditions, and they have been implicated in cases of toxic megacolon and intestinal perforation.

Antimicrobial therapy

The use of antimicrobial agents in infectious diarrhea is a complex and unsettled issue. The physician's and layperson's general inclination is usually that, because it is an infection, the diarrhea should be treated with antibiotics. Whereas antimicrobial therapy can reduce the severity and duration of symptoms of some types of diarrhea (e.g., shigellosis, cholera), a satisfactory outcome can be accomplished in most common gastrointestinal infections with nonspecific symptomatic therapy. Mortality from diarrhea is usually a consequence of volume depletion or dehydration. Antimicrobial therapy has not been proven to affect survival and should not be a substitute for adequate fluid therapy. Another concern about widespread use of antimicrobials for diarrhea is the possibility of induction or selection of antibiotic resistance among bacteria. There has been an alarming increase in detection of fluoroquinolone-resistant *Campylobacter* species that is thought to have resulted from the use of fluoroquinolones in animal husbandry, especially in the poultry industry.

Older reports suggested that antibiotic therapy may prolong the carriage state of *Salmonella*, but this concern has been questioned since the advent of newer antibiotics. There is evidence that in children treated with antibiotics for EHEC the rate of occurrence of hemolytic uremic syndrome is higher than in those not treated.

Undoubtedly, however, antibiotics are indicated for treatment of enteric infections complicated by dysentery, systemic invasion, or dissemination, such as typhoid fever, other invasive *Salmonella* infections, campylobacteriosis, shigellosis, and amebiasis. Moderate-to-severe *C. difficile* colitis is generally treated with antimicrobials. Also, treatment of giardiasis is usually curative, and empiric antibiotic treatment of TD caused by ETEC usually shortens the duration of illness.

Empiric therapy

Empiric antibiotic therapy is considered in a few situations. It is appropriate for patients who have TD; have evidence of inflammatory diarrhea, such as fever, fecal leukocytes, or dysentery; are at high risk for poor outcome, such as elderly and immunocompromised persons; or have persistent watery diarrhea suggestive of giardiasis.

Currently, the antibiotics of choice for the first three indications are the fluoroquinolones, which given for 3 days: ciprofloxacin, 500 mg orally twice a day; levofloxacin, 500 mg orally once daily; ofloxacin, 300 mg orally twice a day; or norfloxacin, 400 mg orally twice a day. These antibiotics are superior to older agents such as erythromycin or trimethoprim-sulfamethoxazole (TMP-SMX). However, the possibility of fluoroquinolone resistance in *Campylobacter* and perhaps in other enteric pathogens must be kept in mind. Metronidazole, 250 mg four times a day for 7 to 10 days, is the recommended empiric treatment when giardiasis is suspected.

Therapy for specific infections

Tables 6.3 and 6.4 list preferred and alternative antibiotic treatments for, respectively, bacterial and parasitic diarrhea.

Shigella Treatment is recommended for all cases. Antimicrobial therapy given early in the course of disease shortens the duration of symptoms, eliminates the carrier state, and decreases the fecal excretion of the organisms, thereby reducing the risk of infection of further contacts of the patient. Most *Shigella* acquired in the United States remain susceptible to TMP-SMX, but shigellosis acquired during international travel currently should be treated with a fluoroquinolone. Studies suggest that azithromycin may also be effective treatment for shigellosis.

Salmonella Most healthy people do well without antibiotic therapy for uncomplicated *Salmonella* diarrhea. Treatment, however, is difficult to withhold and is strongly considered for patients at risk of disseminated infection, such as immunocompromised hosts, infants, the elderly, and persons with a prosthetic vascular graft, artificial heart valve, or aortic aneurysm. Treatment is clearly indicated for *Salmonella* bacteremia, including typhoid fever, and for any infection of extraintestinal organs. Fluoroquinolones are generally the preferred treatment but ceftriaxone, cefixime, or azithromycin may also be effective.

Campylobacter Patients with inflammatory diarrhea should be treated. Given the increasing problem of antibiotic resistance, most notably to macrolides and fluoroquinolones, it is necessary to perform susceptibility testing on *Campylobacter* isolates to guide therapy.

Escherichia coli Most of the diarrheagenic strains of *E. coli* are susceptible to both TMP-SMX and fluoroquinolones, and antibiotic treatment shortens the course

---

TABLE 6.3. Antimicrobial Treatment of Bacterial Diarrhea

Microorganism	Preferred treatment	Alternative treatment
Shigella spp.	TMP/SMX[a] for 3 days, if acquired in the United States	Fluoroquinolone[b] for 3 days, if acquired outside the United States
Salmonella spp.	Fluoroquinolone[b] for 5–7 days	TMP/SMX[a] for 5–7 days
Campylobacter jejuni	Erythromycin[c] for 7 days	Fluoroquinolone[b] for 5–7 days; Azithromycin[c]
Vibrio parahaemolyticus	Fluoroquinolone[b] for 3 days	TMP/SMX[a] or a tetracycline[c] for 3 days
Aeromonas hydrophila *Plesiomonas shigelloides*	Fluoroquinolone[b] for 3 days	TMP/SMX[a]; a tetracycline[c]; chloramphenicol[c]; or third-generation cephalosporin[c] for 3 days
Escherichia coli (except enterohemorrhagic *E. coli*)	TMP/SMX[a] for 3 days	Fluoroquinolone[b] for 3 days
Clostridium difficile	Metronidazole, 500 mg PO t.i.d. for 10 days	Vancomycin, 125 mg PO q.i.d. for 10 days

[a] TMP/SMX: trimethoprim-sulfamethoxazole 160/800 mg PO b.i.d.
[b] Fluoroquinolones: ciprofloxacin, 500 mg PO b.i.d.; levofloxacin, 500 mg q.d. ofloxacin, 300 mg PO b.i.d.; or norfloxacin, 400 mg PO b.i.d.
[c] Erythromycin, 500 mg PO q.i.d. or azithromycin, 250 mg PO q.d. for 5 days; tetracycline, 250–500 mg PO q.i.d. or doxycycline, 100 mg PO b.i.d; furazolidone, 100 mg PO q.i.d.; gentamicin, 5 mg/kg IV or IM q.d.; ceftriaxone, 250 mg IV or IM q.d.; chloramphenicol, 50 mg/kg/day in 4 divided doses PO.

TABLE 6.4.	Antimicrobial Treatment of Parasitic Diarrhea	
Microorganism	Preferred treatment	Alternative
Giardia lamblia	Metronidazole, 250 mg PO t.i.d. for 7 days	Furazolidone, 100 mg PO q.i.d. for 7–10 days
Entamoeba histolytica	Metronidazole, 750 mg PO t.i.d. for 5–10 days followed by either iodoquinol, 650 mg PO t.i.d. for 3 weeks or paromomycin, 500 mg PO t.i.d. for 7 days	Tetracycline, 500 mg PO q.i.d. for 14 days plus dehydroemetine,[a] 0.5–0.75 mg/kg IM b.i.d. for 5 days
Cyclospora cayetanensis	TMP/SMX, 160/800 mg PO b.i.d. for 7 days	

TMP/SMX, trimethoprim-sulfamethoxazole.
[a] Available on special request from Centers for Disease Control and Prevention, (404) 639-3670.

of TD caused by ETEC. EPEC strains are sometimes antibiotic-resistant, so culture and susceptibility testing are indicated when this agent is suspected.

At present, antibiotic treatment for EHEC (e.g., *E. coli* O157:H7) is not recommended because of an observed association between antibiotic treatment and a higher risk of hemolytic uremic syndrome in children.

Clostridium difficile Antibiotic treatment is recommended for those patients whose diarrhea either is severe or does not resolve promptly after the causative antibiotic is discontinued. Although oral vancomycin may be the slightly more effective antibiotic treatment, there are concerns that the indiscriminate use of vancomycin may result in selection of other bacteria that are resistant to vancomycin (e.g., vancomycin-resistant enterococci, glycopeptide-resistant *S. aureus*). Therefore, the current recommendation is that *C. difficile* diarrhea should be treated with metronidazole orally, reserving vancomycin for management of cases in which this treatment fails.

Blastocystis When large numbers of *B. hominis* are found in the stool of patients with severe diarrhea and no other apparent pathogen is found, an attempt to eradicate it with metronidazole may be indicated.

Travelers' diarrhea The foundation of management of TD is oral rehydration, supplemented by use of adsorbents, antisecretory drugs, antimotility drugs, and antibiotics.

The most efficacious drug regimen to date is a combination of an antimicrobial agent and loperamide. A single, large dose of TMP-SMX (2 double-strength tablets) or a fluoroquinolone (e.g., ciprofloxacin 750 mg, levofloxacin 500 mg) may be effective. However, single-dose therapy with fluoroquinolones has been associated with a 40% failure rate in shigellosis and campylobacteriosis, and TMP-SMX has no activity against *Campylobacter* species. A 3-day course of an antibiotic is conventional and more predictably effective than single-dose therapy.

Fluoroquinolones are presently the empiric antibiotics of first choice, because bacterial resistance rates remain relatively low, but a rising incidence of fluoroquinolone-resistant enteric bacterial pathogens in TD can be expected.

Furazolidone is probably not as effective as TMP-SMX or fluoroquinolones, but it is a reasonable therapeutic option for children who travel to an area where TMP-resistant bacteria are common. Aztreonam is poorly absorbed after oral administration and is effective against bacterial enteropathogens, including *Campylobacter*. Aztreonam resistance among enteropathogens has not been a problem, and it may an attractive alternative treatment in the future, but it is not currently available in an oral dosage form.

Prevention of Travelers' Diarrhea
Food-related techniques
Travelers should carefully select, handle, and prepare food and dairy products. Fresh fruits and vegetables are often contaminated with enteric pathogens and should be washed thoroughly and freshly peeled or freshly cooked. Ready-to-eat foods available from street vendors, who lack adequate sanitary facilities, personal hygiene, and refrigeration for perishable food, should be avoided. Expe-

rience in countries where cholera is endemic, particularly in South America bordering the Pacific Ocean, has shown that seafood and undercooked fish (ceviche) are the most risky food products.

Dairy products, especially fresh cheese, cream, milk, and butter, are best avoided, because they can be the vehicle for several enteric pathogens and pasteurization processes are either nonexistent or inconsistent in developing countries.

Safe water

Travelers to destinations where there is a high risk for TD must secure a safe water supply, both for drinking and for brushing teeth. Commercially bottled water and carbonated beverages are generally safe, as is beer. Ice cubes should be regarded as frozen packages of enteric pathogens and avoided. The addition of alcoholic beverages to tap water or ice reduces but does not eliminate the risk of contaminated drinking water.

Water may be made safer by treatment with heat, filtration, or chemicals. Boiling water for 1 minute is most effective, so freshly prepared tea, coffee, and hot soups are safe. Commercially available particle-size purifiers remove bacteria and parasites but not viruses, and they may be cumbersome for travel. Many commercial chemical preparations containing iodine or chlorine are available to make water potable. Iodine treatment kills all three classes of pathogens but is not recommended for pregnant women or for patients with thyroid disease. Chlorine eliminates most microbial agents except for *Giardia* cysts, but its potency is compromised by suspended particulates or cold temperature.

Prophylaxis for travelers' diarrhea

Bismuth subsalicylate, administered as two tablets four times a day, provides 62% to 65% protection against TD. Various antibiotics can be an effective for TD prophylaxis, but are not recommended for most travelers for several reasons. First, only a minority of short-term travelers who do not take prophylaxis acquire TD. Furthermore, prophylactic antibiotic use increases the likelihood of adverse drug reactions or interactions and may select for or induce antibiotic resistance among enteric bacteria. Finally, prompt presumptive short-term antibiotic therapy has been proven to be rapidly effective in treating those travelers who do get diarrhea. Despite these reservations, prophylactic antibiotic therapy may be considered as a rational option for short-term travelers under some circumstances (a) important trip, when even a brief illness cannot be tolerated; (b) increased host susceptibility to diarrhea because of achlorhydria or prior gas-

trectomy; (c) immunosuppression, which may predispose to severe disease or systemic dissemination of enteric pathogens; or (d) chronic renal failure, congestive heart failure, severe angina, insulin-dependent diabetes mellitus, or inflammatory bowel disease, with which the complications of diarrhea might be catastrophic.

The decision regarding antibiotic prophylaxis should be made jointly by the physician and the traveler, who must be educated about the risks and benefits. Prophylaxis is not recommended for pregnant women or for children younger than 2 years old.

Doxycycline is an effective prophylactic agent (85% protective) when administered at a dose of 100 mg daily but not when taken only twice weekly. Photosensitivity, *Candida* overgrowth, and gastrointestinal symptoms have been reported in fewer than 1% of adults treated prophylactically with doxycycline.

TMP-SMX, administered as one double-strength tablet once daily, is 95% effective for the prevention of TD for trips up to 2 weeks long. Skin rash occurs in 1% to 5%. More serious adverse effects, including Stevens-Johnson syndrome and antibiotic-associated colitis, are rare. TMP-SMX is inactive against *Campylobacter*, viruses, and many parasites.

In recent years, when prophylactic antibiotic therapy is considered, the choice has usually been a fluoroquinolone. Common choices include ciprofloxacin 500 mg, ofloxacin 300 mg, levofloxacin 500 mg, or norfloxacin 400 mg, taken once daily. Again, there are risks of photosensitivity and selective colonization by resistant bacteria.

REFERRAL

Primary care practitioners should be comfortable managing most cases of acute diarrhea. Exceptions are cases in which there are signs of severe illness that may be life-threatening or when the patient is compromised by age, frailty, or underlying disease. In general, patients with dysenteric or hemorrhagic diarrhea, especially if it is accompanied by severe volume depletion or signs of systemic sepsis, should be referred to a specialist in infectious diseases or gastroenterology. If there is a suspicion based on the history that an unusual enteric pathogen may be causing the illness, consultation with specialists helps with timely and appropriate selection of diagnostic tests and therapeutic interventions.

KEY POINTS

- First, determine whether the patient has severe illness (Table 6.1).

- Nausea and vomiting are common in toxigenic bacterial food poisoning and viral gastroenteritis.

- Diarrhea lasting longer than 2 weeks should raise suspicion of a parasitic infection or a noninfectious cause of the illness.

- The most common single infectious cause of nosocomial diarrhea is C. difficile.

- Volume repletion is the cornerstone of treatment of acute diarrhea of any cause.

- Nonspecific treatments, especially antimotility drugs, may be helpful in most acute diarrhea syndromes but should be avoided with dysentery or C. difficile–associated diarrhea.

- Antibiotic therapy is indicated in selected cases of infectious diarrhea, including TD.

COMMONLY ASKED QUESTIONS

I am planning a trip to Europe. Am I likely to get diarrhea while there?

No. The risk of acquiring diarrhea in Europe is low; less than 10%. The risk is much higher when traveling to a developing country, especially one in a tropical area.

If I am planning a trip to a tropical, developing country, wouldn't it be better for me to take antibiotics ahead of time to prevent diarrhea rather than waiting until I actually get sick?

Probably not, because most people on brief trips do not get sick. Even if diarrhea does occur, it can usually be treated rapidly and cleared up in a day or so. If the trip is very important, where even a brief illness cannot be tolerated, or if you have a weakened immune system, chronic renal failure, severe angina, or some other serious illness, then your doctor may prescribe prophylactic antibiotics.

When travelling abroad, what warning signs might indicate that I have a serious case of diarrhea and need to seek medical attention?

Diarrhea occurring more than six times per day and lasting more than two days may indicate a more serious problem. Also, fever, blood or pus in the stool, lightheadedness, fainting, severe abdominal cramps, rapid heart rate, or minimal urine output would warrant medical evaluation.

SUGGESTED READINGS

DuPont HL. Review article: infectious diarrhea. *Aliment Pharmacol Ther* 1994;8:3–13.

DuPont HL. Guidelines on acute infectious diarrhea in adults. The Parameters Committee of the American College of Gastroenterology. *Am J Gastroenterol* 1997;92:1962–1975.

Bishai WR, Sears CL. Food poisoning syndromes. *Gastroenterol Clin North Am* 1993;22:570–608.

Gregg CR, Nassar NN. Infectious enteritis. *Curr Treatment Options Gastroenterol* 1999;2:119–126.

Nassar NN, Keiser P, Gregg CR. Keeping travelers healthy. *Am J Med Sci* 1998;315:327–336.

CHAPTER 7

Inflammatory Bowel Disease

David Balis

University of Texas Southwestern Medical Center, Dallas, Texas 75235

DEFINITION

The term *inflammatory bowel disease (IBD)* refers to two chronic inflammatory disorders of the gastrointestinal tract of unknown cause, Crohn's disease (CD) and ulcerative colitis (UC).

UC is characterized by a diffuse, continuous, and superficial inflammation limited to the colon. It involves the rectum and extends proximally in a constant pattern. The hallmark is bloody diarrhea, often with rectal urgency and tenesmus. The clinical course is marked by exacerbations and remissions; removal of the colon is curative.

CD is characterized by a focal, asymmetric, and transmural inflammation that may involve any part of the gastrointestinal tract from mouth to anus. It typically affects the ileum, colon, and perianal region. Clinically, it is manifested by abdominal pain and diarrhea and is often complicated by fistulas or obstruction. Its focal, segmental, transmural, and proximal distribution separates it from UC. CD is neither medically nor surgically curable; there is a tendency for lifelong recurrence, and chronic treatment is required to control symptoms, quality of life, and complications.

UC and CD can occur in any age group but are most common in teenagers and young adults. Whereas the incidence of UC has remained constant, the incidence of CD has clearly been rising; both occur in 5 of every

100,000 persons. Inflammatory bowel disease affects both sexes equally but is more common in Caucasians than in African-Americans, Hispanics, or Asians. For Ashkenazi Jews (from northern Europe), there is a three- to six-fold increased prevalence of IBD (Table 7.1)

CAUSE

Although the exact etiologic cause is unknown, certain features suggest that genetic, infectious, dietary, immunologic, psychosocial, and environmental factors may all interact to cause a defect in the regulation of immune events and to allow persistent amplification of the inflammatory process.

Genetic Predisposition

The strong family clustering as well as the increased incidence in Caucasians and Jews suggests a genetic predisposition. Ten to forty percent of persons with IBD have a relative with IBD. The risk to a child from a parent with IBD is less than 5%; however, if both parents are affected, the risk is 50%. In CD there is a stronger genetic tie, with a 50% concordance between monozygotic twins; siblings of patients with CD are 17 to 35 times more likely to develop CD. Although family studies clearly show a genetic influence, the partial concordance and penetrance suggest that environmental factors play a role in clinical expression.

Infection

The disease's chronic inflammatory nature has prompted a continuing search for an infectious cause. Mycobacteria, measles virus, and *Escherichia coli* have attracted attention, but no specific agent has been isolated.

Regulation of Immune Responses

The response to immunosuppressive agents and the possible representation of the numerous extraintestinal manifestations as autoimmune phenomena suggest that an immune mechanism is involved, with abnormalities in both humoral and cell-mediated immunity. Whereas the normal gut is able to suppress the immune response to the

TABLE 7.1.   Epidemiology of Inflammatory Bowel Disease

15–30 years old
Caucasians
European Jews
Familial aggregation

constant presence of microbial and dietary antigens, the gut in IBD seems unable to shut off the activation of the immune system, resulting in an uncontrolled inflammatory response. This lack of regulation from defective immunosuppression could disrupt homeostasis. However, it is difficult to know whether the enhanced immune response is appropriate to an increased stimulus or indicates an underlying defect in immunoregulation.

Environmental Factors

It is not uncommon for the disease to flare with stress, and it has been suggested that patients with IBD have a characteristic personality that renders them susceptible to stress. Although there is little evidence relating psychological factors to the etiology, there is no doubt that such a chronic disease affecting young persons can cause anger, anxiety, and depression, which are important in modifying the course of the illness.

The constant exposure of the gut to products of ingestion has made food allergy a popular hypothesis. Penetration into the intestinal milieu through increased gut permeability could initiate an unregulated inflammatory response; however, there is no evidence that diet plays an etiologic role.

Environmentally, smoking appears to protect against UC, but it is associated with CD. More than 80% of UC patients are nonsmokers, and UC may begin when a predisposed patient stops smoking; on the other hand, 80% of those with CD are smokers. However, smoking's exact role has yet to be elucidated.

In summary, genetic influences and environmental factors appear to contribute to a defect in the downregulation of immune events, allowing persistent amplification of inflammation and tissue damage.

Initiating Events

Potential initiating events include increased intestinal permeability, aberrant antigen processing, altered immune recognition, and molecular mimicry between antigen and intestine. Once initiated, the amplified immune system leads to the pathophysiologic events of IBD. Cytokines and inflammatory mediators are released, and humoral and cellular immunity is activated, as are complement and kinins. The arachidonic acid cascade is shifted toward the proinflammatory lipoxygenase pathway. Neutrophils accumulate, cause further damage, and amplify the inflammatory response by recruiting additional inflammatory cells. The inflammatory mediators—prostaglandins, leukotrienes, histamine, and vasoactive intestinal peptides—alter epithelial function and contribute to the intestinal secretory process and diarrhea.

PATIENT PRESENTATION

Patients with mild disease have fewer than four stools per day, are ambulatory, tolerate oral feeding, and are without evidence of toxicity, tenderness, or inflammation. Moderate disease is characterized by four to six stools per day with minimal signs of toxicity. Patients with severe disease have more than six bowel movements per day, with fever, weight loss, abdominal pain without peritonitis or obstruction, and anemia. Patients with fulminant disease have more than ten stools per day, evidence of toxicity, obstruction, and rebound tenderness or abscess, and they require transfusion for anemia.

Ulcerative Colitis

The major symptoms of UC are diarrhea with blood and mucus, but the symptoms depend on the extent and severity of inflammation. Patients with proctitis have rectal bleeding with fresh blood, tenesmus, and passage of mucus. They may even be constipated as a result of rectal irritability and decreased compliance. However, the passage of clots is unusual. The more active the disease and the greater the extent beyond the rectum, the more likely it is for the patient to have diarrhea with blood and pus, particularly nocturnal or postprandial diarrhea. Active UC with diarrhea almost always has macroscopic blood as a symptom; the diagnosis should be questioned if this symptom is absent. Although abdominal discomfort and cramping occur, abdominal pain and tenderness are not typical, given the superficial nature of UC. As the severity of inflammation increases, systemic symptoms occur, such as fever, malaise, nausea, vomiting, sweats, arthralgias, weight loss, volume depletion, and tachycardia.

Physical findings vary from mild colon discomfort with palpation and normal vital signs and appearance to evidence of volume depletion, tachycardia, fever, anemia, and a distended, tender abdomen due to fulminant colitis or toxic megacolon.

The clinical course in UC is variable but depends on the extent of involvement and the intensity of inflammation. Although most patients have a relapse within 1 year after the first attack, there may be long periods of remission. Patients with limited involvement of the rectum may have mild disease with bleeding and tenesmus, with minimal systemic or extraintestinal manifestations, and usually do not develop more extensive disease. Eighty-five percent of patients with UC have mild-to-moderate intermittent disease that can be managed without hospitalization. The remainder have more extensive, fulminant disease with severe bloody diarrhea and systemic symptoms and are at higher risk for complications.

Crohn's Disease

The major clinical features of CD include abdominal pain, diarrhea without blood, fatigue, perianal fistulas, and obstruction from strictures, but again these are determined by the site and extent of inflammation.

Although the symptoms of chronic abdominal pain and diarrhea suggest CD, other symptoms may dominate the initial clinical presentation. Patients who are young or aged may present with chronic fevers and weight loss more suggestive of infection or malignancy. Others may initially present with complications such as obstruction, abscess, fistula, or malabsorption.

Patients may appear chronically ill with fatigue, pallor, and systemic symptoms. Weight loss of 10% to 20% of body weight occurs from anorexia, diarrhea, and malabsorption. Fever is usually low grade; high spiking fevers usually signify a complication. A perianal examination may reveal fistulas.

Crohn's disease involving the terminal ileum

Because the terminal ileum is the most commonly involved site, patients often have a history of chronic recurrent right lower quadrant pain, diarrhea, fatigue, and weight loss. The initial presentation may mimic acute appendicitis, but a laparotomy reveals ileitis and a normal appendix. The pain is colicky, associated with passage of material through narrowed, inflamed segments, and is relieved by defecation. The diarrhea is usually moderate, usually without gross blood. Patients may have a right lower quadrant fullness or mass from adherent loops of bowel or abscess. The transmural inflammation leads to edema, fibrosis, and narrowing of the small bowel, causing intestinal obstruction in 20% to 30%, and may manifest with nausea, vomiting, abdominal pain and distention, and reduced stool output.

Colonic Crohn's disease

In patients with colonic CD, abdominal pain and diarrhea are the most frequent symptoms. Rectal bleeding is much less common than in UC, because the rectum is spared and because the disease has a transmural nature with irregular mucosal involvement.

Other presentations of Crohn's disease

Perianal fissures, fistulas, and abscess formation are frequent complications occurring in one third of patients. These signs may be the first indication of CD. The transmural inflammation can burrow through the serosa, resulting in an intraabdominal or psoas abscess with pain, fever, and a tender abdominal mass or psoas sign (pain with hip extension). The fistulas may occur between loops of intestine (enteroenteric fistulas); they may be asymptomatic, or they may cause malabsorption and bacterial overgrowth if from colon to proximal intestine. Fistulas from the bowel may penetrate adjacent organs, most commonly the bladder or, rarely, the vagina or ureter. Enterovesicular fistulas present with recurrent urinary tract infections, pneumaturia, or fecaluria. Enterovaginal fistulas present with a foul-smelling, painful vaginal discharge. Fistulas may penetrate to the skin (enterocutaneous fistula), releasing pus or mucus intermittently. These enterocutaneous fistulas also appear after surgery or drainage of an abscess. They seldom heal spontaneously and often indicate persistent underlying bowel inflammation.

Because CD can involve any portion of the gastrointestinal tract, patients may have oral aphthous ulcers. Gastroduodenal CD mimics peptic ulcer disease with nausea, vomiting, and epigastric pain.

DIAGNOSIS

A high index of suspicion for IBD is required in patients with diarrhea, particularly with bloody diarrhea, abdominal pain, abdominal mass, abscess, rectal bleeding, tenesmus, pus, perianal disease, systemic symptoms, or evidence of inflammation. Atypical presentations include fever of unknown origin and extraintestinal manifestations such as arthritis or liver disease before bowel involvement. CD should also be considered in cases of malabsorption, obstruction, or fistula. If IBD is suspected, the diagnosis is made by the characteristic history, stool examination, endoscopy with biopsy, and radiologic studies while ruling out other causes.

Laboratory Tests

Stool studies are important in excluding an infectious cause and establishing the presence of intestinal inflammation. A cardinal feature is the exudation of inflammatory cells, manifested by fecal leukocytes or red blood cells on stool examination.

Ulcerative colitis
Laboratory results reflect the severity of disease. Patients may have anemia (from iron deficiency, chronic disease, or drug use), leukocytosis, increased sedimentation rate, hypokalemia, or hypoalbuminemia from protein loss. Elevated alkaline phosphatase and gamma-glutamyl transferase (GGT) may indicate biliary involvement.

Crohn's disease
Laboratory features in CD result from blood loss, malabsorption, and the inflammatory process. Patients are usually anemic from deficiency of iron (blood loss or malabsorption), vitamin B_{12} (extensive terminal ileal disease), or folate (anorexia, inhibition by sulfasalazine). Malnutrition, malabsorption, and diarrhea also cause reduced albumin as well as protein and electrolyte abnormalities. Hypocalcemia may reflect calcium malabsorption or vitamin D deficiency and can cause tetany. Malabsorption of fat-soluble vitamins (A, D, E, and K) may cause symptoms of night blindness or prolonged prothrombin time.

Endoscopic Tests

Endoscopy with biopsy is the most important method of establishing the diagnosis.

Ulcerative colitis
Endoscopy reveals inflammation of the mucosa with loss of mucosal vascularity, diffuse erythema, friability, ulcers, and exudate with mucus, blood, and pus. These changes involve the distal rectum (95% of cases) and proceed proximally in a continuous pattern without intervening normal mucosa. The biopsy shows a mucosal inflammatory response with polymorphonuclear leukocytes accumulating near the epithelium, invading the crypts, and forming crypt abscesses which coalescence to form shallow ulcerations. In 40% to 50% of UC patients, the disease is limited to the rectum or rectosigmoid colon; in 30% to 40% the disease is beyond the sigmoid flexure; and 20% have total colitis.

Crohn's disease
Endoscopy reveals focal inflammation with "cobblestone" mucosa from submucosal inflammation. Endoscopic biopsy shows inflammation, but it is limited by its superficial depth and inability to sample the characteristic transmural inflammation, lymphoid hyperplasia, deep fissuring ulcers, and sinus tracts. However, 25% of serial biopsies show the characteristic noncaseating granulomas. Because skip areas, rectal sparing, and small-bowel disease are characteristic of CD, colonoscopy is superior to flexible sigmoidoscopy. Endoscopy is also useful for biopsy of strictures or masses, to evaluate upper gastroduodenal involvement, to dilate strictures, and to perform cancer surveillance.

Radiologic Studies

A radiograph of the abdomen should be obtained if obstruction, toxic megacolon, or perforation is suspected. It may show intestinal edema, dilatation, air-fluid levels, or free air as well as associated nephrolithiasis, cholelithiasis, or arthritis.

In UC, an air-contrast barium enema reveals superficial ulcers, continuous granularity, and absent haustra. In chronic UC, a shortened, narrowed, tubular, "lead pipe" colon is seen. A barium enema is also helpful in showing the proximal extent of involvement in UC (Fig. 7.1).

In CD, barium-contrast studies can confirm the diagnosis, the extent of disease, and the presence of complications. Focal asymmetric penetrating ulcers, cobblestoning, thumbprinting, fistulas, strictures, rectal sparing, skip areas, and terminal ileum and stomach involvement help differentiate CD from UC. Small-bowel barium examination is helpful in CD because it is difficult to gain access to this area with endoscopy. A characteristic finding in terminal ileum CD is the string sign, a thin column of barium caused by luminal narrowing (Fig. 7.2).

Acutely ill patients should be stabilized before endoscopy or barium-contrast studies are performed, because the preparation or procedure may worsen the disease and precipitate toxic dilatation. Oral barium should be avoided in cases of suspected obstruction.

Computed tomography is useful if complications such as abscess are suspected.

Differential Diagnosis

The focus of the differential diagnosis is determined by the presenting features. With rectal bleeding, a colonoscopy or barium enema should be performed to exclude colonic neoplasms, diverticula, arteriovenous malformations, and hemorrhoids. Radiation enteritis should be considered in patients who have undergone pelvic irradiation.

Acute infectious colitis, such as amebiasis, tuberculosis, or infection with *Shigella, Salmonella, Yersinia, Campylobacter, Clostridium difficile,* or *E. coli* 0157:H7, when accompanied by abdominal pain and bloody diarrhea with fecal leukocytes, can be difficult to distinguish at initial presentation and should be excluded with stool cultures. Infection should also be excluded in an exacerbation of known IBD. Although most bacterial pathogens produce acute symptoms, amebiasis causes chronic diarrhea,

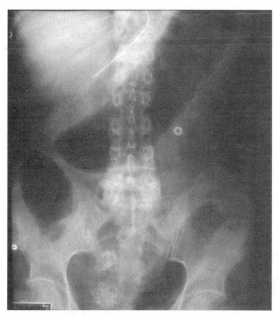

FIGURE 7.1.
Air-contrast barium enema reveals diffuse involvement of the colon with ulcerative colitis manifested by stippled ulcerations as well as loss of haustrations giving the appearance of a "lead pipe." (Radiograph courtesy of William Kilman, M.D., and Amy Balis, M.D., Parkland Hospital, Dallas, Texas.)

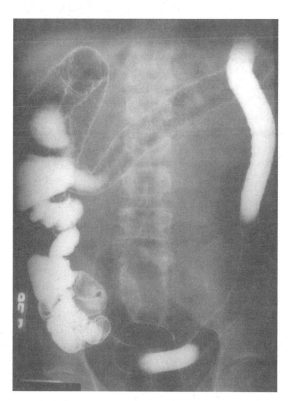

FIGURE 7.2.
Air-contrast barium enema reveals the classic "cobblestone" appearance of the abnormal mucosa of the transverse colon and splenic flexure in a patient with Crohn's disease. Note the normal mucosa proximal and distal to the involved segment. (Radiograph courtesy of William Kilman, M.D., and Amy Balis, M.D., Parkland Hospital, Dallas, Texas.)

rectal bleeding, and cecal ulcers and should be excluded by stool examination, biopsy, and serum antibody for *Entamoeba histolytica* in patients with a history of travel or homosexual exposure. *Yersinia* and tuberculosis particularly infect the terminal ileum, as does CD. Actinomycosis with fistulas can simulate CD. Syphilis, gonorrhea, lymphogranuloma venereum, herpes simplex, and cytomegalovirus all cause proctitis, similar to UC, and should be considered, especially in homosexual men. In immunocompromised hosts such as patients with the acquired immunodeficiency syndrome (AIDS), opportunistic infections must be sought, including *Mycobacterium avium* complex, cytomegalovirus, tuberculosis, and fungal diseases.

In young patients with acute abdominal pain, CD is often diagnosed at laparotomy for presumed appendicitis. In young women, gynecologic diseases should be considered (e.g., endometriosis, pelvic inflammatory disease, ectopic pregnancy, tuboovarian abnormalities). In older patients with abdominal pain, diverticulitis and ischemic colitis should be considered.

Other diseases to consider include ulcers induced by ingestion of nonsteroidal antiinflammatory drugs (NSAIDs), given the high prevalence of use of NSAIDs. Microscopic or collagenous colitis should be considered in an older patient with chronic watery diarrhea. In patients with small-bowel disease, other diseases to consider include sprue, lymphoma, amyloidosis, and eosinophilic gastroenteritis. Systemic vasculitis may also effect the small bowel, including polyarteritis nodosa, systemic lupus erythematosus, rheumatoid arthritis, progressive systemic sclerosis, and cryoglobulinemia, although the underlying disease is usually apparent. Behçet's syndrome can mimic CD with colitis, aphthous ulcers, uveitis, urethritis, arthritis, erythema nodosum, and thrombophlebitis, but oral and genital ulcers usually dominate the picture.

Early in the course, IBD may be difficult to distinguish from irritable bowel disease, but the constitutional symptoms, laboratory abnormalities, presence of fecal blood or leukocytes should alert the clinician to possible IBD.

Once the diagnosis is made, it is usually possible to distinguish between UC and CD, as seen in Table 7.2.

MANAGEMENT

The treatment of UC or CD depends on the extent and severity of intestinal involvement. Initial treatment is medical and is similar for both diseases, with surgery reserved for complications and intractable disease. However, a major difference is that UC can be cured with complete surgical removal, whereas CD is not cured by surgery and tends to recur.

Summary of Diagnosis

- IBD is most common in young adults with chronic, inflammatory diarrhea.
- Stool studies, endoscopy, pathology, and barium studies are obtained for patients with suspected IBD.
- Infection, cancer, ischemia, appendicitis, and vasculitis must be excluded.
- Extent and severity of the disease should be assessed.
- Complications need to be excluded.

Medical Therapy

The aims of therapy are to control symptoms and inflammation, replace nutritional losses, and induce remission. Mild flares can be treated on an outpatient basis, although it must be recognized that the disease may worsen and require hospitalization. Correction of fluid and electrolyte disturbances, as well as transfusions when required, provide improvement. Agents to control diarrhea (diphenoxylate, loperamide, codeine, or anticholinergics) can be helpful in mild-to-moderate cases but should be used with extreme caution in severe cases for fear of precipitating toxic megacolon. Decisions on nutritional therapy are determined by the patient's nutritional status and expected time course. Severely ill patients should receive nothing by mouth to prevent stimulation of intestinal activity, with consideration for parenteral nutrition. Less ill patients can take a light diet or elemental oral feedings for supplemental nutrition with low fecal volume. Iron replacement is necessary with significant blood loss, and folic acid should be supplemented when sulfasalazine is used.

Aminosalicylates

Salicylates act as antiinflammatory agents and are the principal drugs used to treat IBD. Oral salicylates are effective in treating mild to moderate UC and CD and in maintaining remission in both diseases. Oral and rectal formulations can be used together.

Sulfasalazine   Sulfasalazine consists of a salicylate (5-aminosalicylic acid [5-ASA]) linked to a sulfa moiety (sulphapyridine) by an azo bond. This bond is split by colonic bacteria, allowing delivery of 5-ASA in the colon. The liberated 5-ASA remains in the colon and is responsible for the therapeutic effects; the sulphapyridine

| TABLE 7.2. | Differentiating Features of Inflammatory Bowel Disease | |

Feature	Ulcerative colitis	Crohn's disease
Clinical		
Rectal bleeding	++	+
Abdominal pain	+	++
Abdominal mass	–	++
Fissures/fistulas	–	+++
Small bowel disease	+/–	+++
Rectal involvement	+++ (95%)	+ (50%)
Response to antibiotics	–	+
Response to bowel rest	–	+
Recurrence after surgery	–	++
Smoker	–	++
Malignancy	+++	+
Cure with surgery	++	–
Acute symptoms	++	+
Pathologic		
Segmental	–	++
Transmural	–	++
Granulomas	–	+
Aphthous, linear ulcers	–	++
Fibrosis	+	++

+, present; –, absent.

is absorbed from the colon, excreted in the urine, and is solely responsible for the side effects of sulfasalazine. Sulfasalazine is effective, dose-dependent, and inexpensive as a first-line therapy for mild-to-moderate disease and for maintenance of remission.

However, up to one third of the patients develop side effects from sulfasalazine, most commonly headache and gastrointestinal intolerance, which can be minimized by gradual titration and administration with food. Hemolytic anemia, bone marrow suppression, allergic reactions, pancreatitis, pneumonitis, hepatitis, and colitis are rare. Eighty percent of men develop sperm count and function abnormalities, which are reversible. Sulfasalazine also inhibits absorption of folate, and for this reason 1 mg of folate daily is recommended. Sulfazalazine is safe during pregnancy and breast-feeding.

Other 5-ASA preparations Given the side effects and isolated colonic delivery of sulfasalazine, 5-ASA preparations (mesalamine) have been developed. 5-ASA functions topically within the mucosa, necessitating delivery to inflamed sites, but it is absorbed from the proximal gastrointestinal tract (although not from the colon). Therefore, various formulations have been developed to protect 5-ASA from proximal absorption and deliver it distally to sites of inflammation.

Asacol provides delayed release because the preparation is coated with a polymer that dissolves at a pH higher than 7, allowing delivery of 5-ASA to the terminal ileum and colon. Asacol does have a small amount of lactose, so it could potentially worsen diarrhea if the patient is intolerant. Pentasa provides sustained release by encapsulating 5-ASA in microgranules, releasing the drug equally in the small and the large intestine. Olsalazine (Dipentum) consists of two 5-ASA molecules linked together by an azo bond; 5-ASA is released in the colon by colonic bacteria. However, this drug also stimulates small-bowel secretions and can cause diarrhea in 15% to 20% of patients, requiring termination in 6%. 5-ASA is also useful topically as an enema in left-sided colitis or as a suppository in proctitis to treat active disease and maintain remission.

Although mesalamine has fewer side effects than sulfasalazine, they have equal efficacy. Because sulfasalazine (less than $1 per day) is much cheaper than mesalamine (Asacol, $3 per day), it should be used first for colitis, with gradual titration to minimize side effects. Sulfasalazine is started at 500 mg by mouth twice a day and is increased by 1 g every 1 to 2 days until a therapeutic response is seen, usually 4 g per day for active disease and 2 g per day for maintenance. Maintenance therapy should be continued indefinitely at the lowest dose that prevents relapse, with any withdrawal of therapy at a gradual pace. If any symptoms recur, therapeutic doses must be resumed (Table 7.3).

Patients intolerant to sulfasalazine should be switched to a sulfa-free 5-ASA preparation, which is tolerated by 80%. In CD, patients with terminal ileum involvement should use Asacol or Pentasa, and patients with diffuse small-bowel disease should use Pentasa, given their delivery sites.

Corticosteroids

Corticosteroids are the mainstay of therapy for short-term treatment of moderate-to-severe disease to induce remission. However, they should not be used as maintenance therapy because of their inability to prevent relapse and their side effects. In patients who have systemic manifestations or complications or for whom salicylates have failed, oral prednisone, 40 to 60 mg per day, is given initially, with gradual tapering according to the clinical course over 2 to 3 months. Usually, the prednisone is tapered by 5 to 10 mg per week, down to 20 mg per day, then tapered more slowly at 2.5 to 5 mg per week. Parenteral steroids are indicated in more severe cases. If improvement is not observed by 7 to

TABLE 7.3.   Aminosalicylates

Drug	Site of delivery	Active dose	Maintenance dose
Azo-bond			
Sulfasalazine (Azulfadine)	Colon	4–6 g/day	2–4 g/day
Olsalazine (Dipentum)	Colon	1.5–3 g/day	1.5–3 g/day
Delayed-release			
Asacol	Terminal ileum and colon	2.4–4.8 g/day	0.8–4.8 g/day
Sustained-release			
Pentasa	Small intestine and colon	2–4 g/day	1–3 g/day
Topical			
Mesalamine enema	Left colon	1–4 g qhs	1 g qhs
Mesalamine suppository	Rectum	500 mg b.i.d.	500 mg qhs

10 days, more aggressive therapy (surgery or immuno-modulator therapy) should be instituted. The inability to taper or withdraw steroids is an indication for immunosuppressive therapy. Once an acutely ill patient is tolerating oral feeding, a salicylate should be started and administered chronically.

In UC, hydrocortisone enemas (100 mg at bedtime) are useful for distal colitis, and suppositories are given for proctitis. Topical steroids are useful for active disease but not for maintenance, because they are absorbed, which leads to side effects.

Efforts are being made to develop formulations to maximize mucosal effect and minimize absorption. Budesonide is available as an enema and in a controlled-release oral formula that may provide efficacy without the toxicity of other steroid preparations.

Immunomodulators

Azathioprine and 6-mercaptopurine   Azathioprine and 6-mercaptopurine (6-MP) are effective in the long-term management of UC and CD. Azathioprine is converted to 6-MP, which acts as a purine analogue to inhibit DNA synthesis and cell proliferation. These medications possess an antiinflammatory effect and inhibit proliferation of T cells. They are used in patients with UC or CD who are dependent on steroids or whose disease is refractory to standard therapy to induce and maintain remission. The medications allow discontinuation or reduction of steroid therapy; they are also beneficial in healing fistulas and perianal disease in CD. However, they are slow-acting and require 3 to 6 months for maximal effect. The usual starting dose is 50 to 75 mg per day of 6-MP, titrated to 1 to 2 mg per kg per day. Blood counts must be monitored every 1 to 3 months indefinitely, because neutropenia and bone marrow suppression can occur at any time. Bone marrow suppression is usually reversed with a reduction in dose.

Pancreatitis occurs in 3% to 15% of patients after several weeks of therapy. Once pancreatitis has occurred, azathioprine or 6-MP should never be restarted. Although these medications may increase the risk of carcinoma in transplantation patients, long-term monitoring in IBD has not revealed an increase in malignancies.

Cyclosporine   The slow onset of action of 6-MP has led to trials of more potent immunosuppressives. Cyclosporine blocks the immune response by inhibiting T-cell production of interleukin-2. Intravenous cyclosporine (4 mg per kg per day) is used to treat acute, severe, refractory UC and results in improvement in 66% to 75% of patients within 1 to 2 weeks. It is not useful as oral maintenance therapy. Uncontrolled data suggest it may also be useful in severe refractory CD. Given its renal toxicity, however, it may be used only in the short term as a temporizing measure while awaiting other therapy to take effect or awaiting surgery.

Methotrexate   Methotrexate inhibits dihydrofolate reductase and DNA synthesis. In one trial, weekly intramuscular injection of 25 mg of methotrexate in steroid-dependent CD improved symptoms and reduced steroid requirements. More studies are needed, but it may be an alternative to 6-MP as a steroid-sparing agent in CD. Blood counts and liver function tests must be monitored, but folic acid protects against some toxicity. The response of patients with IBD to immune-modifying drugs led to a search for alternative immunosupressive approaches. Inhibition of the proinflammatory cytokine tumor necrosis factor-α has shown particular promise in CD. The new specific immunomodulator therapies should improve treatment and provide insight into the pathogenesis of IBD.

Antibiotics

In CD, metronidazole is as effective as sulfasalazine in mild-to-moderate disease involving the colon, small intestine, or perianal area. It may delay anastomotic recurrence after bowel resection. Long-term therapy is limited by peripheral neuropathy. Ciprofloxacin is used by some in CD, although without controlled data.

Nutritional therapy

A variety of nutritional deficiencies may develop due to anorexia, diarrhea, and malabsorption, particularly in CD. In addition to the enhanced requirement for iron due to blood loss and for protein due to inflammation, patients may malabsorb calcium, magnesium, folate, water-soluble vitamins, fat-soluble vitamins, and vitamin B_{12} and may require supplementation.

Dietary alterations may also help as symptomatic therapy. Patients with diarrhea and cramping can improve with low-fiber diets and the exclusion of non-absorbed carbohydrates (sorbitol, fructose, and lactose if intolerant). Conversely, patients with constipation may improve with increased fiber. Low-fat diets help in fat malabsorption.

Enteral or parenteral nutrition is used as adjunctive therapy in malnourished patients who cannot eat a regular diet due to an exacerbation, in short-bowel syndrome, in obstruction, in growth failure in younger patients, and perioperatively.

Bowel rest with elemental diets or total parenteral nutrition improves the symptoms, inflammation, and nutritional status in CD. In UC, neither bowel rest nor specific nutritional therapy is beneficial as primary therapy.

Elemental formulations contain amino acids, glucose, essential fatty acids, vitamins, minerals, and trace elements that are absorbed in the proximal small bowel, but they often are administered by tube due to their intolerable taste. Total parenteral nutrition is not superior to elemental diets in CD, so it is given to only those patients who are unable to tolerate elemental feedings and those who are severely malnourished.

Surgical Therapy
Ulcerative colitis

UC can be cured by colectomy, which alleviates symptoms, allows discontinuation of medications, and prevents cancer. Absolute indications for surgery in UC are exsanguinating hemorrhage, perforation, carcinoma, and dysplasia. Other indications in UC for surgery are severe colitis unresponsive to maximal medical therapy and less severe but intractable symptoms or intolerable side effects. Only rarely is surgery necessary to control the extraintestinal manifestations of UC.

Surgical alternatives include proctocolectomy with ileostomy or sphincter-saving operations, which create an ileal pouch with ileoanal anastomosis. Eighty percent of patients are fully continent with this procedure, with four to eight liquid bowel movements per day, but they may have complications resulting from inflammation of the residual ileal pouch.

Crohn's disease

Although CD typically recurs after surgical resection, surgery is indicated to treat complications (hemorrhage, perforation, obstruction, persistent fistulas, fulminant disease, or cancer) or refractory disease. Approximately 70% of CD patients require at least one operation. There is a high postoperative rate of recurrence of 10% per year, with 40% of patients undergoing additional surgery within the next 15 years. Surgery should be reserved for complications or symptoms that are intractable despite optimal medical therapy; however, it should not be viewed as a sign of failure, because it can be a fast, effective route to restoration of well-being.

KEY POINTS: MANAGEMENT OF ULCERATIVE COLITIS

- Patients with mild-to-moderate distal colitis (below the splenic flexure)
  They may be treated with topical aminosalicylates, topical steroids, or oral aminosalicylates. If necessary, therapies can be combined. Suppositories are used for disease that is limited to the distal 10 to 20 cm, and enemas are used for disease up to 60 cm.
  Patient preference is important in determining the therapeutic plan.
  Therapy should be continued until bowel movements are normal; then an oral or topical aminosalicylate should be given for maintenance.
  Patients with mild-to-moderate extensive UC (proximal to splenic flexure)
  Oral sulfasalazine, 3 to 6 g per day, should be given. Topical therapy can also be added.

- Patients with refractory disease

  Oral prednisone, 40 to 60 mg per day, should be given.

  Patients who respond to a short course of steroids can usually be maintained on an aminosalicylate, but those who require longer courses or whose disease flares with steroid tapering often require azathioprine or 6-MP for maintenance.

  Azathioprine or 6-MP is effective in patients who do not respond to steroids or who cannot be weaned from steroids but are not so acutely ill as to require intravenous therapy.

- Patients with severe colitis refractory to oral and top-ical aminosalicylates and steroids or with toxicity

  Intravenous hydrocortisone, 300 mg per day, should be given.

  Severely ill patients should be monitored for poten-tial toxic megacolon.

  Serial radiographs of the abdomen should be or-dered if there is evidence of colonic dilatation or clinical deterioration.

  Patients receive nothing by mouth, are given de-compression if an ileus is present, and are given empiric antibiotics.

  If remission is achieved, oral steroids and azathio-prine or 6-MP should be initiated. Failure to im-prove after 7 to 10 days is an indication for colec-tomy or intravenous cyclosporine if the patient is unable to undergo surgery.

  If the patient responds to cyclosporine, it should be switched to an oral dosage of 8 mg per kg per day and tapered, along with steroids, azathioprine, or 6-MP (Table 7.4).

KEY POINTS: MANAGEMENT OF CROHN'S DISEASE

- The medical therapy for CD is similar to that for UC and should be individualized according to the loca-tion, severity, and complications of the disease. Ex-acerbating factors, such as respiratory or enteric infections, smoking, or use of NSAIDs, should be eliminated.

- Mild to moderate CD

  An oral aminosalicylate is given. Sulfasalazine should be used only for CD limited to the colon, with Asacol or Pentasa for small-bowel involvement.

  Metronidazole, 10 to 20 mg per kg per day, can be administered if there is no response to oral amino-salicylate.

- Moderate to severe CD

  Prednisone, 40 to 60 mg per day, is given until res-olution of symptoms and weight gain occur. If there is no response to steroids or the disease flares with tapering, immunosuppression with azathio-prine, 6-MP, or methotrexate may be indicated.

  Because fistulas and abscesses are common in CD, the possibility of infection should be excluded

TABLE 7.4.	**Therapy for Ulcerative Colitis**

Mild or moderate disease
  Distal colitis
    Aminosalicylate (oral or rectal)
    Rectal corticosteroid
  Extensive colitis
    Oral aminosalicylate
Severe disease
  Distal colitis
    Oral corticosteroid
    Rectal corticosteroid
  Extensive colitis
    Oral corticosteroid
    Oral azathioprine or 6-mercaptopurine (6-MP)
Fulminant disease
  Extensive colitis
    Parenteral corticosteroids
    Intravenous cyclosporine
Maintenance
  Distal colitis
    Aminosalicylate (oral or rectal)
    Oral azathioprine or 6-MP
  Extensive colitis
    Oral aminosalicylate
    Oral azathioprine or 6-MP

before initiating steroids, which can mask intra-abdominal sepsis.

  Infections and abscesses require use of appropriate antibiotics and drainage.

  Elemental diets may also be effective.

  If remission is attained, the steroid is tapered and an oral aminosalicylate is added for maintenance of remission.

- Refactory severe CD

  Patients should be hospitalized and, after an ab-scess has been excluded, given parenteral corti-costeroids.

  Surgical consultation is warranted for patients with obstruction or possible peritonitis.

  Nutritional support should be given if the patient is unable to tolerate an oral diet for 5 to 7 days.

  If there is no response to parenteral corticosteriods in 7 to 10 days, resection of the involved intestine should be considered.

  Mesalamine, azathioprine, or 6-MP is effective in maintaining remission in CD, including after surgery.

  Corticosteroids should not be used as long-term agents to prevent the relapse of CD (Table 7.5).

TABLE 7.5.	Therapy for Crohn's Disease

Mild disease
  Oral aminosalicylate
  Metronidazole
Moderate disease
  Oral corticosteroid
  Azathioprine or 6-mercaptopurine (6-MP)
Severe disease
  Parenteral corticosteroids
  Intravenous cyclosporine
Maintenance
  Oral aminosalicylate
  Azathioprine or 6-MP

COMPLICATIONS

Intestinal Manifestations

Toxic megacolon

Toxic megacolon occurs more commonly with UC but also occurs in CD. The dilatation results from the effect of severe inflammation on neuromuscular tone. It is precipitated by severe colitis, hypokalemia, hypomotility agents, or instrumentation for endoscopy or barium enema during severe inflammation. Patients present with signs of toxicity and a tender, distended, and hypoactive abdomen. A radiograph of the abdomen shows colonic dilatation greater than 5 to 6 cm, with loss of haustra and possibly air in the colonic wall. It occurs in 5% of severe attacks of UC. Failure to improve after 24 hours of aggressive medical therapy is an indication for surgery, because otherwise the resulting perforation has a high mortality rate (Fig. 7.3).

Intestinal perforation

Intestinal perforation occurs in 1% to 2% of cases of severe IBD, as extensive ulceration may thin the bowel wall. Patients have evidence of peritonitis with free air under the diaphragm and need immediate colectomy. Peritonitis can also result from rupture of an abscess in CD. However, if the patient is already receiving corticosteroids, the signs of peritonitis may not be obvious, and the patient may have only tachycardia, malaise, and decreased bowel sounds.

Colon cancer

Colon cancer is a long-term complication, particularly in UC, and the risk rises 10 years after the diagnosis. Its development depends on the extent of involvement and

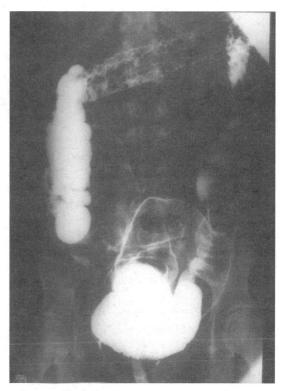

FIGURE 7.3.

A radiograph of the abdomen, with a nasogastric tube in the stomach, shows multiple abnormally dilated segments of colon with diffuse wall irregularity, suggesting toxic megacolon in this woman with ulcerative colitis (incidental calcified uterine leiomyomata). (Radiograph courtesy of William Kilman, M.D., and Amy Balis, M.D., Parkland Hospital, Dallas, Texas.)

duration of disease. The incidence is 0.5% to 1.0% per year after 10 years. Patients with only proctitis do not have an increased risk of cancer.

The development of colon cancer differs in those with IBD from the general population. The symptoms of a cancer (bleeding or change in bowel habits) are difficult to interpret with IBD. In addition, the cancers are distributed more uniformly throughout the colon; they are more often multiple, flat, and infiltrating; and they have a higher grade of malignancy. The frequent ulcers, pseudopolyps, and irregularities in IBD make the diagnosis extremely difficult.

In the past, some physicians recommended prophylactic colectomy for high-risk patients, given their increased risk and the difficulty in early diagnosis. However, the recognition that dysplasia can be identified by colonoscopic surveillance as a precursor of cancer allows selection of those patients at a high enough risk to necessitate prophylactic proctocolectomy. Despite the difficulty in recognizing dysplasia, the unknown natural history of dysplasia, the unknown cost-effectiveness, and the lack of randomized clinical trials, it is recommended that patients who have had extensive disease for more than 10 years undergo screening colonoscopic surveillance every 1 to 2 years with multiple biopsies at 10-cm intervals. The cost has been estimated at about $93,000 per cancer or precancerous lesion detected. If high-grade dysplasia is found, the patient should be referred for prophylactic surgery. If low-grade dysplasia is found, a repeat examination is recommended in 3 to 6 months with multiple biopsies. If dysplasia is confirmed, colectomy is recommended; if no dysplasia is seen, the colonoscopy may be repeated at 6-month intervals (Table 7.6).

Rates of malignancy in CD appear to be higher than normal but less than in UC. Patients with inactive disease should be monitored for a change in symptoms with subsequent colonoscopy. Surveillance guidelines have yet to be defined in CD.

Extraintestinal Manifestations

Extraintestinal manifestations are common and may precede, accompany, or appear independently of IBD (Table 7.7).

Joint manifestations

Joint manifestations occur in 25% of patients in two distinct syndromes. A peripheral arthritis affects the knees, ankles, and wrists with swelling, erythema, and inflammatory synovial fluid. The severity varies with the activity of the IBD and responds to treatment of the underlying bowel disease. Arthritis is more common with colitis than with only small-bowel disease.

In contrast, central arthritis of the spine, ankylosing spondylitis, and sacroiliitis are associated with HLA-B27 and run a course independent from IBD. Symptoms include backache and stiffness with limited range of motion and characteristic radiologic findings such as "bamboo spine."

TABLE 7.6.   Colon Cancer Surveillance Guidelines for Ulcerative Colitis

Colonoscopy with multiple biopsies every 1–2 yr after 10 yr of extensive disease
Colectomy for cancer or high-grade dysplasia
Repeat colonoscopy in 3–6 mo for low-grade dysplasia with colectomy if persistent

TABLE 7.7.   Extraintestinal Manifestations of Inflammatory Bowel Disease

Musculoskeletal
  Peripheral arthritis
  Ankylosing spondylitis, sacroileitis
  Osteoporosis
Skin and mucus membrane
  Erythema nodosum
  Pyoderma gangrenosum
  Aphthous ulcers
Eye
  Iritis, uveitis, episcleritis
Hepatobiliary
  Fatty liver
  Gallstones
  Pericholangitis
  Sclerosing cholangitis
  Cholangiocarcinoma
Renal
  Kidney stones
Venous thrombosis
Metabolic/nutritional
  Weight loss
  Hypoalbuminemia
  Anemia
  Vitamin deficiencies
  Electrolyte deficiencies (potassium, calcium, magnesium)

Skin manifestations

Like peripheral arthritis, skin manifestations, which occur in 15% of patients, are more common with colitis and correlate with activity of the bowel disease. Erythema nodosum manifests as painful, violaceous nodules on the anterior lower leg and may respond to topical or systemic steroids. Pyoderma gangrenosum is a necrotizing, painless ulcer occurring on the legs or trunk. It should not be biopsied because it may break down. It can be treated with topical antibiotics and steroids. Aphthous ulcers occur in CD, and fissuring at the lips may be seen from *Candida* or deficiencies of iron or zinc.

Eye disorders

Ocular manifestations such as iritis, uveitis, and episcleritis occur in 5% of patients in conjunction with active intestinal inflammation. These conditions respond to topical steroids.

Disorders of the liver and gallbladder

Hepatic and biliary complications are frequent. In CD, ileal disease or resection can deplete the bile salt pool due to inadequate absorption and recirculation. Gallstones form because cholesterol is more saturated in the gallbladder as a result of the reduced bile salt pool. Fatty liver may occur due to malnutrition, steroids, or excess carbohydrate in total parenteral nutrition. The spectrum of liver disease ranges from pericholangitis to sclerosing cholangitis with biliary cirrhosis. Pericholangitis is nonprogressive inflammation of intrahepatic bile ductules, manifested by minor elevations of alkaline phosphatase, GGT, and transaminases, with a normal bilirubin. Sclerosing cholangitis occurs in 3% of UC patients and less commonly in CD. It is characterized by progressive inflammation of the bile duct, with elevations of alkaline phosphatase and GGT to two times normal. Endoscopic retrograde cholangiopancreatography (ERCP) reveals the characteristic beading and strictures of intrahepatic and extraphepatic ducts. No proven therapy can limit the inflammation, but ursodeoxycholic acid use is promising. Cholangiocarcinoma is increased in IBD, particularly with sclerosing cholangitis, from which it must be distinguished. All patients with persistent elevations on liver function tests should undergo ERCP to rule out sclerosing cholangitis. Patients with sclerosing cholangitis can develop progressive biliary cirrhosis that is independent of the outcome of the bowel disease.

Kidney stones

Kidney stones are also a common complication. Ileal disease or resection can cause fat malabsorption, which allows calcium to bind to fatty acids, rather than to oxalate as usual. The resulting free oxalate is absorbed and secreted in the urine, increasing the risk for calcium oxalate kidney stones. Uric acid stones also occur more commonly due to dehydration. In addition, patients have low levels of urinary citrate, which normally reduces mineral saturation in the urine. The treatment of kidney stones in IBD includes a low-fat diet, maintenance of fluid intake, low-oxalate diet, supplemental citrate, supplemental calcium to bind intestinal oxalate, and cholestyramine to bind oxalate. In addition, obstructive uropathies can occur from an inflammatory process, and fistulas may cause recurrent urinary tract infections in CD.

Bone disease

Metabolic bone disease commonly occurs as a result of steroid use, malabsorption of calcium and vitamin D, and dairy-free diets. Patients at risk should have bone densitometry studies and should be encouraged to take in 1,500 mg per day of calcium and 400 to 800 U per day of vitamin D.

Malabsorptive syndromes

Diarrhea can be aggravated by malabsorption of fat or bile acids in CD. Diarrhea from fat malabsorption is diagnosed by the presence of more than 5 g per day of fecal fat. It is treated with a low-fat diet and medium-chain triglycerides, which are absorbed proximally without bile salts. Bile salt malabsorption can induce diarrhea by stimulating secretion; the condition can be treated by administration of chlolestyramine to bind bile salts.

Other complications

Other extraintestinal complications include amyloidosis secondary to chronic inflammation, which manifests as nephrotic syndrome, occurs in patients with longstanding suppurative disease, and does not regress with IBD treatment. Thromboembolic complications of the lower extremities and even strokes occur more often and are associated with severe colitis due to elevation of fibrinogen, factor V, and factor VIII and decreased antithrombin III.

PROGNOSIS

The overall prognosis in IBD has improved with the use of glucocorticoids, sulfasalazine, immunosuppressives, and supportive measures. In acute UC, 90% of patients obtain remission and the mortality rate is less than 5%. The prognosis is worse with total colitis, onset when patients is older than 60 years, and toxic megacolon. Most patients have periods of remissions maintained by medical treatment and interrupted by acute exacerbations induced by stress, illness, infection, use of NSAIDs, noncompliance, or cessation of maintenance treatment. Fifteen percent have refractory UC, and 20% to 25% require a colectomy at some time. Death, when it occurs, is usually caused by perforation, postoperative complications, or colon cancer. Left-sided colitis has no increase in mortality, whereas extensive colitis has a 10-year mortality rate of 5% to 10% for severe first attacks—an improvement over the 50% rate that obtained some 15 years ago. Improvement in well-being occurs after colectomy as the patient learns to live with a stoma.

The prognosis in CD is not as favorable as in UC. The course is more chronic and intermittent and responds less well to medical therapy. Some 50% to 75% of patients develop complications requiring surgery. Most deaths are caused by peritonitis, sepsis, or complications of surgery. Patients often have recurrences after surgery. The tendency for relapse and the chronic nature of the disease and therapy can be frustrating to the patient. Nevertheless, therapy results in reasonably stable and productive lives for most CD patients.

REFERRAL

Because IBD is a chronic recurrent illness, a close continuous therapeutic alliance is required between patient and physician to strive for realistic goals. Numerous adjustments in therapy may be necessary. Patient involvement, education, and behavior are key components to effective management. Patients' sharing of their experiences in a support group can be very beneficial. A working relationship with a team of providers is essential, including the primary care physician, gastroenterologist, nutritionist, and surgeon. Referral is often indicated for initial diagnosis, failure of medical therapy, fulminant disease, complications, consideration of immunosuppressive therapy or surgery, cancer surveillance, and nutritional support. In the managed-care era, it is increasingly common for primary care physicians to monitor patients with IBD, especially those receiving maintenance therapy, with consultation as needed for flares or complications.

KEY POINTS

- Most patients with UC present with mild-to-moderate disease characterized by bloody diarrhea due to superficial inflammation involving the distal colon; one third present with severe disease.

- Ten percent of patients have extraintestinal manifestations such as arthralgias, skin disorders, or eye disorders at initial diagnosis.

- In CD, abdominal pain, diarrhea, and weight loss are common as a result of the transmural inflammation.

- Postprandial pain with distention, nausea, and vomiting may indicate obstruction in the small bowel.

- Abdominal x-ray films are indicated if obstruction, toxic megacolon, or perforation is suspected.

- Mesalamine or steroid enemas may control mild distal UC; oral aminosalicylates or prednisone is required for more extensive or severe disease.

- Mild CD can be managed with an aminosalicylate or metronidazole, with the addition of steroids and immunomodulators for more severe disease.

- Maintenance therapy with an aminosalicylate or immunomodulator (azathioprine or 6-MP) is important to prevent relapse in both UC and CD.

- Surveillance colonoscopy for dysplasia or cancer every 1 to 2 years is warranted in patients who have had extensive disease for longer than 10 years.

- Prevention or cure awaits identification of the genetic factors responsible for the failure to downregulate the immune response to an unrecognized environmental agent.

COMMONLY ASKED QUESTIONS

What is inflammatory bowel disease?
IBD refers to two disorders that cause the intestines to be inflamed (red and swollen). Patients may have abdominal pain, diarrhea, weight loss, and bleeding from the intestines. Crohn's disease can cause ulcers in the small intestine and large intestine, whereas ulcerative colitis affects the lower part of the large intestine.

What causes the disease?
The exact cause is unknown. It can run in families, but it is not contagious.

How is it diagnosed?
Once the disease is suspected, a doctor looks inside the intestine with a narrow scope. Barium enema x-rays may also be helpful.

How is the disease treated?
It is important to eat a healthy diet, get plenty of sleep, and effectively manage stress. Medicines are used to suppress the inflammation based on the severity of the illness; they include sulfasalazine (Azulfadine), olsalazine (Dipentum), or mesalamine (Asacol or Pentasa), as well as corticosteroids, azathioprine, or 6-mercaptopurine. If the patient has severe symptoms, hospitalization may be required. Surgery may be needed if medicines are not helping.

Where can I get more information?
Information is available from the Crohn's and Colitis Foundation of America, 386 Park Avenue South (17th floor), New York, NY 10016-8804, telephone 1-800-932-2423. Their website is at www.ccfa.org.

SUGGESTED READINGS

Glickman R. Inflammatory bowel disease: ulcerative colitis and Crohn's disease. In: Fauci, AS, ed. *Harrison's principles of internal medicine,* 14th ed. New York: McGraw-Hill, 1998: 1633–1645.

Hanauer S, Meyers S. Management of Crohn's disease in adults. *Am J Gastroenterol* 1997;92:559–566.

Hanauer S. Inflammatory bowel disease. *N Engl J Med* 1996; 334:841–848.

Hanauer S. Inflammatory bowel disease. In: Bennett JC, Plum F, eds. *Cecil textbook of medicine,* 20th ed. Philadelphia: WB Saunders, 1996:707–715.

Jewell D. Ulcerative colitis. In: Feldman, M, Scharschmidt BF, Sleisenger MW, eds. *Sleisenger and Fordtran's gastrointestinal and liver disease,* 6th ed. Philadelphia: WB Saunders, 1998; 1735–1761.

Katz J. Inflammatory bowel disease. *Med Clin North Am* 1994; 78:1207–1256.

Kornbluth A, Sachar D. Ulcerative colitis practice guidelines in adults. *Am J Gastroenterol* 1997;92:204–211.

Kornbluth A, Sachar D, Salomon P. Crohn's disease. In: Feldman M, Scharschmidt BF, Sleisenger MW, eds. *Sleisenger and Fordtran's gastrointestinal and liver disease,* 6th ed. Philadelphia: WB Saunders, 1998;1708–1734.

Peppercorn M. Inflammatory bowel disease. *Gastroenterol Clin North Am* 1995;24:467–569.

CHAPTER 8

Rational Approach to Colon Cancer Screening

Helen M. Wood

University of Texas Southwestern Medical Center and Veterans Administration Medical Center, Dallas, Texas 75216

DEFINITION

Colorectal cancer (CRC) is a compelling health problem in the United States. It is the third most common form of cancer (not including skin cancer) and the second leading overall cause of cancer-related deaths (14%). In 1997, an estimated 131,200 new cases of CRC were diagnosed, and 55,000 Americans died from CRC. In the United States, the lifetime risk of developing CRC is 5%, and the risk of dying from it is 2.6%. Patients who die from CRC lose, on average, 13 years of life. Although the incidence and mortality rates for CRC have been declining slightly in the United States in recent years, the rates of death from CRC have remained largely unchanged despite advances in medical and surgical treatment. Attention has increasingly focused on the prevention and early detection of CRC through population screening as a means of further reducing the impact of the disease.

KEY POINTS: CLINICAL BURDEN OF DISEASE

- CRC in 1997: more than 130,000 new cases; 55,000 deaths

119

- Second leading cause of cancer death
- Lifetime risk of developing CRC: 5%
- Lifetime risk of dying due from CRC: 2.5%

RISK FACTORS FOR COLORECTAL CANCER

The risk for development of CRC may be influenced by a number of factors (Table 8.1).

Age

Age is one of the strongest risk factors for CRC. Risk increases dramatically with advancing age, beginning slightly at age 40 and then more sharply at age 50 years. This risk doubles with each decade after age 60, apparently peaking after age 75. CRC tends to occur with equal frequency in men and women, but rectal cancer is more frequent in men. African-Americans are more likely to die from CRC than are Caucasians.

Genetic Predisposition

Genetic factors also play an important role in many patients with CRC. Hereditary CRC is categorized into two types. One type, the familial polyposis syndromes, account for about 1% of all CRC and result in an almost 100% chance of developing CRC. The second type, hereditary nonpolyposis colon cancer syndrome, comprises about 5% of all CRC. First-degree relatives of a person with this hereditary type of CRC have a 50% chance of developing CRC.

TABLE 8.1.	**Postulated Risk Factors for Colorectal Cancer.**

Familial polyposis, familial nonpolyposis[a], cancer family syndrome
Prior personal history of ovarian, endometrial, or breast cancer
Prior personal history of colorectal cancer or large adenoma (>1 cm)
Family history of colorectal cancer in one or more first-degree relatives before 55 yr
Family history of adenoma in a first-degree relative before 60 yr
Inflammatory bowel disease
Advanced age
Dietary factors
   Low intake of fiber, fruit, vitamin E, vitamin C, beta-carotene
   High intake of fat, meat, animal protein

[a] An hereditary syndrome with an increased risk of intestinal and exra intestinal malignancies.

A family history of CRC in any first-degree relative, but without a defined genetic syndrome, increases the risk for CRC approximately two-fold, and this group comprises about 15% to 20% of all CRC cases. The risk is increased further if the diagnosis of the first-degree relative was made before the age of 55 years or if more than one first-degree relative was affected. The diagnosis of an adenomatous polyp in a first-degree relative before 60 years of age increases risk, as does a personal history of other types of malignancy, such as ovarian, breast, or endometrial cancer. Patients with a history of either a large colorectal adenoma or CRC are also at subsequent increased risk for CDC.

Inflammatory Bowel Disease

Inflammatory bowel disease (IBD) is associated with an increased risk for CRC, which is related to the extent of colonic involvement, the duration of disease, and age at onset of IBD. Ulcerative colitis and Crohn's disease are associated with similar risks for CRC. Pancolitis associated with ulcerative colitis increases the risk after approximately 8 years, with a cumulative incidence of 30% after 35 years.

Diet

Dietary factors are thought to play an important role in the development of CRC. A number of dietary constituents, including fiber, fruit, vegetables, fat, meat, animal proteins, and certain vitamins, have been suggested as causal factors for CRC, but evidence is strongest for a low intake of dietary fiber and a high intake of animal fat. Although the role of dietary factors in the risk for CRC remains largely uncertain due to complex interactions among food components, current evidence suggests that a modification of diet (increasing fiber and reducing animal fat intake) may protect against the development of CRC.

Idiopathy

Although many factors appear to increase the risk for CRC, some substantially so, about 75% of all new cases of CRC occur in people with no known predisposing factors for the disease other than age.

Modification of Risk Factors

It is not clear whether aspirin or nonsteroidal anti-inflammatory drugs are protective in the development of CRC. Genetic factors are not currently amenable to modification.

NATURAL HISTORY OF COLORECTAL CANCER

It is widely believed that most, if not all, CRCs arise from preexisting adenomatous polyps. Adenomatous polyps occur frequently, and their prevalence increases with age. Colonoscopic studies of average-risk, asymptomatic persons age 50 years and older with negative guaiac (Hemoccult) tests have reported prevalences of 24% to 41%.

Adenoma-Adenocarcinoma Sequence

Direct evidence supporting the belief that CRC arises from preexisting adenomatous polyps is lacking, due to the current standard of practice of excising polyps when they are found, which obscures the natural history of polyps that remain in place. However, indirect evidence supports a multistep process, referred to as the *adenoma-adenocarcinoma sequence,* in which a single epithelial cell from normal colonic mucosa undergoes neoplastic transformation, proliferates, and subsequently results in the formation of an adenoma. Studies show that the process develops slowly over 8 to 10 years, which provides a valuable window of opportunity for the detection and removal of adenomas.

Malignant potential of polyps

Although adenomatous polyps are considered to be the malignant precursors of CRC, not all polyps are adenomatous. Technically, a polyp is defined as any mucosal protrusion into the lumen of the colon. It may be non-neoplastic (e.g., hyperplastic polyp) or neoplastic (either adenomatous or malignant). Although the majority of polyps are neoplastic, about 30% are nonneoplastic and without malignant potential.

Progression to colorectal cancer

Although most CRCs arise from adenomas, only a small proportion of adenomas, as few as 5% to 10%, progress to CRC. The likelihood of malignant progression of an adenoma is related to several factors, the most important of which are size greater than 1 cm, villous as opposed to tubular histologic type, and dysplasia. About 75% of neoplastic polyps are tubular. Only about 5% are villous, with severe dysplasia exhibited in only 5% and invasive carcinoma found in just 3%. In one study that monitored patients for 14 years after the removal of polyps, patients whose polyps were tubulovillous, villous, or greater than 1 cm in size were more than three times as likely to develop CRC than the general population. In contrast, the risk for CRC in patients with small, tubular adenomas was not increased.

Adenocarcinoma

Adenocarcinoma comprises the majority of CRCs, with about one half occurring proximal to the splenic flexure. Some studies now report a greater proportion of CRCs

arising more proximally than was found a decade ago, and that more proximal cancer is associated with increasing age. Although this proximal shift in the site of CRCs, if true, would have implications for CRC screening, because tumors proximal to the descending colon-sigmoid junction are beyond the reach of the sigmoidoscope and therefore not amenable to detection with this method.

Survival Rates

Survival from CRC is predominantly determined by the stage of disease at diagnosis and varies greatly. Localized disease confined to the bowel wall is associated with a 5-year survival rate of 80% to 90%, compared with 35% to 60% once regional lymph nodes are involved, and less than 10% once metastatic disease is present. Sixty percent of patients present with regional or distant metastasis at the time of diagnosis, limiting the efficacy of intervention.

KEY POINTS: NATURAL HISTORY

- The majority of CRCs arise from adenomatous polyps.
- The adenoma-adenocarcinoma sequence evolves over 8 to 10 years.
- Adenomatous polyps are common, but fewer than 10% develop into CRC.
- Approximately 40% to 60% of adenomas and cancers are proximal to the splenic flexure.
- Five-year survival rates for localized disease are 80% to 90%; for regional disease, the rate is 35% to 60%; for metastatic disease, it is less than 10%.
- Sixty percent of patients present with regional or distant metastasis.

GENERAL PRINCIPLES OF SCREENING

CRC screening offers opportunities for both primary screening, the detection and removal of the malignant precursors of cancer (adenomatous polyps), and secondary screening, the detection of CRC at an earlier, more curable stage. The attraction of screening for CRC is obvious. Survival is critically dependent on the stage of disease at diagnosis, but patients usually present with more advanced disease, when current medical and surgical treatments have limited efficacy. In addition, a malignant precursor, adenomas, exists and is amenable to detection and removal as a means of preventing CRC.

Decision to Screen for Colorectal Cancer

Decisions regarding whether to initiate screening for a particular disease are influenced by a number of factors, summarized in Table 8.2. The first three of these four factors are quite characteristic of CRC and favorable for screening. The controversy concerning CRC screening centers on the issues of the appropriate screening test, its use, and the cost-effectiveness of screening.

Screening Performance

The performance of a screening test, in this case for CRC, is measured in several ways.

Sensitivity

The sensitivity, or true-positive rate, of a screening test refers to its ability to detect all of the patients with a particular disease. In other words, sensitivity specifies *the proportion of patients with disease who test positive* on the screening test. Because the goal of any screening program is to detect persons with disease, the sensitivity of the screening test is the primary determinant of the benefit of screening.

Specificity

The specificity, or true-negative rate, of a screening test reflects the ability of the test to specifically identify *only* those patients with disease. In other words, specificity defines the proportion of patients without *disease who have a negative result* on the screening test.

The false-positive rate (defined as 1 minus the specificity) conveys the proportion of patients who do not have disease but for whom further evaluation is pursued due to a positive test result; this evaluation produces no benefit but incurs cost and potential harm. In the context of screening, when there is generally a low likelihood of disease before the test is performed (i.e., a low pretest probability of disease), the false-positive rate of the screening test is often a more useful representation of its performance. Because false-positive results usually account for the majority of evaluations performed, the specificity of the screening test (and its converse, the

TABLE 8.2.	Factors that Favor Screening for a Disease.

Significant clinical burden associated with the disease
Early treatment for disease is more effective than late treatment; can be subsumed under acceptance to patients
Disease characterized by an early, asymptomatic phase
Screening test: simple, accurate, reliable, safe, of reasonable cost, acceptable to patients

false-positive rate), is the principal determinant of the effort of screening.

For almost every screening test, the attempt to increase sensitivity, and therefore the benefit of screening, usually leads to a tradeoff; there is a sacrifice in specificity, which leads to greater effort and cost due to the increased proportion of false-positive tests. This is the case with CRC screening: a false-positive result leads to extensive colonic evaluation, which is costly and carries a risk of complications.

Predictive value

The *predictive value* of a screening test refers to either the proportion of screened persons who have a positive test result and do have CRC (positive predictive value) or the proportion of persons who have a negative test result and do not have CRC (negative predictive value).

The predictive value of a test is greatly influenced by the likelihood of disease before the test is performed. The likelihood of disease is generally low in a screening context, and this tends to reduce the predictive value of a positive test. The impact of a screening test on the outcome of interest is referred to as its *efficacy*, which describes how well the intervention works under ideal circumstances. However, tests are usually performed under less than ideal conditions, and so the *effectiveness* of the screening test is a more realistic reflection of the impact obtained under usual practice conditions.

KEY POINTS: CHARACTERISTICS OF PERFORMANCE OF A SCREENING TEST

- *Sensitivity,* the proportion of diseased persons who test positive, determines the benefit of screening.
- *Specificity,* the proportion of nondiseased persons who test negative, determines the effort and cost of screening.
- *Positive predictive value* refers to the proportion of persons with a positive test who have disease.
- *Negative predictive value* refers to the proportion of persons with a negative test who do not have disease.
- *Efficacy* is the impact of the screening test under ideal conditions.
- *Effectiveness* is the impact of the screening test under typical conditions.

SCREENING TESTS FOR COLORECTAL CANCER

The primary screening modalities for CRC are the digital rectal examination, fecal occult blood test (FOBT), flexible sigmoidoscopy, barium enema, colonoscopy, and various combinations of these tests. Table 8.3 provides a summary of characteristics of these tests.

Digital Rectal Examination

No data specifically addressing the efficacy of the digital rectal examination in reducing the incidence and mortality of CRC are available. However, its limited efficacy can be inferred from the limited extent of the examination (only 6 to 8 cm) and the small proportion of CRCs (only 10%) that are accessible and therefore detectable by digital rectal examination.

Fecal Occult Blood Test

The use of FOBTs to screen for CRC is predicated on the tendency of CRCs and adenomas to bleed and thus enable detection. Guaiac-based tests, such as Hemoccult II and Hemoccult SENSA, are the most commonly used FOBTs. They detect occult blood through a peroxidase-like reaction between the hematin moiety of hemoglobin and the colorless guaiac in the test card.

Other tests include HemoQuant®, which detects blood and blood-derived porphyrin but has a high false-positive rate, and tests that detect intoet hemoglobulin using immunochemical techniques (HemoSelect®). Immunochemical tests are more expensive and more difficult to perform, but they have greater sensitivity and comparable false-positive rates to the guaiac-based tests. The FOBT has been available the longest, is the best studied, and can be performed in the clinician's office.

Procedure

Currently, Hemoccult II is the most frequently recommended FOBT. The standard procedure is to thinly smear small fecal samples from two separate parts of a single stool specimen on each of two windows on the Hemoccult card. This procedure is repeated on three consecutive days, and all three cards must be developed within 7 days of collection. The cards can be developed in the clinician's office; they are assessed for a blue-color reaction at 30 to 60 seconds. A positive screening result is defined as a positive reaction in one or more of the six

TABLE 8.3. Comparison of Screening Tests for Colorectal Neoplasia

Test	Sensitivity (%)	Specificity (%)	Effectiveness (% reduction in CRC mortality)	Strength of evidence	Compliance (%)
FOBT (for CRC)	Varies 50	90–98	15–33	Strongest: 5 CCT (for repeat)	30–50
FS	67 (at best)	Not clear	60–80	Good: high-quality case-control studies	20–50 (may be lower)
FOBT/FS	Unknown	Unknown	40 (vs. FS)	Limited: one small CCT, results NS	FS
DCBE	Estimates:			Limited, but benefit inferred from other evidence	Varies: low to moderate
CRC	55–85	99			
Adenomas (>1 cm)	70–90	90–95			
Adenomas (<1 cm)	50–80	50			
Colonoscopy	Estimates:	98	76	Limited: one case-control study, but benefit inferred from other evidence	One screening study: 15%
CRC	97				
Adenomas (>1 cm)	85				
Adenomas (<1 cm)	78				

CRC, colorectal cancer; FOBT, fecal occult blood test; CCT, controlled clinical trial; FS, flexible sigmoidoscopy; NS, not statistically significant; DCBE, double-contrast barium enema.

windows of the three Hemoccult cards. Testing of a single stool specimen obtained during a digital rectal examination is not recommended.

Many experts recommend dietary restriction from red meat for 2 days before and throughout the testing period to reduce false-positive results.

Performance characteristics

The sensitivity and specificity of the FOBT vary considerably due to study differences.

Sensitivity   The sensitivity of a one-time screening with Hemoccult II for CRC of any stage has ranged from 26% to 92%, but the sensitivity for early-stage, potentially curable CRC, which is the ideal target for screening, is estimated to be 30% to 50%. Repeated screening with FOBT in five controlled clinical trials has had a sensitivity that varied from 72% to 78%, demonstrating the value of repeated screening for detection of CRC.

False-negative FOBT results may occur for several reasons. Most important, this test relies on the tendency of colorectal neoplasias to bleed. However, some cancers do not not bleed, bleed only intermittently, or bleed below the threshold of sensitivity of the test. Adenomas bleed only infrequently, depending on polyp size. As polyp size increases from less than 5 mm to more than 2 cm, the sensitivity of FOBT increases from 6% to 20%. Overall, it is estimated that about two thirds of CRCs, but a much smaller proportion of adenomas, bleed.

Other sources of false-negative tests include sampling errors due to the nonuniform distribution of blood in feces, delay in the development of the slides, and the use of vitamins A, C, and D, which have antioxidant activity that may interfere with the peroxidase-like reaction of guaiac-based tests.

Specificity   The specificity of FOBT for CRC has also varied, ranging from 90% to 98%. What does this mean clinically?

Although only about 0.5% of all asymptomatic, average-risk persons 50 years of age and older harbor CRC, 1% to 4% test positive on initial screening with nonrehydrated Hemoccult II. In clinical trials of FOBT, the predictive value of a positive FOBT result was about 3% to 14% for early-stage CRC and 20% to 40% for adenoma.

In other words, taking the midrange of this predictive value, out of every 1,000 persons who test positive, about 300 have adenomas or an early stage of CRC, of which only 2 to 3 are CRC. For each cancer detected, nine patients would need to undergo colonoscopy or double-contrast barium enema.

Attempts to increase sensitivity by the use of a rehydrated Hemoccult slide, where a drop of water is added to each window, have resulted in a four-fold increase in the false-positive rate, from 2% to 8%, and a parallel increase in the rate of extensive colonic evaluation. The tradeoff becomes one between missed cancer and a higher rate of unnecessary colonic evaluation; small changes in the specificity of the test (and the false-positive rate) have a much greater impact on the latter and therefore on the cost and effort of screening.

Sources of false-positive tests for occult blood in stool are numerous. The most important stems from the fact that FOBT is not a test for cancer; it is a test for blood in the stool. Bleeding from other causes, such as hemorrhoids, may result in false-positive tests, as may dietary factors, such as hemoglobin in uncooked red meat, poultry, and dark fish and the peroxidase activity of certain raw fruits and vegetables. Dietary restriction is recommended to reduce the number of false-positive tests.

The use of nonsteroidal antiinflammatory drugs and even warfarin may also result in false-positive tests; these findings may be caused by bleeding from other gastrointestinal lesions, which are not always significant, and cancer may be absent. Actual data are limited, which makes the interpretation of a positive test in the face of one of these agents difficult. To avoid the complexity of interpreting a positive test, it may be prudent for the patient to avoid these agents for 1 week before the FOBT, unless stopping use of these agents would be unduly uncomfortable (inadequate pain relief) or risky because of possible thromboembolism.

Effectiveness of early detection

Reduction in morbidity and mortality   There is growing direct evidence that FOBT, followed by diagnostic and therapeutic colonic evaluation, reduces CRC mortality.

Although case-control studies have reported reductions of 30% to 60% in mortality from CRC associated with annual or biennial screening, their interpretation is limited due to several potential biases associated with case-control design.

The most compelling evidence that FOBT is a means of reducing CRC mortality comes from five long-term clinical trials, four of which were randomized. These trials differed with respect to many important variables, including population studied, ages of patients, screening interval, duration of follow-up, and type of FOBT, as well as factors such as rehydration and dietary restriction, type of colorectal evaluation, and patient compliance with the testing regimen. Nevertheless, a shift to an earlier, more curable stage of CRC at diagnosis and reductions in mortality from CRC of 15% to 33% have been found consistently, although the greatest reduction was found in a study using rehydrated FOBT. In absolute terms, these reductions translate into a relatively small survival benefit of 1 to 3 persons for every 1,000 patients screened.

The small absolute benefit of screening may result from a number of factors: the relatively small sample sizes in comparison with the baseline incidence and mortality of CRC, the limited duration of follow-up in comparison with the long dwell time for cancer, the low sensitivity of FOBT for detecting adenomas, and the low overall compliance with screening. However, it is possible that the benefit of screening may have been overestimated for other reasons. In these trials, some of the benefit of screening may have resulted from the high rate of colonoscopy performed to evaluate the large number of false-positive tests. In addition, although death rates from CRC were reduced, the incidence of death due to all causes was not. It is important to demonstrate this latter end point to ensure that a screening intervention does not inadvertently increase death due to another cause. Although it is commonly believed that detection and removal of adenomas reduces the incidence of CRC, this presumed benefit was not demonstrated in these clinical trials.

Screening intervals   Annual screening with FOBT is recommended because it is associated with greater, more consistent reductions in CRC mortality than is biennial screening.

POSITIVE RESULTS   Patients with a positive FOBT should undergo complete evaluation of the colon, preferably with colonoscopy. A combination of air-contrast barium enema and flexible sigmoidoscopy is an acceptable alternative if examination by colonoscopy is incomplete, if there are contraindications to colonoscopy, or if resources for colonoscopy are limited. The latter strategy is associated with lower cost and risk, but it is limited by a low sensitivity for detection of adenomas smaller than 1 cm and the need for colonoscopy in the 15% of patients who have abnormal examinations.

Although colonoscopy requires sedation and incurs a small risk of complications, such as a perforation rate of 0.8% for biopsy and polypectomy, it allows for both diagnosis and treatment of colonic neoplasia.

Several studies have shown that patients who test positive on FOBT but who have a negative colon evaluation are at lower risk for CRC, although the time interval of low risk has not been precisely defined. Subsequent screening can be deferred for at least 5 years and perhaps for as long as 10 years.

NEGATIVE RESULTS   Patients who test negative on FOBT should undergo repeat screening in 1 year, but if signs or symptoms develop in the ensuing interval, the patient should undergo evaluation sooner. Although the negative predictive value of FOBT in an asymptomatic population has been estimated to be 99% based on limited data, it is much lower in the presence of symptoms.

Compliance   Long-term compliance with repeated screening in clinical trials is low, 30% to 50%, and limits the efficacy of FOBT, despite specific attempts to ensure compliance that would not generally be characteristic of routine practice.

Drawbacks   The impact of FOBT translates into about 1 to 3 lives saved per 1,000 persons screened over at least 10 years. It is imperfect as a screening strategy due to its low sensitivity; it is unable to detect all cancers, its ability to detect adenomas is particularly poor, and its false-positive rate is high, which results in large numbers of unnecessary colon evaluations. In the future, stool tumor markers, immunochemical tests, and fecal mutagen assays may increase the sensitivity of fecal tests for CRC, but these tests are still under investigation.

Sigmoidoscopy

Sigmoidoscopy as a screening test for CRC offers distinct advantages over FOBT in allowing direct visualization of colorectal mucosa, the capability to biopsy lesions during the procedure, and a greater sensitivity for adenomas. It is therefore aimed not only at detecting early-stage CRC but also at detecting and removing the malignant precursor lesions.

Procedure

Rigid sigmoidoscopes 30 cm in length have largely been replaced by 35- or 60-cm flexible instruments that allow better visualization of a larger portion of the bowel and are better tolerated by patients. An enema is given 1 to 2 hours before the procedure to prepare the distal bowel. Antibiotic prophylaxis for endocarditis is indicated for patients who are at high risk. The examination takes an average of 8 minutes in experienced hands and is generally well tolerated without sedation. Although biopsy specimens can be obtained, polypectomy with electrocautery is not safe because it requires full bowel preparation. Nonphysician health care professionals have been successfully trained to perform flexible sigmoidoscopy.

Performance characteristics

Defining a positive test   Controversy exists as to which lesions constitute a positive test on flexible sigmoidoscopy and require follow-up with colonoscopy. There is a general consensus that patients found to have cancer or any polyp larger than 1 cm should be referred for colonoscopy and that those patients found to have only hyperplastic polyps do not require further evaluation. However, agreement with regard to the management of adenomatous polyps smaller than 1 cm has not been reached, largely because there is insufficient evidence to precisely define the risks related to specific prognostic features and because there are enormous costs associated with evaluating all persons with these lesions.

Limited studies suggest that the finding of a single, tubular adenoma smaller than 1 cm conveys no more risk for development of CRC than is found in the general population. A small, distal tubular adenoma carries substantially less than a 1% risk of more advanced proximal lesions, whereas the risk associated with an adenoma that is larger than 1 cm or contains villous elements is greater than 10%. Because most polyps found on flexible sigmoidoscopy are tubular and less than 1 cm in size, ignoring such low-risk lesions would dramatically reduce referrals for colonoscopy and result in substantial savings. However, the decision concerning referral for colonoscopy currently remains an individual one.

Sensitivity   The sensitivity of flexible sigmoidoscopy depends on whether the criterion for accuracy is the ability to detect neoplasia within reach of the instrument or the ability to detect neoplasia anywhere in the colon. Studies in which flexible sigmoidoscopy and colonoscopy were performed in the same patients have shown that 40% to 60% of all adenomas are detected in the distal 60 cm by colonoscopy and would presumably be detectable by flexible sigmoidoscopy. However, depending on the examiner's experience, only about 80% of 60-cm examinations visualize the entire sigmoid colon, and, on average, only about one half of examinations achieve a 60-cm depth of insertion. Although many flexible sigmoidoscopy examinations lead to a follow-up colonoscopy that would detect additional lesions, about one third of patients have isolated proximal adenomas without distal polyps to signal their presence. At best, then, the sensitivity of a 60-cm flexible sigmoidoscopy, even if combined with a follow-up colonoscopy when distal adenomas are found, can be estimated to be about 66%.

Specificity   What constitutes a false-positive examination on flexible sigmoidoscopy is controversial. Some authors suggest that referral for colonoscopy based on the detection of small adenomas that may not have led to CRC may be considered a false-positive result; because of the prevalence of these lesions, the false-positive rate would be high. If referral is restricted to patients with CRC or large adenomas, then the false-positive rate is negligible.

Effectiveness of early detection

Data from high-quality case-control studies suggest that screening with flexible sigmoidoscopy would detect 1 to 4 cases of CRC per 1,000 patients and that mortality from CRC would be substantially reduced.

Reduction in morbidity and mortality   The strongest evidence to date supporting sigmoidoscopy as a screening test for CRC comes from two case-control studies of large managed-care populations. Both studies found much lower rates of rigid sigmoidoscopy (about 10%) among HMO members who died of distal CRC than among age- and gender-matched controls (about 24% to 30%). Patients who had undergone at least one screening examination experienced a 60% to 80% reduction in the risk of death due to distal colon or rectal cancer. In both studies, the benefit of screening was apparently limited to the portion of the colon screened.

These studies provide the most compelling evidence to date to support the role of sigmoidoscopy in screening for CRC. Although the cost-control design of these studies introduces the potential for significant bias, this effect was significantly reduced by the population-based sample of patients, the large magnitude of benefits confirmed by screening with sigmoidoscopy, and the site-specific nature of the benefit. Other case-control studies have confirmed these findings, including one in the veteran population that demonstrated the benefit of polypectomy in reducing the risk for CRC.

Specific data regarding the impact of screening with flexible sigmoidoscopy on CRC mortality are lacking. However, flexible sigmoidoscopy allows for a greater length of the colon to be examined and provides a higher-quality examination than does rigid sigmoidoscopy. In addition, it has been shown to be more acceptable to patients, and the rates of colonic perforation (1.4 per 10,000 examinations) and serious bleeding (1 per 1,000) for this test compare favorably with those for rigid sigmoidoscopy. For these reasons, the benefits of screening with rigid sigmoidoscopy would be generalizable to a flexible examination.

Screening intervals   The optimal interval for screening must be inferred, because no controlled clinical trial has evaluated the impact of screening interval. Mathematical modeling based on the estimate that adenomas progress to malignant cancer over 7 to 10 years has suggested an interval of 3 to 5 years between examinations. In one study, only 6% of patients typical of a screening population developed small adenomas (but no cancers or large adenomas) within an average of 3.4 years after a negative flexible sigmoidoscopy examination; the authors recommended increasing the interval of flexible sigmoidoscopy to every 5 years. One case-control study demonstrated that serial examinations occurring as infrequently as every 10 years are as effective as those with shorter intervals. However, establishing the appropriate interval for screening with flexible sigmoidoscopy rests on a subjective determination of an acceptable threshold for missed adenomas.

Compliance   Compliance with flexible sigmoidoscopy screening has varied considerably and is influenced by a number of factors, including the risk status of the patient, efforts to educate and remind the patient, and health professional recommendations. The best estimates are the rates of compliance in screening populations, which have been as low as a few percent and as high as 30% to 50% when screening is funded by and performed in the workplace.

Drawbacks   Despite the lack of information on the sensitivity, specificity, and predictive value of flexible sigmoidoscopy for detecting CRC, its greatest limitation is obvious: it screens only half of the colon. This approach may be considered analogous to screening for breast cancer by performing mammography on only one breast. Flexible sigmoidoscopy as a strategy is entertained primarily because it is much less costly than colonoscopy.

Combination of Fecal Occult Blood Test and Sigmoidoscopy

Theoretically, the addition of sigmoidoscopy to FOBT could improve the detection of rectosigmoid neoplasia, particularly of polyps. Two controlled clinical trials have evaluated the benefit of combining FOBT with sigmoidoscopy. In one, screening annually with FOBT and rigid sigmoidoscopy reduced mortality from CRC by about 40%, compared with annual rigid sigmoidoscopy alone, although the results did not reach statistical significance. In another trial, a combination of FOBT and flexible sigmoidoscopy yielded a greater detection rate for neoplasia than did FOBT alone, but this trial was too small to assess mortality from CRC.

Barium Enema

Barium enema offers the advantage of imaging the entire colon, but little is known about its use as a screening test for CRC.

Procedure
In general, a double-contrast barium enema, in which air is instilled into the colon after the barium has been removed, is preferred over a single-contrast examination for screening; the double-contrast barium enema provides better delineation of polyps. Bowel preparation is achieved with a low-residue diet and laxatives and enemas during the 24 hours preceding the examination. Double-contrast barium enema takes about 20 to 30 minutes and can be performed without sedation.

Performance characteristics
The performance of double-contrast barium enema has not been adequately assessed in a screening population. However, information is available concerning its detection rate for polyps and cancers, although these studies generally involved patients who were symptomatic. These studies have reported sensitivities of 50% to 80% for polyps smaller than 1 cm, 70% to 90% for those larger than 1 cm, and 55% to 85% for localized CRC. False-positive tests, caused mainly by retained stool in portions of the colon, vary in a similar manner: 1% for cancers, 5% to 10% for large polyps, and 50% for small polyps.

Effectiveness of early detection
No studies have addressed the impact of screening double-contrast barium enema on the mortality or incidence of CRC. Conclusions concerning its effectiveness must be inferred from the assumed reduction in mortality associated with its ability to detect early-stage cancer and the malignant precursor lesions, adenomas. The optimal screening interval also has not been studied, although experts have suggested 5 to 10 years. Compliance in a screening population has not been assessed; in symptomatic patients, it varies greatly. In general, the rate of complications is exceeding low.

Colonoscopy

Colonoscopy represents the optimal choice for screening, because it combines investigation of the entire colon with the capability to definitively treat most neoplasias with polypectomy.

Procedure
Colonoscopy requires full-bowel preparation with either an oral cathartic solution or laxatives and enemas. As with flexible sigmoidoscopy, antibiotic prophylaxis for endocarditis is indicated for those patients who are at high risk for endocarditis. Although some discomfort is associated with the examination due to the practice of distending the bowel with air, patients undergo parenteral analgesia and sedation that maintains consciousness,

enabling them to provide feedback during the examination but minimizing discomfort. Polypectomy by a number of methods can be performed. A colonoscopy can be performed on an outpatient basis in about 15 to 20 minutes by an experienced endoscopist.

Performance characteristics

The sensitivity of colonoscopy for colorectal neoplasia has been assessed in studies in which back-to-back colonoscopies were performed in the same patients. In general, the miss rate for large adenomas was low (less than 5%), but for small adenomas it ranged from 15% to 27% in studies of patients at higher risk for CRC and 25% in a screening population of persons with negative FOBT results.

However, the use of a second colonoscopy as the gold standard is less than ideal. A miss rate for large adenomas of 3% is reported by autopsy studies that compared the pathologic finding of the colon on autopsy with colonoscopy. The examiner's competence varies considerably and influences the sensitivity of the examination, particularly with regard to the depth of penetration, which reaches the cecum in about 80% to 95% examinations.

Effectiveness of early detection

Reduction in morbidity and mortality   Only indirect evidence is available to assess the effectiveness of colonoscopy with polypectomy in reducing CRC mortality, because the current standard of care is to remove polyps when they are detected. This practice makes studying the impact of not performing polypectomy difficult.

Patients with polyps who do not undergo polypectomy have a higher rate of death from CRC than do general-population controls. The best evidence to date is a case-control study that reanalyzed data from the National Polyp Study, a large prospective study of the impact of colonoscopy and polypectomy, which demonstrated a 76% reduction in CRC mortality in its patients, compared with the standardized incidence rate of the general population.

Although the uncontrolled nature of these studies may have introduced bias and overestimated the benefit of colonoscopy, the demonstrated reduction in incidence and mortality of CRC is probably too large to attribute to bias alone and most likely represents real benefit. However, more precise quantification of the benefits of screening colonoscopy with polypectomy is limited; this quantification is a pivotal issue in cost-effectiveness analyses.

Screening intervals   No studies have directly addressed the optimal screening interval for colonoscopy. Based on the high sensitivity of the test, the time required for CRC to develop from an adenoma, and studies of proctosigmoidoscopy, experts have recommended an interval of 10 years.

A detailed discussion of subsequent surveillance of persons found to have adenomatous polyps on colonoscopy is beyond the scope of this chapter. In general, based on data from the National Polyp Study, after the colon has been cleared of all adenomas, a repeat colonoscopy is recommended as surveillance for new polyps in 3 years. After one negative 3-year examination, surveillance colonoscopy every 5 years is recommended.

Complications   Prospective studies of colonoscopy have reported the following rates of complications: perforation, 1 per 1,000 examinations; major bleeding, 3 per 1,000; and death, 1 to 3 per 10,000.

Compliance   Few data are available concerning compliance with colonoscopy as a screening examination. Eighty percent of patients in the National Polyp Study complied with a repeat colonoscopy, but these patients probably were more motivated because a polyp had already been detected. One study that offered free screening with colonoscopy had only a 15% participation rate.

SCREENING RECOMMENDATIONS

Average-Risk Asymptomatic Adults

Asymptomatic persons who are at risk by virtue of age alone (i.e., who have no other associated high-risk factors) are considered to be at average or standard risk. Table 8.4 summarizes the recommendations of various organizations for colorectal screening in asymptomatic, average-risk persons.

The change in the position of the U.S. Preventive Services Task Force (USPSTF) in December 1995 to recommend screening for CRC has been interpreted as key in establishing the merit of such screening, because the USPSTF uses evidence-based methods to establish its guidelines. The USPSTF recommends screening for adults aged 50 years and older, with either annual FOBT or periodic flexible sigmoidoscopy, although the interval for flexible sigmoidoscopy screening was not specified. Because of insufficient evidence, no preference for FOBT, flexible sigmoidoscopy, or a combination of these two tests could be stated, nor could routine screening with digital rectal examination, barium enema, or colonoscopy be recommended.

TABLE 8.4.	Recommendations for Colorectal Cancer Screening in Asymptomatic Average-risk Adults			
Organization	Screening test	Interval	When to begin	When to stop
USPSTF (perform one)	FOBT or FS	Yearly Every 3–5 yr	age 50 yr age 50 yr	
ACS (perform all three)	DRE and FOBT and FS	Yearly Yearly Every 3–5 yr	age 40 yr age 50 yr age 50 yr	
ACP (perform one)	DCBE, FS, or colonoscopy; FOBT if one of above is refused	Every 10 yr Yearly	age 50 yr	age 70 yr
AHCPR (perform one)	FOBT or FS or combination FOBT/FS or DCBE or Colonoscopy	Yearly Every 5 yr Every 5–10 yr Every 10 yr		

USPSTF, United States Preventive Services Task Force; ACS, American Cancer Society; ACP, American College of Physicians; AHCPR, Agency for Health Care Policy and Research; FOBT, fecal occult blood test; FS, flexible sigmoidoscopy; DRE, digital rectal examination; DCBE, double-contrast barium enema.

Most recently, an expert panel convened for the Agency for Health Care Policy and Research (AHCPR) published its recommendations, which were endorsed by a large number of organizations, including the American Cancer Society (ACS), the American Gastroenterological Association, the American Society for Gastrointestinal Endoscopy, and the American College of Obstetricians and Gynecologists. Like the USPSTF, this panel recommends annual FOBT but recommends combining it with either flexible sigmoidoscopy, double-contrast barium enema, or colonoscopy. The ACS continues to recommend that several screening tests be used in conjunction with one another: digital rectal examination, FOBT, flexible sigmoidoscopy.

Although there now appears to be consensus in recommending screening for CRC, differences remain concerning which test to recommend, when to start screening, and the optimal interval for screening. Several important issues are not well addressed, such as when to discontinue screening, the appropriate follow-up of positive screening tests, and the role of surveillance colonoscopy.

High-Risk Asymptomatic Adults

Patients at high risk for CRC because of a genetic predisposition or preexisting colorectal adenomas or CRCs require earlier and more intensive surveillance. However, data addressing the optimal screening strategies in these patients are limited and vary with the factor conferring additional risk. The benefits of screening with sigmoid- oscopy in patients with familial polyposis coli and of surveillance colonoscopy in patients with IBD are well established. No direct data are available to guide recommendations for patients with a family history of CRC in a first-degree relative, previously treated CRC, or large adenoma.

Current recommendations are based on descriptive studies and a presumed higher survival benefit than is demonstrated with screening of average-risk patients. Most organizations, including the USPSTF, the AHCPR, and the ACS, recommend periodic colonoscopy or double-contrast barium enema for persons with familial polyposis, hereditary nonpolyposis colon cancer syndrome, extensive IBD of long duration, or previous large adenomas or CRC. Table 8.5 summarizes the recommendations of the AHCPR for these and other high-risk groups, although experts vary in their recommendations for surveillance in several of the groups. The ACS recommends colonoscopy or double-contrast barium enema beginning at age 35 or 40 years, or 5 to 10 years before the age of onset of cancer in the affected relative, for persons with one or more first-degree relatives with CRC in whom the age at onset was 55 years or younger.

COST-EFFECTIVENESS OF SCREENING

The evaluation of cost-effectiveness is a complex methodology in which a well-defined mathematical model is applied to a specified set of assumptions with regard both to CRC (probabilities related to the incidence, mortality,

Risk factor	Recommendation
Familial polyposis	Refer for genetic testing: if gene present or indeterminate, FS yearly beginning at puberty; consider colectomy once polyps are found
HNPCRC	Refer for genetic testing; colonoscopy every 1–2 yr starting ages 20–30 yr, then yearly after age 40 yr
Family history of CRC in first-degree relative (before age 55) or adenoma (before age 60)	Same screening tests as in average-risk persons but begin at age 40
Prior large (>1 cm) or multiple adenomas	Repeat colonoscopy in 3 yr; subsequent follow-up interval at discretion of patient and physician
Prior CRC	Colonoscopy after 3 yr, then every 5 yr
Inflammatory bowel disease	Colonoscopy every 1–2 yr after 8 yr of pancolitis, or after 15 yr of left-sided colitis

TABLE 8.5. Screening and Surveillance for CRC in Asymptomatic Persons at High Risk: Recommendations of AHCPR

CRC, colorectal cancer; AHCPR, Agency for Health Care Policy and Research; FS, flexible sigmoidoscopy; HNPCRC, hereditary nonpolyposiscolorectal cancer.

and impact of treatment) and to the screening tests (performance characteristics, cost, and probabilities related to complications, effectiveness of early detection, and compliance) and diagnostic and surveillance tests that are performed after screening. The results of this evaluation are highly dependent on the assumptions of the model, and although these assumptions can be varied to encompass the range of possibilities thought to be reasonable for each factor considered, data on some probabilities are often unavailable.

A number of cost-effectiveness evaluations have addressed CRC screening. In general, screening with either FOBT, flexible sigmoidoscopy, double-contrast barium enema, or colonoscopy is reasonable when compared

with other widely accepted screening tests or medical interventions, which is usually the standard of comparison used in deciding whether to accept a new intervention. However, the widespread implementation of repeated screening, when less than a third of the eligible population is currently being screened, would result in an enormous immediate increase in health care expenditures, for which the benefit would accrue only in subsequent years. Much of the controversy surrounding CRC screening stems from this effect.

Although flexible sigmoidoscopy alone appears to be slightly less cost-effective than other strategies, many of the assumptions of the cost-effectiveness models are too uncertain to recommend one test strongly over another. The cost-effectiveness of CRC screening is particularly affected by assumptions regarding the natural history of polyps, false-positive rates associated with the screening tests, screening intervals, compliance with screening, mortality reduction, patient age, and costs associated with testing, particularly for colonoscopy.

The cost of colonoscopy is expected to drop dramatically, which would make this procedure highly attractive as a screening strategy, but compliance may continue to be a barrier.

FINAL RECOMMENDATIONS

Screening for CRC is almost uniformly recommended for average-risk asymptomatic persons aged 50 years and older, and it may reduce the relative mortality from CRC substantially. However, consensus is lacking about the type of screening test, the testing interval, the point at which screening should be discontinued, and the appropriate follow-up for detected neoplasia.

A number of reasonable screening tests, including FOBT, flexible sigmoidoscopy, and double-contrast barium enema, can be considered based on the evidence to date. Some tests, particularly FOBT and flexible sigmoidoscopy, may complement one another. Although sizable relative reductions in CRC mortality may be possible with CRC screening, these translate into an absolute impact of about 1 to 5 lives saved as the result of long-term screening of 1,000 persons. In the context of screening for disease, small magnitudes of benefit are typical, although this benefit is multiplied on a public-health level by its application to a large general population. Therefore, cost and availability of resources are important factors when considering screening for CRC.

Colonoscopy with polypectomy may ultimately become the preferred strategy, but its initial cost and patient compliance are barriers. Many questions remain, the answers to which will contribute to improvements in screening for CRC in the future.

KEY POINTS

- Screening for CRC is uniformly recommended for average-risk asymptomatic persons aged 50 years and older.

- Recommendations lack consensus for type of screening test, testing interval, and appropriate follow-up when neoplasia is detected.

- Reasonable screening tests include FOBT, flexible sigmoidoscopy, and double-contrast barium enema.

- The absolute impact of screening is estimated to be 1 to 5 lives saved for every 1,000 persons screened.

- Cost and availability of resources are important factors to consider in screening for CRC.

- Colonoscopy with polypectomy may become the preferred screening strategy if the cost of colonoscopy can be significantly reduced.

COMMONLY ASKED QUESTIONS

Why do I need to have a screening test for colon cancer?
Colorectal cancer is a common cause of death in older persons, but it usually does not cause symptoms until later in the disease, when cure is not as likely. Screening before symptoms develop detects disease earlier and results in a greater chance of cure.

What is flexible sigmoidoscopy and will it hurt?
Flexible sigmoidoscopy involves inserting a flexible tube-like instrument through the anus into the rectum. The instrument is passed forward through approximately half of the colon, allowing for direct examination of the lining of this portion of the colon for any abnormalities. There is often some mild discomfort caused by moving the sigmoidoscope through the colon, but it is generally well tolerated without any sedation. A small number of persons need to stop the test due to significant discomfort.

What are the risks of flexible sigmoidoscopy?
Flexible sigmoidoscopy is a very safe test. Only a few persons out of 10,000 who undergo this test develop serious bleeding or damage to the colon.

How likely is it that the test will be positive and what does it mean?
Tests for fecal occult blood are positive in 10 to 40 of every 1,000 persons who undergo the test. On additional testing of these persons, only 1 or 2 are actually found to have colon cancer. For every 1,000 persons undergoing a single flexible sigmoidoscopy, 1 to 4 are found to have colon cancer. However, up to 80 have growths in the colon, called polyps, of a certain type that may lead to colon cancer.

How often will I need the test?
For persons 50 years of age and older without symptoms, most experts recommend fecal occult blood tests every year and flexible sigmoidoscopy every 3 to 5 years.

SUGGESTED READINGS

American College of Physicians. Clinical guideline: part I. Suggested technique for fecal occult blood testing and interpretation in colorectal cancer screening. *Ann Intern Med* 1997;126:808–810.

Berry DP, Clarke P, Hardcastle JD, Vellacott KD. Randomized trial of the addition of flexible sigmoidoscopy to faecal occult blood testing for colorectal neoplasia population screening. *Br J Surg* 1997;84:1274–1726.

Bond JH, for the Practice Parameters Committee of the American College of Gastroenterology. Polyp guideline: diagnosis, treatment, and surveillance for patients with nonfamilial colorectal polyps. *Ann Intern Med* 1993;119:836–843.

Kim EC, Lance P. Colorectal polyps and their relationship to cancer. Colorectal neoplasia, part II: diagnosis and treatment. *Gastroenterol Clin North Am* 1997;26:1–17.

Lieberman DA. Cost effectiveness model for colon cancer screening. *Gastroenterology* 1995;109:1781–1790.

Mandel JS, Bond JH, Church TR, Snover DC, et al. The Minnesota Colon Cancer Control Study. Reducing mortality from colorectal cancer by screening for fecal occult blood. *N Engl J Med* 1993;328:1365–1371.

Sackett DL, Haynes RB, Guyatt, GH, Tugwell P. *Clinical epidemiology: a basic sciences for clinical medicine,* 2nd ed. Boston: Little, Brown, 1991.

Selby JV, Friedman GD, Quesenberry CP, Weiss NS. A case-control study of screening sigmoidoscopy and mortality from colorectal cancer. *N Engl J Med* 1992;326:653–657.

Selby JV, Friedman GD, Quesenberry CP, Weiss NS. Effect of fecal occult blood testing on mortality from colorectal cancer: a case-control study. *Ann Intern Med* 1993;118:1–6.

Wilmink AB. Overview of the epidemiology of colorectal cancer. *Dis Colon Rectum* 1997;40:483–493.

Winawer SJ, Fletcher RH, Miller L, Godlee F, et al. Colorectal cancer screening: clinical guidelines and rationale. *Gastroenterology* 1997;112:594–642.

Winawer SJ, Zauber AG, Ho MN, et al. Prevention of colorectal cancer by colonoscopic polypectomy. *N Engl J Med* 1993;329:1977–1981.

9

Irritable Bowel Syndrome

Shalini Reddy

University of Texas Southwestern Medical Center, Dallas, Texas 75235

DEFINITION

Gastrointestinal complaints without clear organic causes are a common reason for patients to present to a primary care physician. One estimate of the frequency of functional gastrointestinal disorders showed them to be present in up to 69% of the national population; only 39% of these patients sought medical attention for these disorders (I). Patients frequently present with nonspecific complaints such as nausea, vomiting, abdominal pain, diarrhea, and constipation, for which they may have received a number of previous diagnostic procedures and treatments. Physicians are subsequently challenged by patient complaints of subjective severity without apparent anatomic explanation.

Functional Gastrointestinal Disorders

In order to standardize the diagnosis of these disorders for the purposes of treatment and research, a multinational working team consisting of prominent investigators in the field has assembled a symptom— and organ-system—based classification of functional gastrointestinal disorders. This diagnostic classification is shown in Table 9.I.

TABLE 9.1. Functional Gastrointestinal Disorders

A. Esophageal disorders
  A1. Globus
  A2. Rumination syndrome
  A3. Functional chest pain of presumed esophageal origin
  A4. Functional heartburn
  A5. Functional dysphagia
  A6. Unspecified functional esophageal disorder
B. Gastroduodenal disorders
  B1. Functional dyspepsia
    B1a A1. Ulcer-like dyspepsia
    B1b A2. Dysmotility-like dyspepsia
    B1c A3. Unspecified dyspepsia
  B2. Aerophagia
C. Bowel disorders
  C1. Irritable bowel syndrome
  C2. Functional abdominal bloating
  C3. Functional constipation
  C4. Functional diarrhea
  C5. Unspecified functional bowel disorder
D. Functional abdominal pain
  D1. Functional abdominal pain syndrome
  D2. Unspecified functional abdominal pain
E. Biliary disorders
  E1. Gallbladder dysfunction
  E2. Sphincter of Oddi dysfunction
F. Anorectal disorders
  F1. Functional incontinence
  F2. Functional anorectal pain
    F2a B1. Levator ani syndrome
    F2b B2. Proctalgia fugax
  F3. Dyschezia
    F3a C1. Pelvic floor dyssynergia
    F3b C2. Internal anal sphincter dysfunction
  F4. Unspecified functional anorectal disorder

Reprinted with permission from Drossman Da. *The functional gastrointestinal disorders.* Boston: Little, Brown, 1994, Table 1-1, p. 9.)

The functional gastrointestinal disorders associated with pain (functional bowel disorders, functional chest pain, functional dyspepsia, chronic functional abdominal pain, and functional biliary pain) have the highest rates of medical visits of all the functional gastrointestinal disorders (1). Estimates of visits to physicians for irritable bowel syndrome (IBS) range from 2.4 to 3.5 million per year (2).

Functional Bowel Disorders

The functional bowel disorders are a subset of disorders with symptoms referable to the middle to lower gastro-intestinal system. Table 9.2 lists the diagnostic criteria for the functional bowel disorders. The term *unspecified functional bowel disorder* refers to disorders that do not fit into another category of functional bowel disorders. A review of all of the functional gastrointestinal disorders is beyond the scope of this chapter, which focuses primarily on the clinical features and treatment of IBS. References that discuss other functional gastrointestinal disorders are noted at the end of the chapter.

Irritable Bowel Syndrome

The diagnosis of IBS requires the presence of abdominal pain related to defecation or altered bowel habits. Disordered defecation and abdominal distention must also be present (3). The other functional bowel disorders lack all of the diagnostic criteria necessary for the diagnosis of IBS. IBS has been called "mucous colitis" or "spastic colon"; for the sake of uniformity of diag-

TABLE 9.2. Diagnostic Criteria for the Functional Bowel Disorders from the Rome Multinational Consensus Panel

Diagnostic criteria for functional abdominal bloating—all of the following:
  Symptoms of abdominal fullness, bloating, or distention
  Symptoms are unrelated to obvious maldigestion
  Insufficient criteria for diagnosis of functional dyspepsia, irritable bowel syndrome, or other functional disorders

Diagnostic criteria for functional constipation—two or more of the following:
  Straining at defecation at least one fourth of the time
  Lumpy and/or hard stools at least one fourth of the time
  Sensation of incomplete evacuation at least one fourth of the time
  Two or fewer bowel movements in a week

Diagnostic criteria for functional diarrhea—two or more of the following:
  Unformed ("mushy" or watery) stool more than three fourths of the time
  Three or more bowel movements per day more than half of the time
  Increase stool weights greater than 200 g/day, but no more than 500 g/day.

Reprinted with permission from Drossman DA. *The functional gastrointestinal disorders.* Boston: Little, Brown, 1994, Appendix C–D.

nosis, these terms have been replaced with the term irritable bowel syndrome.

Standard criteria for diagnosis

In an attempt to refine the diagnosis of IBS, Manning and colleagues compared 15 symptoms in patients with IBS and patients with organic disease (4). They found that six symptoms correlated with the presence of IBS versus organic disease and that the risk of having IBS increased proportionally to the number of symptoms present. The Manning criteria are listed in Table 9.3.

These diagnostic criteria were evaluated for validity by separate authors and were found to be of greatest value in young children and women. The relative sensitivity of the Manning criteria for distinguishing IBS from non-IBS gastrointestinal disorders was 42% to 58%, and the specificity was 74% to 85% (5). Kruis and coworkers further defined IBS symptoms in 1982. They evaluated a series of patients with gastrointestinal complaints and found that the presence of the symptoms listed in Table 9.4 were highly correlated with a diagnosis of IBS (6).

The Manning and Kruis diagnostic criteria were further modified by a subgroup of the Rome Multinational Consensus Panel. This group of gastroenterologists developed symptom-based diagnostic criteria by reviewing available literature on IBS. The diagnostic criteria focus on the presence of chronic abdominal pain associated with altered gut physiology. The Rome diagnostic criteria are listed in Table 9.5. The absence of altered gut physiology (disordered defecation or pain associated with defecation) suggests an alternative diagnosis such as chronic functional abdominal pain.

Epidemiology

Estimates of the prevalence of IBS in the general population range from 7.1% to 20.0% (1,7–10). Of these, 50% consult a physician for symptoms of IBS (11). Women are more likely to consult a physician in Western societies; in India and Sri Lanka, men are more likely to consult a physician. Factors that influence consulting behavior include the number of IBS symptoms, the pres-

TABLE 9.3. **Manning Criteria for the Diagnosis of Irritable Bowel Syndrome**

Looser stools at onset of pain
More frequent stools at onset of pain
Pain eased after bowel movement
Abdominal distention
Passage of mucus per rectum
Sense of incomplete evacuation

TABLE 9.4. **Kruis Criteria for Diagnosis of Irritable Bowel Syndrome**

Abdominal pain plus flatulence plus irregularity
Symptoms duration >2 yr
Diarrhea and constipation

ence of psychosocial stressors, and the presence of perceived pain (11,12).

CAUSE

The search for the cause of IBS has been frustrating, in large part because of the varied definitions of it. Before the development of symptom-based diagnostic criteria for IBS, there were multiple conflicting reports about its pathogenesis. Use of the Rome criteria for the diagnosis of patients should standardize research techniques. The major categories of causes focus on abnormalities in gut motility, disordered pain perception and processing, local gastrointestinal irritants, and psychological stressors. In reality, IBS is probably a heterogenous group of disorders of multifactorial origin. Each of these factors is examined in this chapter.

Motility Abnormalities

Numerous studies have suggested that the defect in the irritable bowel is an abnormality in colonic and/or small-bowel motility. The first studies, done by Thomas Almy in the 1940s, demonstrated that normal subjects experienced symptoms of IBS and showed proctoscopic

TABLE 9.5. **Rome Diagnostic Criteria for Irritable Bowel Syndrome**

Continuous or recurrent symptoms for at least 3 months of both of the following:
1. Abdominal pain or discomfort that is
   Relieved with defecation *and/or*
   Associated with a change in frequency of stool *and/or*
   Associated with a change in consistency of stool
2. Three or more of the following, at least one fourth of occasions or days:
   Altered stool frequency (more than three bowel movements per day or fewer than three bowel movements per week)
   Altered stool form
   Altered stool passage
   Passage of mucus
   Bloating or feeling of abdominal distention

Reprinted with permission from Drossman DA. *The functional gastrointestinal disorders.* Boston: Little, Brown, 1994.

evidence of colonic spasm when subjected to various stressors (13) and that patients with IBS were more susceptible to the physical manifestations of stress, including the "normal" colonic reactions to stress (14). Later studies confirmed that patients with IBS have greater colonic motor reactivity in response to various provocative stimuli such as stress, cholinergic drugs, and balloon distention than do normal controls (15).

Altered Pain Perception or Processing

Patients with IBS also have increased perception of abdominal pain. Various studies have confirmed that patients with IBS are hypersensitive to distention anywhere in the gastrointestinal tract. This increased sensitivity to visceral pain does not, however, extend to somatic pain. Patients with IBS appear to be hypersensitive to rectal balloon distention but have normal or supranormal tolerance for somatic pain such as ice-water immersion (16). Although not all patients with IBS are hypersensitive to colonic distension, all patients with IBS have some abnormality of visceral pain processing. This may take the form of altered patterns of pain referral or increased intensity of pain perception, compared with normal controls. Hypersensitivity to pain may be secondary to abnormal visceral signal processing by afferent neurons. Figure 9.1 demonstrates normal visceral pain perception.

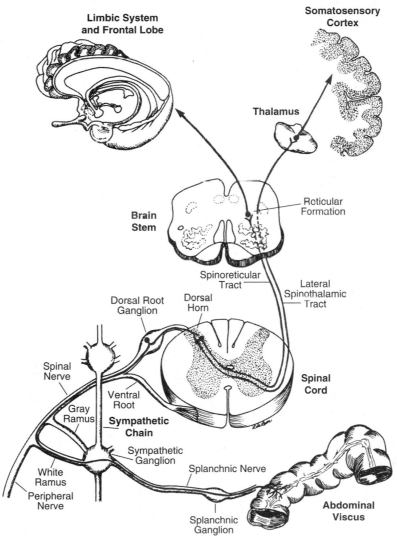

FIGURE 9.1.

Neuroanatomic pathway of visceral pain perception. (From Klein KB. Approach to the patient with abdominal pain. In: Yamada T, ed. *Textbook of gastroenterology.* Philadelphia: JB Lippincott, 1995:752.)

Modulation of the pain stimulus is accomplished at each level of transmission from afferent neurons in the gut to spinal cord tracts and the somatosensory cortex. Accentuation of pain at the visceral level may be secondary to tissue injury or inflammation. Recurrent peripheral stimulation may downregulate normal pain control mechanisms. Modulation at the spinal cord probably occurs through a combination of inhibitory stimuli from the periphery and the central nervous system. Figure 9.2 demonstrates the gate-control theory of visceral pain modification (17). Afferent first-order neurons may either inhibit or stimulate inhibitory sensory interneurons that modulate second-order nerve transmission. Central nervous system modulation occurs through the endorphin-mediated analgesia system, which is thought to originate in the cortex with links to the periaqueductal gray matter and the nucleus raphe magnus. Serotonin and norepinephrine appear to facilitate endorphin activity (18). Abnormalities in pain processing may occur at any of the sites of modulation. In addition to the biochemical abnormalities, the patient's hypervigilance may contribute to the increased perception of pain.

Luminal Factors

Various luminal irritants have been suggested as culprits in IBS. Many studies have examined dietary malabsorption of lactose, fructose, and sorbitol. There are conflicting data on the importance of sugar malabsorption as an agent for IBS. A few studies have suggested, with minimal supportive evidence, that food allergies may play a role in IBS. Hypersensitivity to bile acids may ac-

count for the diarrhea seen in some IBS patients (19). Infectious diarrhea may be a contributing or initiating factor for the onset of IBS symptoms (20).

Psychological Factors

IBS patients have a higher incidence of psychopathology when compared with IBS nonpatients and normal controls (21). The most common psychiatric illnesses reported in conjunction with IBS are somatization, anxiety, and depression (22). Patients with severe IBS commonly have a history of traumatic life events such as sexual or physical abuse (23). Psychological stress is a frequent trigger for worsening of IBS symptoms. Conflicting data exist as to whether psychological factors contribute predominantly to symptomatology or to consulting behavior.

Although the exact mechanisms for IBS have not been elucidated, it is becoming increasingly clear that autonomic dysfunction, abnormal central nervous system functioning, psychological factors, and motility factors all contribute.

PATIENT PRESENTATION

IBS patients note the onset of symptoms between 15 and 35 years of age but generally report difficulties with abdominal pain and disordered defecation since early childhood. Patients may present after an acutely stressful life situation with "new" symptoms suggestive of IBS; detailed questioning reveals that the symptoms have been present for much longer. They may present with coexistent symptoms referable to other areas of the gastro-

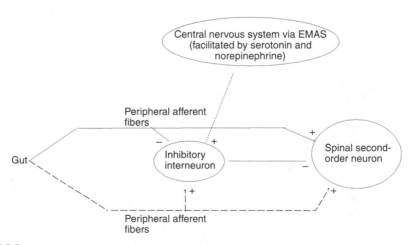

FIGURE 9.2.

Gate-control theory of visceral pain modification. EMAS, endorphin-mediated analgesia system. (Modified from Klein KB. Approach to the patient with abdominal pain. In: Yamada T, ed. *Textbook of gastroenterology.* Philadelphia: JB Lippincott, 1995:752.)

intestinal tract as well as chronic nongastrointestinal complaints. Common nongastrointestinal complaints include pelvic pain, dysmenorrhea, dyspareunia, irritative voiding symptoms, myofascial pain, fatigue, and sleep disturbances (24). Patients frequently give a history of having multiple, frequently negative tests or abdominal/pelvic surgeries for the evaluation of their gastrointestinal complaints.

The course of the disease tends to be of a chronic, intermittent nature with varying degrees of diarrhea, constipation, abdominal bloating, and pain. Remission occurs in about one third of patients over a 2-year follow-up period (25).

History

The general approach to the patient with IBS begins with a careful history, with particular attention to the nature of the abdominal pain, associated symptoms, family history of cancers, psychosocial issues, and history of abuse. The physician should ask about the existence of childhood bowel disorders. The patient should be extensively queried about symptoms that may suggest organic disease. Table 9.6 summarizes historical clues to the presence of organic disease. A thorough medication history should also be obtained. Selected medications that can cause symptoms of IBS are listed in Table 9.7. Numerous other medications may cause symptoms compatible with IBS. The temporal relation between initiation of the medication and onset of symptoms should be elicited.

In addition to the symptoms specified in the Rome criteria (Table 9.3) or the Manning criteria (Table 9.5), symptoms suggesting IBS include alternating diarrhea and constipation, longstanding symptoms, and waxing and waning symptoms. In addition, patients with IBS frequently have poorly localized migratory abdominal

Findings Suggestive of Organic Disease   **TABLE 9.6.**

Pain on awakening from sleep
Pain that interferes with normal sleep patterns
Diarrhea that awakens the patient
Weight loss
Fever
Steatorrhea
Blood in the stools
Physical examination abnormalities
New onset of symptoms in elderly patient
History of steadily worsening symptoms

Medications that May Simulate Irritable Bowel Syndrome   **TABLE 9.7.**

Diarrhea	Constipation
Magnesium-containing antacids	Antacids containing aluminum or calcium
Antibiotics	Anticholinergics
Colchicine/allopurinol	Anticonvulsants
Digoxin	Diuretics
Sorbitol-containing medications	Iron
Theophylline	Verapamil
Thyroxine	Opiod analgesics
Metoclopramide	Phenothiazine
Metformin	Tricyclic antidepressants
Acarbose	Monoamine oxidase inhibitors

Lynn RB, Friedman LS. Irritable bowel syndrome: managing the patient with abdominal pain and altered bowel habits. *Med Clin North Am* 1995;79:373–390.

pain with variable levels of pain. Bowel movements relieve the pain, and food frequently exacerbates the symptoms (27).

A thorough dietary history should be obtained, specifically evaluating for foods that exacerbate symptoms. Food allergy does not seem to play a significant role in patients with IBS; in fact, true food allergy is quite rare. However, patients with a history of atopy should be evaluated for food allergies (28). Although carbohydrate malabsorption is not more prevalent in IBS patients than in normal controls, the former group is more likely to develop abdominal distress from carbohydrate malabsorption. The combination of fructose and sorbitol appears to be particularly causative (29). Table 9.8 lists common foods that contain fructose and sorbitol.

Common Foods Containing Fructose and Sorbitol   **TABLE 9.8.**

Sorbitol	Fructose
Diet foods	Soft drinks
Sugarfree gum	Honey
Fruit juices	Apples/pears
Pears/peaches/prunes	Grapes
Wine	Prunes/cherries
Vinegar	Dried figs/dates

New symptoms or exacerbating factors should be asked about, as well as recent psychosocial difficulties (12). Inquiries related to narcotic use, disability, and secondary gain should be made.

Physical Examination

The physical examination is generally normal in patients with IBS, with perhaps the exception of a palpable, tender sigmoid colon or discomfort with rectal examination (3). Because these findings are not specific for IBS, the physical examination primarily serves to reassure the patient with the "laying on of hands" and to rule out any gross abnormalities (30). Any abnormality on the physical examination should prompt the examiner to pursue organic disease as the cause of the patient's complaints.

DIAGNOSIS

Because the differential diagnosis for the symptoms of IBS is broad, IBS has historically been diagnosed by exclusion of other organic diseases. This results in ordering a number of tests and subjecting the patient to multiple diagnostic procedures with potential risks.

Positive diagnosis of IBS by use of the Rome criteria (Table 9.5) obviates the need to pursue a detailed, nonspecific workup in every patient with symptoms suggestive of IBS. Figure 9.3 illustrates a general strategy for assessing a patient with symptoms suggestive of IBS (30).

Based on the history, patients may be divided into one of three IBS subgroups: diarrhea-predominant, constipation-predominant, or bloating-predominant.

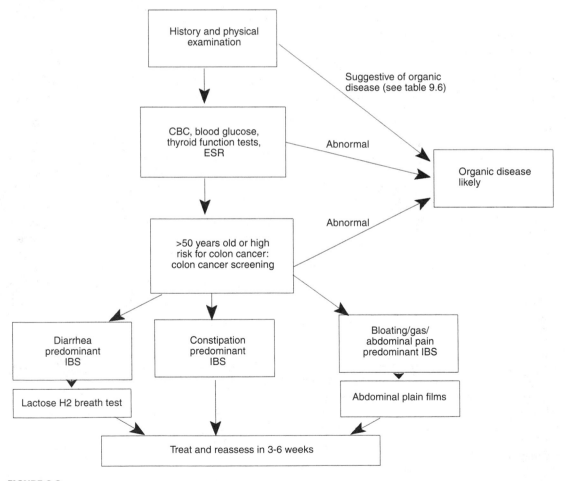

FIGURE 9.3.

Initial diagnostic approach to the patient with symptoms of irritable bowel syndrome (IBS). CBC, complete blood count; ESR, erythrocyte sedimentation rate.

The differential diagnosis for patients with symptoms of IBS is broad; a selected differential diagnosis for the symptoms of IBS is listed in Table 9.9.

Laboratory Testing

Initial screening

The initial screens for patients with IBS should be limited to general ones for common, potentially treatable organic diseases. Blood chemistry analyses, a complete blood count, erythrocyte sedimentation rate, and thyroid function tests should be done for all patients (31). Screening for colon cancer should be performed for all patients older than 50 years of age and for those patients with risk factors for colon cancer. (See Chapter 8 for a review of colon cancer risk factors and recommendations for colon cancer screening.)

Testing based on subgroups

Additional initial screening tests should be done based on the subgroup of IBS.

For patients with diarrhea-predominant IBS, lactose intolerance should be sought with a lactose H_2 breath test (27). Lactose intolerance may also be evaluated by

a brief lactose exclusion diet. Patients who do not have improvement in their symptoms with a lactose-free diet should not stay on such an exclusionary diet because they risk long-term reduction in calcium intake (32). Stool studies looking for ova and parasites or leukocytes should be considered in the appropriate clinical settings (e.g., travel history, history of antibiotic use).

Patients with gas- or bloating-predominant IBS should have an abdominal plain radiographic film made during an acute painful episode to rule out bowel obstruction.

Follow-Up Screening

For symptoms present at the 3- to 6-week reassessment, further studies should be considered.

If diarrheal symptoms persist, further studies can be ordered to assess the quantity and quality of the diarrhea. A timed-stool collection for volume, osmolarity, electrolytes, laxatives, and fecal fat can be performed. Stool volumes greater than 400 cc per day suggest malabsorptive or secretory diarrhea. Other examinations that can be considered in diarrhea-predominant IBS are jejunal aspirates for ova and parasites, transit tests of the small bowel and colon, and colonoscopy with biopsies to exclude collagenous colitis. Generally, these tests are performed by a gastroenterologist in consultation.

For patients with constipation-predominant IBS, tests of colonic functioning should be considered, such as colonic transit testing or anorectal manometry.

For those patients with bloating-predominant IBS, carbohydrate malabsorption, bacterial overgrowth, and mechanical obstruction must be considered.

Figure 9.4 summarizes the evaluation of patients with initial treatment failure.

Selected Differential Diagnosis for Irritable Bowel Syndrome (IBS)	TABLE 9.9.

General

  Psychiatric disorders (depression, anxiety, somatization disorder)
  Medications

Constipation-predominant IBS

  Intestinal pseudo-obstruction (Ogilve's syndrome)
  Intestinal obstruction
  Diabetic autonomic neuropathy
  Hypothyroidism
  Scleroderma

Diarrhea predominant IBS

  Colonic abnormalities (villous adenoma, collagenous colitis)
  Lactose malabsorption
  Inflammatory bowel disorders
  Endocrine disorders (hyperthyroidism, hormone-producing tumors)
  Chronic pancreatitis, sprue
  Postgastrectomy syndromes
  Infectious diarrhea
  Diabetic autonomic neuropathy

Summary of Diagnosis

- Does the patient fulfill the Rome criteria for the diagnosis of IBS?
- What is the patient's family, psychosocial, and past history?
- Are there any signs of organic disease?
- Do any foods exacerbate the symptoms?
- Is the patient taking any medications that may mimic or worsen IBS symptoms?
- Why is the patient seeking medical attention now?

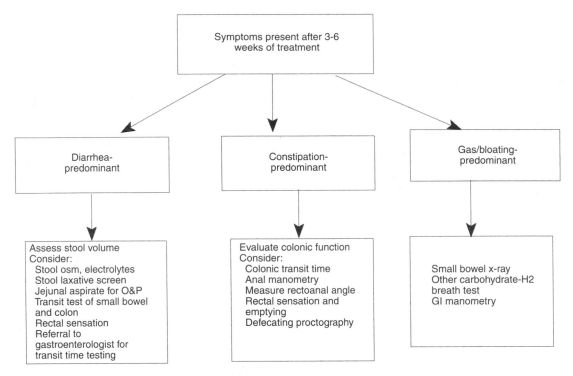

FIGURE 9.4.

Diagnostic evaluation of irritable bowel syndrome after failure of initial management strategy. GI, gastrointestinal; O&P, ova and parasites. (From Drossman DA, Camilleri M. Irritable bowel syndrome: a technical review for practice guideline development. *Gastroenterology* 1997;112:2120–2137.)

MANAGEMENT

Once initial screening tests are completed, the clinician should treat the patient empirically according to the IBS subgroup. Treatment should be continued for 3 to 6 weeks, after which the patient should be given a return appointment for reevaluation of symptoms. This allows the practitioner to collect clinical data from more than one point in time and begins to establish the doctor-patient relationship that is necessary for IBS treatment.

The lack of a defined physiologic basis for IBS has frustrated attempts to definitively "cure" the disease. Studies of medications for the treatment of IBS have been hampered by nonstandardized diagnostic criteria for patient inclusion, variations in symptom-severity reporting, and variable placebo response. Therefore, most medications are recommended based on largely anecdotal evidence. The principal modalities of management include an effective doctor-patient relationship, minimal dietary changes, self-monitoring of symptoms, and few medications.

Management of IBS is a prolonged process that can be exhausting and unrewarding for the primary care physi-

cian. The focus of treatment should be on the management of a chronic illness, rather than its cure.

Treatment Classification

To help with the management of IBS, patients should be classified as having mild, moderate, or severe IBS based on the severity of their symptoms, physiologic and psychosocial associations, illness behavior, and activity disruption (12). Table 9.10 summarizes the spectrum of clinical features in various subgroups of IBS.

Mild disease

Most patients with IBS seen in a primary care practice have mild disease that can be managed satisfactorily without extensive referral. Figure 9.5 shows the treatments available for differing severities of IBS. This graduated approach allows the practitioner to tailor therapy to the patient's specific symptoms (12). The various treatment options are discussed later.

Patients with mild disease have infrequent symptoms that do not result in significant psychological or func-

Spectrum of Clinical Features Among Patients with Irritable Bowel Syndrome (IBS)

TABLE 9.10.

Clinical Feature	Mild IBS	Moderate IBS	Severe IBS
Estimated prevalence (%)	70	25	5
Clinical setting	Primary	Secondary	Tertiary
Correlation with altered gut physiology	+++	++	+
Constant symptoms	0	++++	
Activity disruption	0	+	+++
Health care use	+	++	+++
Psychiatric diagnoses	0	+	+++

Reprinted with permission from Drossman DA. The irritable bowel syndrome: review and a graduated multicomponent treatment approach. Ann Intern Med 1992;116:1009–1016.

tional impairment. These patients can be treated with education, reassurance, and a few dietary changes.

Moderate disease

Patients who have moderate symptoms have intermittent functional impairments and more psychological distress from their symptoms. They are frequently able to relate symptoms to psychological stressors or to specific dietary indiscretions. These patients may require directed pharmacotherapy, behavioral therapy, and psy-

chotherapy in addition to the treatments described for patients with mild symptoms.

Severe disease

Patients with severe disease have frequent disruption of daily activities and cannot relate symptoms to specific physiologic changes such as diet or activity. These patients have the highest rates of psychological disturbances and frequently are displeased with physicians' attempts to treat them. They seek a diagnosis and are skeptical about possible psychological contributions to their disease.

Education and Reassurance

The cornerstone for the effective treatment of any patient with IBS is establishment of a therapeutic, trusting, long-term doctor-patient relationship. During the initial visit, the physician should apply symptom-based criteria so that the positively obtained diagnosis of IBS can be conveyed to the patient confidently. The clinician should validate the patient's symptoms without suggesting that the disease is "all in your head." Once the diagnosis is established, the nature of the disease should be explained to the patient. This involves recognizing that IBS is a chronic disease of multifactorial origin and that remissions and relapses are common. The clinician should provide information about the role of psychosocial stress in exacerbating the disease. It is sometimes helpful to explain that the cause of the disease has not been completely defined but that physiologic abnormalities in pain perception play a role. This helps to support any future decisions to use medications that alter neurohormonal mechanisms of pain perception (e.g., anti-

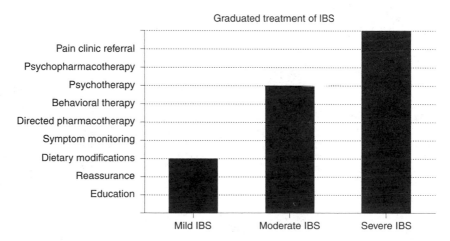

FIGURE 9.5.
A graduated treatment approach to irritable bowel syndrome (IBS) based on severity of symptoms.

depressants). Patient education regarding the nonmalignant nature of the disease and the good overall prognosis may help to reassure the patient. Education also helps to justify extensive testing and the setting of limits on narcotic use (12).

The patient's expectations should be discussed and tempered by realistic expectations. Attainable long-term goals should be established, with a focus on alleviating symptoms and improving quality of life. This can be done by establishing a therapeutic partnership with the patient and involving the patient in the development of a plan of care. Treatment for IBS is most satisfactory if the doctor-patient relationship is of an ongoing, continuous nature. Patients with IBS may benefit from frequent office visits, as indicated by the patient's response to therapy and psychosocial factors.

Dietary Therapy

Modification of diet

Dietary modification is controversial. A progressively restrictive diet may lead to "fear of food" and subsequent malnutrition without significant improvement in symptoms. With that caveat, certain foods and medicines may be evaluated by the patient's symptom diary as specific causative agents. As discussed earlier, Tables 9.7 and 9.8 list specific foods and medicines that are troublesome. There is no clear consensus about increased dietary fiber. Some studies report an improvement in symptoms with increased fiber in the diet; however, in these studies there were almost equivalent improvements with placebo (33).

Increased dietary fiber

Increased dietary fiber or bulking agents may be used with constipation-dominant IBS, with the caveat that increased gas may be produced. Bran, in doses of 20 to 30 g per day, may be most useful for patients with constipation-predominant IBS (34) but should be used with caution in other IBS patients because of its propensity to cause increased bowel gas from bacterial fermentation. This can be particularly troublesome because most patients with IBS are sensitive to colonic distention.

Symptom Monitoring

Symptom monitoring can be accomplished by having the patient keep a simple diary listing symptoms, symptom severity, associated dietary or psychosocial factors, emotional responses to the pain, and thoughts about the symptoms (30).

Psychotherapy

Various psychological treatment modalities are available for patients with moderate to severe IBS. These include interpersonal psychotherapy, relaxation training, hypnotherapy, and cognitive-behavioral therapy. Although studies of psychotherapy for IBS patients have been criticized for methodologic inadequacies (35), there appears to be some value for these forms of therapy in reducing psychological stress from the illness and improving quality-of-life scores (36).

Pharmacotherapy

Treatment of abnormal gut motility

Pharmacotherapy should be directed at the predominant symptom of IBS and should follow the general principles of initiating therapy and reassessing the patient after 3 to 6 weeks. Figure 9.6 summarizes this directed pharmacologic treatment approach.

Diarrhea-predominant disease   Specific therapy directed at diarrhea-predominant IBS involves primarily symptomatic drug treatment. Loperamide results in decreased stool frequency and passage of unformed stools. It is preferred over other opioids because it does not have addictive potential (37). When initial treatment with loperamide fails, cholestyramine is available to empirically treat patients who may have idiopathic malabsorption of bile acid rather than IBS.

Constipation-predominant disease   As discussed previously, bran can be used to increase the intake of dietary fiber. However, calcium polycarbophil, psyllium, and methylcellulose result in less bloating than bran (38).

Osmotic laxatives such as magnesium preparations may be helpful as well. If these initial treatments are not successful, polyethylene glycol (PEG)–based laxatives or cisapride may be used. One to two glasses per day of a PEG-based laxative may be tried. Cisapride has been reported to be helpful in patients with constipation-predominant IBS (39).

Distention-, bloating-, or pain-predominant disease Because IBS has been considered a motility disorder, it seems logical that agents that improve the mechanics of gut motility and decrease disordered muscle contractions would be helpful. With this rationale in mind, antispasmodics and gut smooth-muscle relaxants have been used empirically to treat IBS. Antispasmodic agents that are approved for use in the United States are the anticholinergic agents hyoscyamine and dicyclomine. De-

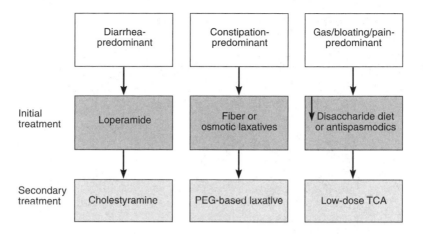

FIGURE 9.6.

Directed pharmacotherapy for initial and secondary therapy of irritable bowel syndrome (IBS). PEG, polyethylene glycol; TCA, tricyclic antidepressant.

spite the fact that these two agents were no better than placebo for the treatment of IBS, they remain in widespread use and may be effective in individual patients. A 1994 meta-analysis (40) found five drugs to be effective in treating abdominal pain, but not bloating or constipation, with no significant adverse reactions: cimetropium bromide, pinaverium bromide, trimebutine, octilium bromide, and mebeverine (40). None of these agents is approved for use in the United States.

Antispasmodics can be used for acute exacerbations of IBS; chronic use may result in rapid declines in efficacy. The use of hyoscyamine and dicylomine in combination with barbiturates or benzodiazepines can result in long-term addiction to the latter substances. Sublingual preparations of hyoscyamine are available and may be used for their rapid onset of action.

Antidepressants

Tricyclic antidepressants have been classically used in IBS because of the high proportion of patients with co-existent depression. A retrospective study done in 1994, however, suggested that they are efficacious in patients without significant psychiatric features. Patients with diarrhea- or bloating-predominant IBS benefitted the most from tricyclic antidepressants, probably related to the neuromodulatory effects of these agents on visceral pain perception. In addition, the effective doses used in IBS were lower than those required for treatment of depression (41). Symptom improvement can be seen in patients within the first 7 to 10 days of treatment. The prescription of a tricyclic antidepressant should be ac-

companied by education for the patient about the neuromodulatory effect of the drug and its use in controlling disease-induced depressive symptoms. Common antidepressants and their doses are listed in Table 9.11.

Patients with concomitant depression require higher doses. Tricyclic antidepressants appear to be less effective for constipation-predominant IBS.

There have been no controlled trials to support the use of selective serotonin reuptake inhibitors in IBS, but anecdotal evidence suggests that they are also effective. They may theoretically be better for constipation-predominant IBS because of their frequent side effect of diarrhea.

Pain Management Centers

Pain management centers provide a comprehensive approach to patients with chronic pain syndromes. This form of therapy should be reserved for patients with severe symptoms that are refractory to other treatments.

REFERRAL

Referrals should be kept to a minimum for patients with IBS, so as to maintain an optimal doctor-patient relationship and minimize doctor shopping. An IBS patient who visits multiple physicians is more likely to undergo repetitive or unnecessary tests that are not necessary once a symptom-based diagnosis is obtained. Those patients for whom initial therapy has failed (as outlined previously) and who continue to have intractable symptoms should be evaluated by a gastroenterologist to pursue further diagnostic procedures as indicated. Referral

		Effects			
Generic Name	Gastrointestinal dose/day	Anticholinergic	Drowsiness	Insomnia	Other
Amitriptyline	10–150	++++	++++	0	—
Clomipramine	25–100	+++	++	++	Good for obsessive-compulsive disorder
Desipramine	10–150	+	+	+	Panic disorder higher doses
Doxepin	10–200	+++	++++	0	disorder
Imipramine	10–150	+++	+++	+	—
Nefazodone	25–100	0	+++	0	—
Trazadone	25–50	0	++++	0	1% priapism

TABLE 9.11. Antidepressants Used in Irritable Bowel Syndrome

to a psychologist or psychiatrist should be considered early for patients with moderate IBS symptoms. In addition, patients with concomitant major depression, somatization, or panic disorder should be referred to a psychiatrist early in the course of treating the disease.

KEY POINTS

- A positive diagnosis of IBS can be made with the use of the Rome criteria.

- Guide diagnostic testing and treatment in accordance with the strategy outlined in Figure 9.3.

- Minimize referrals.

- A therapeutic, trusting doctor-patient relationship is the cornerstone of treatment.

- Classify and treat IBS individually by predominant symptom (diarrhea, constipation, or gas and bloating).

COMMONLY ASKED QUESTIONS

What is irritable bowel syndrome?
It is a common, non–life-threatening disturbance of the bowels. The main symptoms are pain in the abdomen and abnormal bowel movement. People with IBS may experience bloating, diarrhea, constipation, or a combination of these symptoms. Some people also experience a feeling of incomplete emptying after having a bowel movement.

What causes irritable bowel syndrome?
The cause of IBS is not well understood. It may result from abnormal muscle functioning of the intestines. There also seems to be an increased sensitivity to pain in patients with IBS.

Am I going to have problems all my life?
You will probably experience symptoms that come and go correlating with various stresses throughout your life.

How is irritable bowel syndrome diagnosed?
Your physician will do a complete history and physical examination. The diagnosis of IBS can often be made after a careful review of your history. Your doctor may also do blood tests, x-ray studies, or colon tests. Tests on your stools may also be done. These tests are done to look for inflammation, infection, or other abnormalities. The tests may show no visible abnormalities in your intestines. This does not mean there is nothing wrong with your colon. Remember that IBS is abnormal functioning of the bowels.

Do foods affect irritable bowel syndrome?
Some people with IBS have a difficult time eating certain foods, such as fatty foods, alcoholic beverages, and caffeinated beverages. Because different foods affect different people, it is useful for you to keep a food and symptom diary for a few weeks. You can use this to find out which foods worsen your symptoms. Then you can work with your doctor to decide which foods to eliminate from your diet. Most people with IBS seem to have improvement in their symptoms with a low-fat, high-fiber diet.

What treatments are available?
The most important aspect of treatment is determining the situations that seem to worsen symptoms. Keeping a symptom diary and recording situations, diet, and symptoms can help you determine the pattern for your bowel symptoms. Stress management might help. Your doctor may prescribe medications for you to use if your symptoms are moderate to severe. If you have a great deal of diarrhea, the doctor may give you an antidiarrheal medicine. If you have constipation, you may be given a fiber-containing diet or laxative. Your doctor may prescribe an antidepressant medication if you have problems with pain; these types of medicines help block pain from being sensed by the brain. There are some medicines called antispasmodics that may also help with pain; examples are hyoscyamine and dicyclomine.

REFERENCES

1. Drossman DA. U.S. householder survey of functional gastrointestinal disorders. *Dig Dis Sci* 1993;38:1569–1580.

2. Sandler RS. Epidemiology of irritable bowel syndrome in the United States. *Gastroenterology* 1990;99:409–415.

3. Drossman DA. *The functional gastrointestinal disorders.* Boston: Little, Brown, 1994.

4. Manning AP, Thompson WG, Heaton KW, Morris AF. Towards positive diagnosis of the irritable bowel. *Br Med J* 1978;2:653–654.

5. Talley NJ. Diagnostic value of the Manning criteria in irritable bowel syndrome. *Gut* 1990;31:77–81.

6. Kruis W. A diagnostic score for the irritable bowel syndrome. Its value in the exclusion of organic disease. *Gastroenterology* 1984;87:1–7.

7. Whitehead W, Crowell MD. Existence of irritable bowel syndrome supported by factor analysis of symptoms in two community samples. *Gastroenterology* 1990;98:336–340.

8. Jones R, Lydeard S. Irritable bowel syndrome in the general population. *Br Med J* 1992;304:87–90.

9. Thompson WG, Heaton KW. Functional bowel disorders in apparently healthy people. *Gastroenterology* 1980; 79: 283–288.

10. O'Talley NJ. Epidemiology of colonic symptoms and the irritable bowel syndrome. *Gastroenterology* 1991;101: 927–934.

11. Heaton KW, O'Donnell LJD. Symptoms of irritable bowel syndrome in a British urban community: consulters and nonconsulters. *Gastroenterology* 1992;102:1962–1967.

12. Drossman DA. The irritable bowel syndrome: review and a graduated multicomponent treatment approach. *Ann Intern Med* 1992;116:1009–1016.

13. Almy T. Alterations in colonic function in man under stress: experimental production of changes simulating the "irritable colon." *Gastroenterology* 1947;8:616–626.

14. Almy T. Alterations in colonic function in man under stress III: experimental production of sigmoid spasm in patients with spastic constipation. *Gastroenterology* 1949; 22:437–449.

15. Whitehead WE, Engel BT, Schuster MM. Irritable bowel syndrome: physiological and psychological differences between diarrhea-predominant and constipation-predominant patients. *Dig Dis Sci* 1980;25:404–413.

16. Cook IJ. Patients with irritable bowel syndrome have greater pain tolerance than normal subjects. *Gastroenterology* 1987;93:727–733.

17. Klein KB. Approach to the patient with abdominal pain. In: Yamada T, ed. *Textbook of gastroenterology.* Philadelphia: JB Lippincott, 1995:752.

18. Drossman DA. Chronic functional abdominal pain. *Am J Gastroenterol* 1996;91:2270–2281.

19. Oddson E. A secretory epithelium of the small intestine with increased sensitivity to bile acids in irritable bowel syndrome associated with diarrhea. *Scand J Gastroenterol* 1978;13:409–416.

20. Neal KR, Hebden J. Prevalence of gastrointestinal symptoms six months after bacterial gastroenteritis and risk factors for development of the irritable bowel syndrome: postal survey of patients. *Br Med J* 1997;314:7083: 779–782.

21. Drossman DA. Psychosocial aspects of functional gastrointestinal disorders. *Gastroenterol Int* 1995;8:47–90.

22. Walker EA. Irritable bowel syndrome and psychiatric illness. *Am J Psychiatry* 1990;147:565–572.

23. Drossman DA. Sexual and physical abuse in women with functional or organic gastrointestinal disorders. *Ann Intern Med* 1990;113:828–833.

24. Whorwell PJ, McCallum M, Creed FH. Non colonic features of irritable bowel syndrome. *Gut* 1986;27:37–40.

25. Talley NJ, Weaver AL. Onset and disappearance of gastrointestinal symptoms and functional gastrointestinal disorders. *Am J Epidemiol* 1992;136:165–177.

26. Lynn RB, Friedman LS. Irritable bowel syndrome: managing the patient with abdominal pain and altered bowel habits. *Med Clin North Am* 1995;79:373–390.

27. Lynn RB, Friedman LS. Irritable bowel syndrome. *N Engl J Med* 1993;329:1940–1945.

28. Awetchkenbaum JF, Burakoff R. Food allergy and the irritable bowel syndrome. *Am J Gastroenterol* 1988;83: 901–904.

29. Fernandez-Banares F, Esteve-Pardo M. Sugar malabsorption in functional bowel disease: clinical implications. *Am J Gastroenterol* 1993;88:2044–2050.

30. Drossman DA. Diagnosing and treating patients with refractory functional GI disorders. *Ann Intern Med* 1995; 123: 688–697.

31. Drossman DA, Camilleri M. Irritable bowel syndrome: a technical review for practice guideline development. *Gastroenterology* 1997;112:2120–2137.

32. Longsreth, G. Irritable bowel syndrome: diagnosis in the managed care era. *Dig Dis Sci* 1997;42:1105–1111.

33. Lucey MR, Clark ML. Is bran efficacious in irritable bowel syndrome? A double blind placebo controlled crossover study. *Gut* 1987;28:221–226.

34. Cann PA, Read NW. What is the benefit of coarse wheat bran in patients with irritable bowel syndrome? *Gut* 1984; 25:168–173.

35. Talley NJ, Owen BK. Psychological treatments for irritable bowel syndrome: a critique of controlled treatment trials. *Am J Gastroenterol* 1995;91:277–286.

36. Walker EA, Roy-Byrne P, Katon WJ. Irritable bowel syndrome and psychiatric illness. *Am J Psychiatry* 1990; 147:565–572.

37. Cann PA, Read NW. Role of loperamide and placebo in management of IBS. *Dig Dis Sci* 1984;29:239–247.

38. Toskes PP, Connery KL, Ritchey TW. Calcium polycarbophil compared with placebo in IBS. *Dig Dis Sci* 1984; 29:239–247.

39. Van Outryve M, Milo R. Prokinetic treatment of constipation predominant IBS: a placebo controlled study of cisapride. *J Clin Gastroenterol* 1991;13:49–57.

40. Poynard T, Naveau S. Meta-analysis of smooth muscle relaxants in the treatment of IBS. *Aliment Pharmacol Ther* 1994;8:499–510.

41. Clouse RE, Lustman PJ. Antidepressant therapy in 138 patients with irritable bowel syndrome: a five-year clinical experience. *Aliment Pharmacol Ther* 1994;8:409–441.

SUGGESTED READINGS

American Gastroenterological Association Web site. Available at: http://www.gastro.org. (9/21/99).

Drossman DA. The irritable bowel syndrome: review and a graduated multicomponent treatment approach. *Ann Intern Med* 1992;116:1009–1016.

Drossman DA. *The functional gastrointestinal disorders.* Boston: Little, Brown, 1994.

Drossman DA. Irritable bowel syndrome: a technical review for practice guideline development. *Gastroenterology* 1997;112: 2120–2137.

International Foundation for Functional Gastrointestinal Disorders (IFFGD) Web site. Available at: http://www.execpc.com/iffgd/. (9/21/99)

CHAPTER 10

Gastrointestinal Disease in Patients Infected with the Human Immunodeficiency Virus

Daniel J. Skiest and Peter J. Kaplan
University of Texas Southwestern Medical Center, Dallas, Texas 75235

DEFINITION

The management of patients infected with the human immunodeficiency virus (HIV) has changed dramatically in the past few years in the developed world. Since 1995, morbidity and mortality related to the acquired immunodeficiency syndrome (AIDS) have decreased substantially. Much of the improvement can be attributed to the widespread use of combination antiretrovirals, commonly known as highly active antiretroviral therapy (HAART). Other reasons for decreased morbidity include improvements in the prevention and treatment of opportunistic infections and malignancies. As patients live longer and HIV infection comes to be thought of as a chronic disease, primary care physicians are more likely to encounter these patients in their practices.

Gastrointestinal Disorders in HIV-Infected Patients

The gastrointestinal tract is an important target of HIV. Early in disease, HIV may infect various aspects of the gastrointestinal tract directly. The acute retroviral syndrome, which is associated with very high levels of plasma *viremia* and widespread seeding of lymphoid organs, is characterized by fever, pharyngitis, headache, lymphadenopathy, arthralgias, myalgias, and rash. Many patients with this syndrome also have gastrointestinal symptoms including diarrhea, nausea, vomiting, and anorexia. In addition, numerous opportunistic infections and other AIDS-related conditions can affect the gastrointestinal tract.

When evaluating the HIV-infected patient with gastrointestinal symptoms, the physician must be aware of the immunosuppressive state of the patient. Patients who are early in their infection and are without evidence of substantial immunosuppression can be assessed and treated similarly to the patient without HIV infection, because they are unlikely to acquire an opportunistic infection or other AIDS-related condition. The differential diagnosis widens significantly for the immunosuppressed HIV-infected patient—that is, one whose CD4-positive T-lymphocyte count (CD4 count) is less than 200 cells/μL.

Many patients treated with HAART undergo marked increases in the numbers of circulating CD4 cells and reductions in HIV viral load. This has led to fewer opportunistic infections, but, occasionally, unusual manifestations of opportunistic infections may occur. These unusual manifestations of clinical disease are associated with an exuberant inflammatory response caused by HAART-induced "immune reconstitution." Some of these may manifestations involve gastrointestinal pathology that may be encountered by the primary care physician.

Effect of Anti-HIV Medications on the Gastrointestinal System

Studies have shown that HIV replication occurs at very high levels from the onset of infection and continues unabated unless antiretroviral medication is administered. Because destruction of the immune system results from unchecked HIV replication, most experienced clinicians recommend antiretroviral treatment early in disease, long before there is any clinical evidence of immunosuppression. Although patients may benefit from early antiretroviral therapy, they are also exposed to potentially toxic medications with numerous side effects for longer periods.

Antiretroviral medications and medications used for the treatment and prophylaxis of opportunistic infections are important causes of gastrointestinal problems in HIV-infected persons. Three classes of antiretrovirals are currently available. The nucleoside analogues include zidovudine (Retrovir, AZT, ZDV), didanosine (Videx, ddI), zalcitabine (Hivid, ddC), stavudine (Zerit, D4T), lamivudine (Epivir, 3TC), and abacavir (Ziagen). The nonnucleoside reverse transcriptase inhibitors include nevirapine (Viramune), delavirdine (Rescriptor), and efavirenz (Sustiva). The protease inhibitors include saquinavir hard gel capsule (Invirase), saquinavir soft gel capsule (Fortovase), ritonavir (Norvir), indinavir (Crixivan), nelfinavir (Viracept) and amprenavir (Agenerase). Current recommendations are to use three drugs in combination—usually two nucleoside analogues with either a protease inhibitor or a nonnucleoside agent.

Although all of the antiretroviral medications can cause gastrointestinal side effects, the most important offenders are zidovudine (nausea), didanosine (diarrhea and pancreatitis), nelfinavir (diarrhea), ritonavir (nausea and vomiting), saquinavir soft gel capsules (nausea and diarrhea), and amprenavir (nausea and diarrhea). Abacavir causes a severe hypersensitivity reaction in approximately 3% of patients. It is characterized by fever, nausea, vomiting, and malaise with or without a rash. It usually occurs within 4 weeks after initiation of therapy. If abacavir hypersensitivity is suspected, the medication should be stopped immediately, because continued use has occasionally resulted in death. The most common gastrointestinal side effects of the antiretroviral agents are listed in Table 10.1. Other medications used in the treatment of HIV may also cause gastrointestinal side effects, including conventional agents prescribed by treating clinicians and alternative medications, which HIV-infected patients commonly take; these are listed in Table 10.2.

ORAL COMPLICATIONS

Oropharyngeal manifestations of HIV are an important cause of morbidity because of pain and resultant decreased oral intake.

Candida

Infection of the oral cavity with *Candida* species (usually *Candida albicans*) is common in HIV-infected persons and may be the earliest sign of immunosuppression.

Patient presentation

There are four well-recognized forms of oral candidiasis in HIV-infected patients. The most common form is

Major Gastrointestinal Side Effects of Antiretroviral Agents Used for Treatment of HIV Infection	**TABLE 10.1.**

Medication	Side Effect[a]
Abacavir	Hypersensitivity ~3%: nausea, vomiting diarrhea, fever, ± rash
Amprenavir	Nausea, diarrhea
Didanosine	Pancreatitis, diarrhea, increased LFTs
Efavirenz	Increased LFTs
Lamivudine	Pancreatitis (mainly in children)
Stavudine	Increased LFTs, pancreatitis (rare)
Zalcitabine	Oral and esophageal ulcers, pancreatitis, vomiting
Zidovudine	Nausea, vomiting, hepatitis
Delavirdine	None
Nevirapine	Increased LFTs
Indinvavir	Nausea, vomiting, diarrhea, increased indirect bilirubin, hepatitis
Nelfinavir	Nausea, diarrhea
Ritonavir	Nausea, vomiting, diarrhea, hepatitis, altered taste
Saquinavir soft gel capsule (Fortovase)	Nausea, diarrhea, dyspepsia, increased LFTs, abdominal pain
Saquinavir hard gel capsule (Invirase)	Nausea, diarrhea, increased LFTs

LFTs, liver function tests.
[a] The most prominent side effects are listed in bold typeface.

Medication in HIV Infection that are Associated with Gastrointestinal Side Effects	**TABLE 10.2.**

Elevated LFTs	Diarrhea	Pancreatitis
Atovaquone	Didanosine	Didanosine
Azithromycin	Nelfinavir	Zalcitabine
Clarithromycin	Ritonavir	Lamivudine (rare)
Clindamycin	Saquinavir	Stavudine (rare)
Ciprofloxacin	Clarithromycin	Pentamidine
Dapsone	Azithromycin	Trimethoprim-sulfamethoxazole
Delavirdine	Erythromycin	
Didanosine	Itraconazole	
Efaulrenz		
Ethionamide	Quinolone	
Fluconazole	Any antibiotic (*Clostridium difficite*–associated)	
Flucytosine	Abacavir	
Ganciclovir	Amprenavir	
Indinavir		
Itraconazole		
Isoniazid		
Ketoconazole		
Metronidazole		
Nelfinavir		
Nevirapine		
Pentaminide		
Pyrazinamide		
Rifabutin		
Rifampin		
Ritonavir		
Saquinavir		
Sulfadiazine		
Trimethoprim-sulfamethoxazole		
Trimetrexate		
Zidovudine		

LFTs, liver function tests.

pseudomembranous candidiasis (thrush), which manifests as white plaques. The plaques can be scraped off, leaving an erythematous, sometimes bleeding surface. The atrophic (erythematous) form appears as smooth red patches on the tongue and buccal mucosa. Angular cheilitis is an erythematous cracking and fissuring of the corners of the mouth. Finally, a hyperkeratotic form, which cannot be scraped off, can be confused with leukoplakia.

Diagnosis

The diagnosis of oral candidiasis is usually empiric. However, if the diagnosis is unclear, scrapings can be taken and viewed under the microscope after treatment with potassium hydroxide for the presence of hyphae, pseudo-

hyphae, and budding yeast. In addition, fungal cultures can be done. Although *C. albicans* is the most common species implicated, occasionally other *Candida* species may be isolated, either alone or in conjunction with *C. albicans*.

Management

Topical agents should be used initially. These include nystatin oral suspension, clotrimazole troches, and nystatin vaginal tablets.

Systemic therapy should be reserved for those not re-sponding to topical therapy, in order to minimize cost, side effects, drug interactions, and fungal resistance. The mainstay of systemic therapy is the oral azoles. Keto-conazole is active against most *Candida* species that cause oral candidiasis; however, it has limited use in HIV-infected patients because of drug interactions and poor absorption (gastric acid is required for ketoconazole ab-sorption, and HIV-infected patients may have achlor-hydria). Fluconazole, 100 mg per day, is effective and well tolerated and is the most widely used form of sys-temic treatment. Itraconazole, 100 mg twice a day, is also effective, although it may be associated with more drug-drug interactions than fluconazole, and it requires gastric acid for maximal absorption.

Occasionally, severely immunosuppressed patients who have significant fluconazole exposure develop oral candidiasis that is resistant to fluconazole. In these cases, a new formulation of itraconazole (solution), which does not require acid for absorption, may be successful. An oral form of amphotericin B suspension is also avail-able. In cases with complete resistance to the azoles, in-travenous amphotericin B is the treatment of choice.

Aphthous Ulcers

Patient presentation
Recurrent aphthous ulcerations are common in HIV-infected persons. They appear similar to the aphthous ulcers seen in patients with Behçet's disease. They are painful and usually occur on the buccal mucosa but are also found on the tongue, soft palate, tonsillar pillars, and oropharynx. Similar ulcers may occur in the esophagus. They may begin as small (3 mm) ulcers, but often become quite large (up to 1 to 3 cm). There is usually a well-defined base with a yellow central area surrounded by a zone of erythema. They may last from a few weeks to up to 1 month in HIV-infected patients, and they often occur in crops. These ulcerations can be a significant source of morbidity because they result in decreased oral intake.

Cause
The cause of recurrent aphthous ulcers is not known, al-though some researchers have postulated a role for in-flammatory cytokines such as tumor necrosis factor-α (TNF-α); others have suggested that HIV itself is causative.

Diagnosis
Herpetic lesions, caused by herpes simplex virus (HSV), are common in the differential diagnosis. If the diagnosis is in doubt, viral cultures for HSV should be obtained.

Biopsy may occasionally be necessary to exclude other causes of oral ulcerations, such as malignancy, *Histoplasma capsulatum, Cryptococcus neoformans, Geotrichum* spp., *Mycobacterium tuberculosis,* and cytomegalovirus (CMV).

Management
Topical agents   Initial therapy for aphthous ulcers is with topical agents. Triamcinolone acetonide (Orabase) may be combined in a oral solution with various combi-nations of antibiotics (e.g., tetracycline) and an antihist-amine (e.g., diphenhydramine).

Systemic therapy   Large ulcers often do not respond to topical therapy and require systemic treatment with prednisone (40 to 60 mg per day tapered over 4 to 6 weeks) or thalidomide, an inhibitor of TNF-α. The dose of thalidomide used in clinical trials has been 100 to 200 mg per day for 4 to 6 weeks.

Approximately one half to two thirds of patients im-prove with thalidomide; however, the drug has serious toxicities (especially teratogenicity in pregnancy), and its use is regulated closely.

Other Conditions

Gingivitis and periodontal disease
Gingivitis and peridontal disease may be severe in HIV-infected persons. Patients with advanced HIV disease may have a necrotizing gingivitis with severe pain, loss of soft tissue, and bone exposure. Topical and, sometimes, oral antibiotics such as penicillin or clindamycin may be required.

Xerostomia
Xerostomia is a frequent finding in patients with HIV. It may be associated with salivary gland disease or with the sicca syndrome (dry eyes and dry mouth) in some patients. Treatment is symptomatic with saline rinses and salivary substitutes.

Oral hairy leukoplakia
Oral hairy leukoplakia is a benign condition character-ized by painless, white, corrugated lesions on the ante-rior lateral aspect of the tongue. The lesions are thought to be caused by the Epstein-Barr virus. Treatment with acyclovir may be successful, but because lesions recur soon after the medication is discontinued it is not recommended.

Viral infections
HSV is an important cause of recurrent vesicles and ul-cerations in this patient population. Occasionally, CMV or herpes zoster virus can also cause ulcerations.

Treatment of recurrences of HSV-related oral ulcers is accomplished with an oral nucleoside analogue, given for 5 days, such as acyclovir, 400 mg three times a day; valacyclovir, 500 mg twice a day; or famciclovir, 125 mg twice a day.

Cancer

Malignancies of the gastrointestinal tract, including the oral cavity, are commonly encountered in patients with AIDS.

Kaposi's sarcoma This is the most common oral malignancy, and it is commonly associated with the well-recognized cutaneous manifestations. It usually occurs on the palate, although the gingiva and oropharynx can also be involved. Treatment is with intralesional chemotherapy, systemic chemotherapy, radiation, or excision.

Non-Hodgkin's lymphoma This disease, usually a high-grade B-cell lymphoma, may involve the oral cavity, most commonly the gingiva and alveolar ridges. The tonsils may also be involved. Treatment usually consists of systemic chemotherapy.

Squamous cell carcinoma Squamous cell carcinoma of the tongue may be more common in homosexual men with AIDS. Early biopsy of suggestive lesions should be considered.

ESOPHAGEAL COMPLICATIONS

Symptoms of esophageal disease are the second most common gastrointestinal complaint encountered in the patient with AIDS. Up to 40% of such patients may present with esophageal disease during their illness.

Cause

The usual causes of esophageal disease in the HIV-infected patient include, in order of decreasing frequency, *Candida,* CMV, idiopathic (aphthous) ulcers, HSV, and pill-induced disease (Table 10.3). Less common conditions resulting in esophageal pathology are Kaposi's sarcoma, mycobacterial disease including *Mycobacterium avium* complex (MAC) or *M. tuberculosis* infection, non-Hodgkin's lymphoma, histoplasmosis, and gastroesophageal reflux disease (GERD).

Patients may present with more than one cause; specifically, they may have concomitant infection with *Candida* and either CMV or HSV.

Patient Presentation

Typical presentation

The usual symptoms of esophagitis include substernal chest pain, odynophagia, and dysphagia. These symp-

Esophageal Disease in HIV Infection		TABLE 10.3.
Cause	Incidence (%)	Treatment
Candida	50–90	Fluconazole, itraconazole, amphotericin B
Cytomegalovirus	6–16	Ganciclovir or foscarnet
Herpes simplex virus	6–16	Acyclovir
Idiopathic (aphthous)	4–12	Prednisone or thalidomide
Pill-induced disease	?	Stop medication (e.g., zalcitabine, zidovudine)
Gastroesophageal reflux disease	0–4	H₂ blockers, proton pump inhibitors

toms may be accompanied by weight loss, vomiting, and dehydration. Symptoms may be present for several days to weeks.

Candidal infection

Candida accounts for the majority of esophageal disease and may be symptomatic or asymptomatic. Oral candidal infection does not necessarily predict candidal esophagitis. Patients with candidal esophagitis often have oral thrush; however, patients without thrush may have *Candida* involving the esophagus, and patients with noncandidal esophageal disease may have thrush.

Cytomegalovirus esophagitis

Patients with CMV esophagitis, which is the most common cause of esophageal ulcerations, usually present with odynophagia or substernal pain, or both. An esophageal stricture may occur as a complication of longstanding CMV esophagitis.

Herpes simplex virus

HSV accounts for approximately 5% to 15% of esophageal disease. Patients with esophageal ulcers due to HSV may also have oral ulcers. The presentation and findings are similar to those of CMV.

Other

Idiopathic (aphthous) esophageal ulcers manifest similarly to other causes of esophageal ulceration. Patients with GERD may present with burning, chest pain, or dysphagia.

Pill-induced pathology

Medications are occasionally associated with esophageal ulcerations. The nucleoside analogues, zalcitabine (ddC) and zidovudine (ZDV or AZT), have been reported to cause esophageal ulcerations. Other drugs that may occasionally cause esophageal ulcerations include doxycycline, potassium, and nonsteroidal antiinflammatory drugs.

Diagnosis

The approach to the diagnosis of esophageal disease in the patient with HIV infection depends on several factors. An algorithm for the workup of such patients is shown in Figure 10.1.

Initial workup

First, the degree of immunosuppression should be noted. If the CD4 count is higher than 250 cells/µL, significant HIV-related pathology is less likely and other causes should be considered (e.g., GERD, pill-induced esophagitis). If the CD4 count is lower than 200 to 250 cells/µL, an opportunistic illness is more likely and the workup should proceed accordingly.

If thrush is present and the patient is not acutely ill, then a therapeutic trial with a systemic antifungal agent is warranted, because candidal esophagitis is the most likely diagnosis.

Radiographic and endoscopic studies

If there is no response to the therapeutic trial in 1 week, further workup is required.

Radiographic studies (i.e., barium swallow) are not sufficiently sensitive or specific and do not allow the collection of specimens for culture and histopathology. Therefore, they are generally not useful.

Endoscopy is the procedure of choice and should be the initial step if the patient is systemically ill or appears toxic. The characteristic finding of CMV esophagitis on endoscopy or esophagography is a large, solitary ulcer in the middle or distal esophagus, usually with clearly defined margins. However, many patients have multiple ulcers, and any portion of the esophagus can be involved. Occasionally diffuse esophagitis, upper gastrointestinal bleeding, and a distal esophageal mass are found.

Brushings and biopsies should be obtained for definitive diagnosis (multiple biopsies may be required to establish the diagnosis of CMV). Cultures for *Candida*, CMV, and HSV should be done, although some patients with AIDS are CMV-viremic and there may be

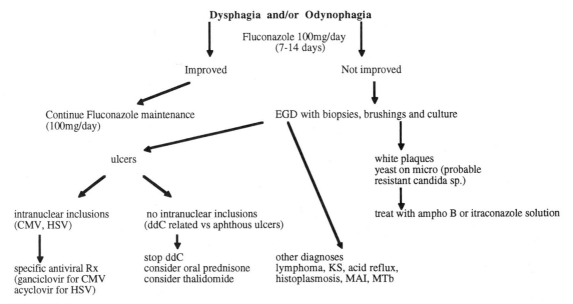

FIGURE 10.1.

Workup for the AIDS patient with esophageal symptoms, ampho B, amphotericin B; CMV, cytomegalovirus; ddC, zalcitabine; EGD, esophagogastroduodenoscopy; HSV, herpes simplex virus; KS, Kaposi's sarcoma; MAI, Mycobacterium avium-intracellulare; MTb, Mycobacterium tuberculosis; Rx, drug.

"blood contamination" of ulcers with CMV, resulting in a false-positive result.

The diagnosis of idiopathic ulceration is made when biopsies fail to demonstrate any histopathologic evidence of a viral cause.

Drug-induced esophagitis may be more likely if the offending medication is taken at bedtime (see Chapter 1).

Management

Treatment

Treatment should be directed at the specific cause (Table 10.3).

Candidal esophagitis   The first-line treatment for candidal esophagitis is fluconazole, 100 mg per day. If there is evidence of fungal resistance, a second-line agent, such as itraconazole solution (100 mg twice per day) or intravenous amphotericin B (0.3 to 0.5 mg/kg per day) can be used. If there is evidence of azole-resistant *Candida* esophagitis, a clinician with expertise in treating HIV-infected patients should be consulted.

Cytomegalovirus   Treatment of CMV is with intravenous ganciclovir, 5 mg/kg every 12 hours, or foscarnet, 90 mg/kg every 12 hours.

Herpes simplex virus   HSV infection can be treated with acyclovir, 400 mg three times a day orally or 5 mg/kg intravenously every 8 hours.

Gastroesophageal reflux disease   If GERD is the main cause, then histamine type 2 (H_2) blockers or proton pump inhibitors can be used; however, use of these medications may result in decreased absorption of concomitant medications used in the treatment of HIV, such as ketoconazole and itraconazole.

Aphthous ulcer   In the case of a negative ulcer biopsy (i.e., aphthous ulcer), treatment with corticosteroids or thalidomide should be given, as discussed previously. Symptomatic treatment may also be needed with oral narcotic analgesics and topical anesthetics, such as viscous lidocaine.

Follow-up

The need for maintenance therapy after induction treatment for *Candida*, CMV, or HSV is somewhat controversial. Although recurrence of symptoms with each of these causes is frequent, continued maintenance therapy with fluconazole, ganciclovir, or acyclovir, respectively, is associated with increased toxicity, cost, inconvenience, and the potential for development of resistance.

Nevertheless, patients with frequent recurrences should probably receive continuous maintenance therapy. Patients with excellent responses to HAART, with increases in CD4 counts and decreases in HIV viral load to levels at or near the limit of detection, may be at lower risk for recurrence and probably do not require lifelong maintenance therapy.

PANCREATITIS

Pancreatic involvement in HIV is relatively common but is often asymptomatic. Hyperamylasemia is common and may be caused by salivary gland disease, macroamylasemia, or pancreatitis.

Cause

The causes of pancreatitis in HIV-infected patients include the usual non-HIV related causes (i.e., gallstones and alcohol) as well as specific HIV-related conditions.

Medication-induced pancreatitis is not uncommon; the most common offending agents are didanosine, zalcitabine, pentamidine, trimethroprim-sulfamethoxazole (TMP-SMX), and, occasionally, stavudine. More recently, the protease inhibitors have been associated with hypertriglyceridemia, a potential cause of pancreatitis.

Opportunistic infections that may occasionally involve the pancreas include CMV, disseminated MAC, *M. tuberculosis*, *Toxoplasma gondii*, *C. neoformans*, extrapulmonary pneumocystis, *Cryptosporidium parvum*, and possibly HIV itself.

AIDS-related malignancies (Kaposi's sarcoma or non-Hodgkin's lymphoma) occasionally involve the pancreas as part of disseminated disease.

Pancreatitis may also occur as part of the AIDS cholangiopathy syndrome (discussed later).

Patient Presentation

The presentation of pacreatitis is similar in patients with or without AIDS (see Chapter 5).

Management

Management of AIDS-related pancreatitis is similar to management in non-AIDS patients (see Chapter 5). HIV-infected patients with pancreatitis may be quite ill and often require hospitalization. Offending medications should be discontinued. The patient should be given nothing by mouth and should receive intravenous hydration and pain medication while a specific cause is sought.

DIARRHEAL ILLNESSES

Diarrhea has been reported to occur in more than half of AIDS patients and is a major source of morbidity. Diarrhea in the HIV-infected patient can be from a myriad of causes, several of which may occur simultaneously.

Diarrhea may be seen in the earliest phase of HIV disease as part of the acute retroviral syndrome. Numerous medications can be associated with diarrhea (Table 10.2); HIV itself can produce a chronic enteropathy, and many opportunistic pathogens may cause a diarrheal illness.

Acute Diarrhea

Cause

For most patients with AIDS and diarrhea, a careful workup will identify at least one pathogen. In one study of 141 AIDS patients with diarrhea who were referred by primary care physicians to a gastroenterologist, 83% had at least one enteric pathogen identified. The most common pathogens detected were microsporidia species, *C. parvum*, CMV, and MAC, and 28% of patients had more than one pathogen identified.

Patient presentation

The history is the most important aspect in the initial evaluation of the HIV-infected patient with diarrhea. Certain aspects of the history are helpful in determining the likelihood of various causes of acute diarrhea and the need for empiric treatment. Important aspects of the history include duration of symptoms, degree of immunocompromise (as measured by the CD4 count), prior opportunistic infections, recent travel history, recent ingestion of antibiotics, presence of hematochezia or pus in the stool, and specific accompanying symptomatology.

An evaluation of all medications (both physician-prescribed and alternative) and diet may reveal a possible cause. A brief avoidance of the suspected etiologic agent may reveal its role. In a patient with a CD4 count consistently higher than 200 cells/µL and no prior opportunistic illnesses, the most likely causes are those endemic to the local community; the workup for such a patient should proceed as for diarrhea in the immunocompetent host (see Chapter 6). Patients with a CD4 lower than 200 cells/µL are susceptible to a multitude of infectious and noninfectious causes of diarrhea, and the workup outlined in Figure 10.2 should be used.

Diagnosis

It is important to distinguish whether the diarrhea is acute or chronic (longer than 2 weeks).

A diagnostic workup limited to the suspected pathogens may be most appropriate and cost-effective. Recent hospitalization or use of antibiotics predisposes to *Clostridium* colitis, whereas recent travel to an underdeveloped country puts the patient at risk for enterotoxigenic strains of *Escherichia coli*, as well as amebiasis. *Campylobacter jejuni* is a frequent cause of diarrhea in HIV-infected patients and often causes invasive disease. An acute dysentery with blood and/or pus in the stool is suggestive of shigellosis or salmonellosis. Patients with HIV infection have a high incidence of invasive disease caused by *Salmonella species*.

Stool samples should be sent for culture and examination for parasites, and an assay for the presence of *C. difficile* toxin should be performed initially. Bacterial blood cultures are indicated for the febrile or toxic-appearing patient because of the high rate of bacteremia due to *Salmonella* species and *Campylobacter* species (see Chapter 6).

Chronic Diarrhea

Chronic diarrhea in AIDS patients causes malnutrition, weight loss, and premature death. Therefore, discovery of its cause and implementation of therapy is important. This is particularly true of the patient who has had one or more prior opportunistic infections or immunocompromise reflected by a CD4 count lower than 200 cells/µL. Detection and differentiation among the many opportunistic protozoa, mycobacteria, fungi, and viruses depend on a systematic approach.

Diagnosis

Some patients with chronic diarrhea have a symptom complex that favors a particular pathogen. For example, a patient with diarrhea, fever and night sweats, abdominal pain, pancytopenia, and elevation of the serum alkaline phosphatase whose CD4 count is less than 50 cells/µL is most likely to have infection with MAC.

Laboratory testing   For the patient who has AIDS and a CD4 nadir of fewer than 200 cells/µL and is clinically stable for outpatient evaluation, a systematic workup of chronic diarrhea includes the following. An initial stool specimen should be collected for culture of *Salmonella*, *Shigella*, and *Campylobacter* and to assay for the presence of *C. difficile* toxin (if there is history of recent antibiotic use). Stool should be examined with specific stains for parasites, including *Isospora*, *Cyclospora*, *Cryptosporidium*, and microsporidia. Cultures for *Mycobacterium* should also be done. Lysis centrifugation (Isolator) blood culture for fungus and mycobacteria are useful in the appropriate circumstances (i.e., when disseminated MAC

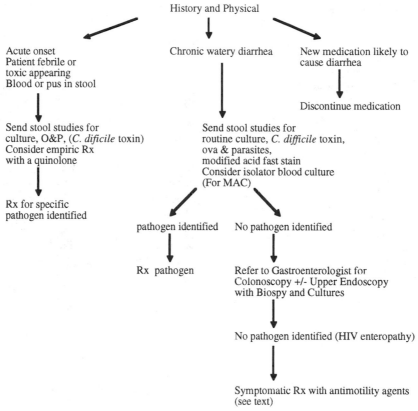

FIGURE 10.2.
Workup for the AIDS patient with diarrhea. C. difficile, Clostridium difficile; HIV, human immuno-deficiency virus; MAC, Mycobacterium avium complex; O&P, ova and parasites; Rx, drug treatment.

is suspected). Up to three stool specimens may be required for the diagnosis of certain pathogens.

It is also important to assess the volume and electrolyte status of the patient with diarrhea.

Radiologic and endoscopic studies If symptoms persist and no cause is identified on the initial workup, referral to a gastroenterologist for endoscopy is indicated.

Radiologic studies, such as upper gastrointestinal studies with small-bowel follow-through and barium enema, may demonstrate abnormalities but are relatively nonspecific and do not identify a specific pathogen.

Generally, full colonoscopy should be done instead of flexible sigmoidoscopy, because certain causes of colitis (e.g., CMV) may be isolated to the right colon. Mucosal biopsies of the duodenum, jejunum, ileum, or colon should be sent for histologic study and for staining and culture for *Mycobacterium, Cyclospora, Cryptosporidium*, microsporidia, and CMV.

Management of diarrhea

Empiric treatment In most instances empiric therapy is best deferred until a specific cause is found. However, if the patient appears toxic and is likely to have an invasive organism such as *Salmonella* or *Shigella*, empiric treatment may be warranted. This usually consists of a quinolone such as ciprofloxacin, 500 mg by mouth twice a day for 10 days. If *C. difficile* colitis is likely, an empiric course of metronidazole may be indicated.

Antimotility agents These agents should be avoided in most cases until the cause of the diarrhea has been determined and treated with specific antimicrobials. However, if no specific cause can be found after a careful workup, then symptomatic treatment with an antidiarrheal agent should be commenced. Luminal agents such as kaolin-pectin, bismuth subsalicylate, cholestyramine, or psyllium may help with mild diarrhea, but for significant diarrhea, symptomatic therapy with an antimotility agent such as loperamide or diphenoxylate is initiated.

Persistent diarrhea   If diarrhea persists, then a narcotic medication such as tincture of opium, paregoric, or codeine can be tried. Octreotide, a somatostatin analogue, has been used to treat chronic, voluminous diarrhea that is refractory to all other agents. In initial small trials, it was moderately successful in controlling diarrhea. A more recent randomized, placebo-controlled trial did not show any benefit, however.

Repletion of both volume and electrolytes can be given orally for mild volume depletion. However, patients with moderate-to-severe dehydration require intravenous rehydration. Occasionally, patients with evidence of malabsorption and severe malnutrition require hyperalimentation.

HIV Enteropathy

Despite a careful workup, no specific cause is found for a significant minority of patients with chronic diarrhea. Some of these patients may have a pathogen that is undetectable by current methods, but many have HIV enteropathy.

Cause

Several mechanisms of enteropathy have been proposed, including HIV infection of the gut, autonomic denervation, lactase deficiency, dysregulation of the enteric immune system, local lymphokine production, and bacterial overgrowth in the small bowel. However, none of these has been definitively proven.

Patient presentation

This syndrome is characterized by chronic diarrhea, accompanied by wasting and malnutrition, in the absence of an identifiable pathogen. Pathologically, villus atrophy with or without crypt hyperplasia is present, resembling the changes resulting from chemotherapy, radiotherapy, celiac disease, or severe malnutrition.

Management

Therapy is directed toward symptom control with antimotility agents and optimization of the antiretroviral regimen. It is important that patients be given this diagnosis only after a thorough workup for treatable pathogens.

Pathogens Unique to HIV-Infected Patients

Mycobacterium avium complex

MAC is an atypical mycobacterial infection that causes disseminated disease in up to 40% of late-stage AIDS patients (CD4 count less than 50 cells/μL). After colonization of the respiratory or gastrointestinal tract, the organism multiplies in the foamy macrophages of the mucosa of the small and large bowel, commonly disseminating hematogenously to the reticuloendothelial system, including the liver, spleen, bone marrow, and lymph nodes.

Patient presentation   The clinical manifestations of disseminated MAC are nonspecific. Commonly, the patient presents with crampy abdominal pain, nonbloody diarrhea, fever, night sweats, nausea, and weight loss. Some patients may have evidence of malabsorption. A subset of patients present with obstructive jaundice due to periportal lymphadenopathy. Findings on physical examination are nonspecific but may reveal hepatosplenomegaly and abdominal tenderness in addition to fever.

Diagnosis   The diagnosis of disseminated MAC is made by culture of the organism from the blood or from another normally sterile site (especially bone marrow). A finding of acid-fast bacilli in the stool supports the diagnosis but is not sufficient in most cases to establish the cause. Therefore, one or more isolator blood cultures (lysis-centrifugation) should be done. The hepatic alkaline phosphatase is often elevated, and a normocytic anemia is common.

Occasionally, other methods are required to make the diagnosis when blood cultures are negative. These include bone marrow biopsy, enteroscopic mucosal biopsy, liver biopsy, and splenic and lymph node aspirates.

Histologic examination of infected tissues usually reveals macrophages with large numbers of acid-fast bacilli. Granulomas, if present, are usually poorly formed, probably because of the patient's poor immune response.

With involvement of the small intestine (especially duodenum), endoscopy may reveal erythema, edema, friability of the mucosa, erosions, and white nodules.

Computed tomographic scans of the abdomen may reveal intraabdominal adenopathy.

Management
Untreated disseminated MAC is associated with substantial morbidity and decreased survival. The mainstay of MAC treatment is a macrolide antibiotic (clarithromycin or azithromycin). A second agent (usually ethambutol) is added to prevent the emergence of resistance. Some authorities would include rifabutin as a third agent; however, this strategy has not been shown to improve outcome, and there are concerns about drug interactions

of rifabutin with the azole antifungal agents and with protease inhibitors. The use of *in vitro* susceptibility testing is not routinely recommended due to lack of standardization. However in selected instances when macrolide resistance is suspected, such testing may be useful. The majority of patients who respond to therapy usually show clinical improvement within 4 to 6 months after beginning appropriate therapy.

In the pre-HAART era, patients with disseminated MAC required lifelong maintenance therapy with the same regimen used initially. It is possible that patients receiving HAART may experience significant "immune reconstitution," sufficient to obviate the need for lifelong maintenance therapy. However, until clinical data are available to support this strategy, patients with MAC infection should receive maintenance therapy.

Cryptosporidiosis

C. parvum, a protozoan, may be found in the stools of 10% to 20% of patients with AIDS and diarrhea. The organism can be acquired from contaminated drinking water, or it can be transmitted by the fecal-oral route.

Patient presentation At CD4 counts near normal, the diarrheal symptoms are generally acute and self-limited to 1 to 3 weeks. Patients with low CD4 counts (less than 100 cells/μl) may present with chronic, watery, nonbloody diarrhea, abdominal cramping, weight loss, anorexia, and malaise. Fever is usually absent or, if present, is of low grade. The organism may be found as a cause of HIV-cholangiopathy and acalculous cholecystitis in some patients (see the later discussion of cholangiopathy).

Diagnosis If the organism is suspected, the initial step should be examination of stool with the modified acid-fast stain, *Cryptosporidium*-specific ELISA, or monoclonal antibody-based immunofluorescent staining. If this is unrevealing, the next step is a biopsy of the colon or, occasionally, biopsy of the small bowel.

Typically, this protozoan is found in the small or large bowel, but it may also be detected in the biliary tract, stomach, esophagus, and pharynx. Organisms are round, 2 to 5 μm in size, and basophilic; they are found in and around the villous crypts.

Management
TREATMENT Treatment is supportive and symptomatic.

Initial anecdotal data suggested that paromomycin, an oral nonabsorbable aminoglycoside, was efficacious. However, a double-blind, placebo-controlled prospective trial did not demonstrate a benefit from paromomycin.

There is anecdotal evidence suggesting that azithromycin or atovaquone may be beneficial. One study reported benefit from a combination therapy with azithromycin and paromomycin.

Some patients with cryptosporidial diarrhea may respond to HAART alone with complete resolution of symptoms.

PREVENTION HIV-infected persons can reduce the risk of waterborne cryptosporidiosis by boiling for 1 minute all water intended for drinking, or by using microstraining filters that can remove particles that are 0.1 to 1.0 mm in size.

Microsporidiosis

Microsporidial disease is caused by one of several species of an obligate-intracellular protozoa, 1 to 2 μm in size. Ninety percent of cases are caused by *Enterocytozoon bieneusi*, and the majority of the rest are caused by *Encephalitozoon (Septata) intestinalis*. In one study of AIDS patients referred to a gastroenterologist for evaluation of chronic diarrhea, microsporidiosis was the most common cause and was found in 39% of patients. *E. intestinalis* is usually disseminated, whereas *E. bieneusi* is usually confined to the gastrointestinal tract. The primary site of infection is the small intestine, with the highest intensity of infection seen in the jejunum.

Patient presentation Typical symptoms include chronic diarrhea, malabsorption, and wasting in an AIDS patient with a cell count lower than 100 cells/μL. Malabsorption may be more common in the patient with microsporidiosis, compared with those infected by other pathogens (e.g., *Cryptosporidium*, MAC, CMV). Other manifestations may include HIV cholangiopathy and distant sites of infection.

Diagnosis The diagnosis of microsporidiosis is difficult because of the small size and poor staining characteristics of the organism. Previously, small-bowel biopsy and analysis of the mucosa by electron microscopy was required. Light microscopy of biopsy material with various staining techniques has also been used. In centers with experience in diagnosing microsporidiosis, concentrated stool can be examined with the modified trichrome stain or the chromotrope B stain.

Management Treatment with albendazole, 400 mg twice a day for 2 to 4 weeks, has been effective in clearing *E. intestinalis* infections. Chronic maintenance therapy may be required to prevent relapses.

No effective treatment is available for *E. bieneusi*, the more common isolate. There are anecdotal reports of response to albendazole, TMP-SMX, thalidomide, pyrimethamine, and metronidazole. Some infections may respond to HAART.

Cyclospora

Cyclospora cayetanensis is a coccidial organism intermediate in size between *Cryptosporidium* and *Isospora belli*. Patients typically have chronic watery diarrhea, crampy abdominal pain, and possibly fever. The clinical syndrome cannot be distinguished from infection with *Cryptosporidium* or *I. belli*. Diagnosis is made by examination of stool with the modified acid-fast stain. Treatment is with TMP-SMX, twice a day for 10 days. Long-term maintenance therapy with TMP-SMX DS three times per week or once a day may be required.

Blastocystis hominis

This organism may frequently be found in the stool of HIV-infected patients with diarrhea; however, the organism has not conclusively been proven to cause diarrhea. It is often found as a copathogen along with organisms known to cause infectious diarrhea, so in most instances, treatment is not recommended. However, in selected instances in which no other pathogen is found after an extensive workup, a trial of metronidazole may be considered.

Giardia lamblia

Infection with this organism is an important cause of diarrhea in HIV-infected patients, especially in homosexual men, in whom oral-anal contact is an important means of transmission. There is no evidence that infection with *G. lamblia* is more severe in HIV-infected persons than in others; however, the usual course of treatment (i.e., metronidazole for 5 days) may be inadequate, and longer courses (10 to 14 days) may be indicated.

Isospora belli

Infection with *I. belli* has been reported to occur in approximately 3% of AIDS patients from the United States and in up to 15% of patients in developing countries. The illness is characterized by watery diarrhea, often with volume depletion. Weight loss, nausea, and abdominal cramping may also be present. The diagnosis of infection with *I. belli* is made by identification of the large oocysts in the stool by the modified acid-fast stain. Treatment is with double-strength TMP-SMX four times daily for 10 days. Chronic suppressive therapy is recommended with either TMP-SMX or sulfadoxine-pyrimethamine (Fansidar), owing to the high rate of relapse.

Amebiasis

Infection with *Entamoeba histolytica* is similar in the HIV-infected and immunocompetent persons. The clinical manifestations of infection with this parasite vary from asymptomatic colonization to self-limited diarrhea to invasive colitis manifesting with bloody diarrhea. Extraintestinal involvement most commonly infects the liver.

Endolimax nana, *Entamoeba coli*, and *Entamoeba hartmanni* are often found in the stool of patients with diarrhea. These organisms are not pathogens and do not require treatment.

Cytomegalovirus

Before the HAART era, CMV disease was diagnosed in 10% to 45% of patients with late-stage AIDS, and some autopsy series documented CMV in up to 90% of patients. Several studies have demonstrated a declining incidence of CMV disease since the advent of HAART. Homosexual men have the highest rates of CMV seroprevalence and disease. CMV disease occurs as a result of reactivation of latent virus in highly immunosuppressed patients. Most patients have a CD4 count of less than 100 cells/µL, usually less than 50 cells/µL.

Patient presentation   After retinitis, the most common manifestation of CMV disease in patients with AIDS is in the gastrointestinal tract. Almost any portion of the gastrointestinal tract may be involved, most commonly the colon and esophagus. Other manifestations include oral ulcerations, gastritis, small-bowel involvement, and HIV cholangiopathy. Occasional manifestations include anorectal ulcerations, hepatitis, pancreatitis, and involvement of the appendix.

The gross appearance of lesions is relatively similar in any portion of the gastrointestinal tract. Ulcerations, erosions, and mucosal hemorrhage are commonly found.

Patients diagnosed with CMV of the gastrointestinal tract should be assessed for retinal involvement by a ophthalmologist experienced in treating HIV-infected patients.

The presentation of CMV esophagitis has already been discussed (see Esophageal Complications).

Patients with gastric involvement may present with epigastric discomfort, nausea, and vomiting and may have ulcerations as seen in patients with esophagitis. Involvement of the small bowel can result in ulcerations, diarrhea, fever, and occasionally perforation.

Patients with colonic involvement may have a relatively insidious presentation, or they may be acutely ill and toxic appearing. Common signs and symptoms include diarrhea (bloody or nonbloody), fever, abdominal pain, nausea, tenesmus, weight loss, and anorexia. Ulcerations are most commonly diffuse and may be complicated by bleeding and, not uncommonly, perforation. Colonic obstruction has also occurred in the setting of CMV colitis.

Diagnosis   The diagnosis of CMV disease requires histopathologic confirmation. Histopathology reveals enlarged cells with intranuclear and intracytoplasmic inclusions. The intranuclear inclusions are often surrounded by a clear halo, the pathognomonic "owl's eye" cell.

Routine histopathology can be aided by other techniques such as immunohistochemistry, in situ hybridization, and in situ polymerase chain reaction of biopsy specimens, although some experts state that a careful search of biopsy specimens for cytomegalic cells is adequate. Viral culture of biopsy specimens may be helpful, but culture have been reported to be positive in some patients without proven CMV disease.

Radiographic findings for luminal CMV involvement are nonspecific; therefore, endoscopy with biopsy of ulcerations or other abnormalities is required for diagnosis. In cases with normal-appearing mucosa, random biopsies should be taken.

In those with suspected CMV colitis, full colonoscopy is recommended: many patients have only right-sided disease, which would be missed by sigmoidoscopy. The endoscopic appearance of CMV colitis is highly variable. It may be localized or diffuse, and in some cases the colon may appear normal.

Serology is not useful because asymptomatic patients with HIV (especially homosexual men) are usually positive for CMV immunoglobulin G antibody.

Management   The treatment of gastrointestinal CMV infection (as well as other causes of diarrhea) is outlined in Table 10.4.

Induction therapy for CMV-related diarrhea should be given for 3 weeks (occasionally longer) with intravenous ganciclovir 5 mg/kg twice a day or foscarnet 90 mg/kg twice a day. A beneficial response is seen in approximately 70% to 80% of patients.

The role of maintenance therapy for patients with gastrointestinal CMV involvement is not as clear as it is for retinitis. In some studies, maintenance therapy did not significantly prolong time to relapse. In addition, both ganciclovir and foscarnet are associated with significant treatment-limiting toxicities and require use of an indwelling central venous catheter. Oral ganciclovir is an attractive option for maintenance therapy, but no trials have been reported. Cidofovir, a nucleotide analogue with a prolonged half-life permitting once-weekly

dosing, has been approved for treatment of CMV retinitis. It may be efficacious for gastrointestinal CMV; however, published data are lacking, and the drug has significant dose-limiting nephrotoxicity.

HEPATOBILIARY COMPLICATIONS

Liver Disease

Liver disease is common in HIV-infected persons. Most AIDS patients have abnormal liver function tests and hepatomegaly, which may result from a myriad of causes in this population.

Cause

The four main categories of liver abnormalities in HIV infection are viral infections, drug-induced changes, opportunistic infections, and opportunistic malignancies. HIV itself may result in hepatomegaly associated with nonspecific histologic changes.

Hepatitis   Hepatitis A is frequently seen in homosexual men, although the clinical manifestations in HIV are not thought to be different from those seen in the normal population.

Because of similar modes of transmission (sexual and parenteral), HIV-seropositive persons are frequently coinfected with hepatitis B virus (HBV) or hepatitis C virus (HCV), or both. HIV-infected patients who acquire HBV are more likely to develop chronic hepatitis than would be the case in the normal population. Conversely, because liver damage in chronic HBV requires intact cell-mediated immunity, patients with AIDS usually have less evidence of hepatic damage and lower transaminase levels than do patients without HIV infection. Cirrhosis may be less common as the degree of immunosuppression increases. Concurrent infection with HBV and hepatitis delta virus may result in fulminant hepatitis.

Concomitant infection with HCV and HIV is especially common among intravenous drug users. Data are conflicting on whether the course of hepatitis C is altered in HIV-infected persons. Some studies have reported an increased likelihood of progression to cirrhosis and liver failure, but other studies have not confirmed this finding.

Other viruses   Other viruses may infect the liver, including CMV, HSV, adenovirus, varicella-zoster virus, Epstein-Barr virus, human herpesvirus 6, although the frequency of clinically significant liver involvement is low.

Treatment of Diarrhea in HIV-Infected Patients

Organism	Therapy
Bacteria	
Campylobacter jejuni	Ciprofloxacin 500 mg PO b.i.d. × 5 days OR erythromycin 250–500 mg q.i.d. for 7–14 days
Clostridium difficile	Metronidazole 250 mg PO q.i.d. × 10 days
Salmonella spp.	Ciprofloxacin 500–750 mg PO b.i.d. × 7–10 days
Shigella spp.	Ciprofloxacin 500–750 mg PO b.i.d. × 7–10 days
Fungi	
Histoplasma capsulatum	Amphotericin B 10–15 mg/kg total dose divided into daily doses of 0.5–1.0 mg/kg followed by maintenance with itraconazole 200 mg PO b.i.d.
Mycobacteria	
Mycobacterium tuberculosis	Three- or four-drug regimen including isonlazid and rifampin
Mycobacterium avium complex	Clarithromycin 500 mg PO b.i.d. + ethambutol 15–20 mg/kg/day indefinitely
Parasites	
Entamoeba histolytica	Metronidazole 750 mg PO t.i.d. × 10 days followed by luminal agent (iodoquinol 650 mg PO t.i.d. × 20 days or paromomycin 500 mg t.i.d. × 7 days)
Giardia lamblia	Metronidazole 250–500 mg PO t.i.d. × 5–10 days
Cyclospora cayetanesis	TMP-SMX 1 DS tablet PO b.i.d. × 10 days followed by maintenance
Isospora belli	TMP-SMX 1 DS tablet PO q.i.d. × 10 days followed by suppression with 1 DS tablet daily or TIW
Microsporidia	
Enterocytozoon bieneusi	No effective treatment
Septata intestinalis	Albendazole 400 mg PO b.i.d. for 2–4 wk
Blastocystis hominis	Treatment usually not indicated
Cryptosporidium parvum	Azithromycin plus paromomycin may be beneficial
Viruses	
Cytomegalovirus	Ganciclovir 5 mg/kg IV b.i.d. × 21 days OR foscarnet 90 mg/kg IV b.i.d. for 21 days; need for maintenance therapy is controversial

TMP-SMX, trimethoprim-sulfamethoxazole; DS, double-strength.

Medications   Medications commonly used to treat HIV and its complications may result in hepatotoxic effects. The most important drugs with hepatotoxic effects are listed in Table 10.2. Other toxins, especially alcohol, should be considered as a cause of liver disease in HIV-infected persons, as should non-HIV related illnesses.

Infections and malignancies   Numerous opportunistic infections and malignancies may involve the liver. Mycobacterial infection, usually by MAC or *M. tuberculosis*, are among the most common causes of granulomatous hepatitis in this patient population. Fungal infections, including *Cryptococcus, H. capsulatum, Candida* spp., and *Coccidioides immitis*, may involve the liver as well.

Infection with *Bartonella henselae* (the agent of bacillary angiomatosis and cat-scratch disease), a gram-negative bacteria, may result in peliosis hepatitis. This condition is characterized by cystic blood-filled spaces in the liver that can be seen on computed tomographic scans. It may manifest with fever, abdominal pain, hepatomegaly, and elevated liver function values.

The most common malignancies involving the liver in AIDS patients are Kaposi's sarcoma and non-Hodgkin's lymphoma. Non-HIV–related illnesses may cause liver disease as well.

Diagnosis

The role of liver biopsy in the workup of the HIV-infected patient with liver abnormalities is controversial.

Most studies have not shown an enhanced yield of liver biopsy over extensive, less invasive testing.

Many of the processes affecting the liver (e.g., MAC, *M. tuberculosis*, lymphoma) involve other organs as well. Therefore, culture of blood, including lysis centrifugation cultures, and culture and biopsy of lymph nodes and/or bone marrow may establish the diagnosis. Likewise, discontinuation of a potentially hepatotoxic medication may result in improvement.

However, if the initial workup is negative, then the patient should be referred for liver biopsy, especially if the alkaline phosphatase level is significantly increased or if there are localized lesions. The yield of liver biopsy has generally been about 50% to 75% in most series, with MAC being the most common diagnosis.

Management

Treatment with interferon has been disappointing for both HBV and HCV infection in this population. Lamivudine, an antiretroviral agent, also has activity against HBV and is often included in the antiretroviral regiments of HIV-HBV coinfected patients. Ribavirin-interferon combinations appear promising for non-HIV–infected persons with HCV, but studies in HCV-HIV coinfected patients are lacking.

The management of liver disease is discussed in Chapter 4.

Biliary Tract Disease

Disease of the biliary tract is usually a late manifestation of HIV disease (CD4 count less than 100 cells/μL) and is caused by infection with an opportunistic pathogen.

Cause

The most common causes are include *Cryptosporidium* spp., CMV, and microsporidia. Less commonly, disseminated MAC, *I. belli*, or malignancy may result in cholangiopathy. In many cases, no specific cause can be found.

Patient presentation

Biliary tract disease in HIV may manifest as acalculous cholecystitis, AIDS-associated sclerosing cholangitis, papillary stenosis (cholangiopathy), or a combination of these.

AIDS-associated sclerosing cholangitis and acalculous cholecystitis may both cause right upper quadrant or epigastric pain and fever. Nausea, vomiting, weight loss, and diarrhea are often present.

Diagnosis

Initially, stool studies should be sent, because the causative pathogen may be identified in stool.

Alkaline phosphatase levels are usually markedly increased (especially in AIDS-associated sclerosing cholangitis), with mildly increased transaminases and a normal to minimally elevated bilirubin value. Right upper quadrant ultrasound may show a dilated gallbladder, with or without wall thickening (acalculous cholecystitis), or dilated intrahepatic or extrahepatic ducts with thickening of ductal walls (AIDS associated sclerosing cholangitis).

The diagnosis of HIV-related cholangiopathy is suggested by the constellation of symptoms, laboratory findings, and radiosonographic findings in a patient with a CD4 count lower than 100 cells/μL.

Lysis centrifugation cultures of blood should be ordered to rule out MAC disease of the liver, which may also manifest with a markedly elevated alkaline phosphatase concentration, fevers, and diarrhea.

If these studies are unrevealing, the patient with these findings should be referred to a gastroenterologist for endoscopic retrograde cholangiopancreatography (ERCP). Even if the ultrasound examination is normal, ERCP should be pursued if there is a high index suspicion for HIV cholangiopathy, because a significant minority of patients with HIV cholangiopathy have a normal ultrasound examination. The ERCP, which is the cornerstone of diagnosis, may reveal sclerosing cholangitis (focal strictures and dilatation of the intrahepatic and extrahepatic ducts) or papillary stenosis, or both. Another pattern that may be seen on ERCP is extrahepatic strictures alone. The gastroenterologist performing the ERCP should obtain tissue for culture and biopsy, bile aspirates, and brushings for cytologic examination.

Management

If a specific cause is found (i.e., MAC or CMV), then treatment should be directed toward the known pathogen. If papillary stenosis is present, sphincterotomy should be performed; this often results in amelioration of pain. Biliary stents may also lead to improvement in some patients. If cholecystitis is present, the patient should be referred to a surgeon for cholecystectomy.

AIDS WASTING SYNDROME

Progressive weight loss is independently associated with death; therefore, identification of reversible causes and aggressive treatment is important.

Cause

The pathogenesis of HIV wasting is probably multifactorial, including reduced food intake during periods of infection or stress, altered lipid metabolism, endocrine abnormalities including low testosterone levels, malabsorption, cytokine effects, and increase in resting energy expenditure.

Patient Presentation

AIDS wasting syndrome is defined as unexplained loss of 10% of premorbid body weight, accompanied by either diarrhea or chronic weakness, with fever greater than 38.3°C (101°F), for longer than 1 month, in the absence of identifiable causes. It is usually seen as a late complication of HIV infection.

Management

Many patients who respond to HAART with a reduction in viral load and a increase in the CD4 count have reversal of weight loss. If there is no reversal in wasting after antiretroviral therapy is started or changed, specific therapy for wasting is indicated.

Therapy is directed at increasing appetite or reversing the catabolic state, or both. Initial therapy is with high-caloric enteral supplements such as Advera or Ensure. Megestrol acetate, 800 mg per day, has been shown to result in increased body weight; however, most of the increased weight is fat, rather than lean body mass. Dronabinol, 2.5 to 5.0 mg twice a day, is effective in stimulating appetite but has not consistently been associated with weight gain. Anabolic agents, including anabolic steroids (available parenterally, transdermally, or orally) and human growth hormone, have produced significant increases in lean body mass, but therapy is costly and weight loss may recur after discontinuation of treatment.

REFERRAL

Evaluation and management of the HIV-infected patient with gastrointestinal symptoms remain challenging for the primary care physician because of the broad differential diagnosis and the wide array of presentations and pathogens. With the advent of HAART, new, previously unrecognized clinical presentations are possible. However, if a careful and methodic approach is taken, most patients can be treated satisfactorily either by their primary care physician or with an appropriate referral to a gastroenterologist.

Patients with symptoms of esophagitis, HIV cholangiopathy, or chronic diarrhea should be referred to a gastroenterologist for evaluation by upper endoscopy, ERCP, or colonoscopy, respectively.

KEY POINTS

- Gastrointestinal symptoms and HIV
  The CD4 count determines the diagnostic possibilities.
  Medications are frequent causes of gastrointestinal symptoms.
  Non-HIV–related problems should be considered.

- AIDS-related diarrhea
  A pathogen can be identified for most patients.
  Any offending medications should be discontinued.
  The workup should include routine culture, tests for ova and parasites (including *Cryptosporidium,* microsporidia, and *Cyclospora*), and isolator culture for MAC.
  If diarrhea is persistent, colonoscopy should be performed.
  Patients with no diagnosis may have HIV enteropathy.
  Symptomatic treatment may be necessary if no pathogen is identified.

COMMONLY ASKED QUESTIONS

Should I stop my HIV medicines if I get sick?

In general, you should not stop your antiretroviral therapy, because inadequate dosing of antiretroviral agents, especially the protease inhibitors, may lead to the development of viral resistance. If an antiretroviral agent is suspected to be the cause of significant diarrhea and symptomatic treatment is ineffectual, then it may be better to stop all antiretrovirals together, rather than retaining only one or two drugs, because of the possibility of development of resistance. The one exception is abacavir (Ziagen). If you develop symptoms of hypersensitivity to abacavir, characterized by fever, nausea, and malaise with or without rash, you should stop this medication immediately and call your doctor.

SUGGESTED READINGS

Bonacini M. Hepatobiliary complications in patients with in human immunodeficiency virus infection. *Am J Med* 1992; 92:404–411.

Coodley GO, Loveless MO, Merrill TM. The HIV wasting syndrome: a review. *J Acquir Immune Defic Syndr* 1994;7:681–694.

Greenspan JS, Greenspan D, Winkler JR. Diagnosis and management of oral manifestations of HIV infection and AIDS. *Infect Dis Clin North Am* 1988;2:373–385.

Jacobson JM, Greenspan JS, Spritzler J, et al. Thalidomide for the treatment of oral aphthous ulcers in patients with human immunodeficiency virus infection. *N Engl J Med* 1997;336: 1487–1493.

Kiviat NB. Human papillomavirus and hepatitis viral infections in human immunodeficiency virus-infected persons. In: Devita VT, Hellman S, Rosenberg SA, eds. *AIDS: biology, diag-*

nosis, treatment and prevention, 4th ed. Philadelphia: Lippincott-Raven Publishers, 1997.

Kotler DP, ed. HIV infection and the gastrointestinal tract. *Gastroenterol Clin North Am* 1997;26:1–455.

Laine L, Bonacini M. Esophageal disease in human immunodeficiency virus infection. *Arch Intern Med* 1994;154: 1577–1582.

Schwartz MS, Brandt LJ. The spectrum of pancreatic disorders in patients with acquired immune deficiency syndrome. *Am J Gastroenterol* 1989;84:459–462.

Smith PD, Quinn TC, Strober W, Janoff EN, Masur H. National Institutes of Health conference: Gastrointestinal infections in AIDS. *Ann Intern Med* 1992;116:63–77.

Wilcox CM. Esophageal disease in the acquired immunodeficiency syndrome: etiology, diagnosis, and management. *Am J Med* 1992;92:412–421.

Wilcox CM, Monkemuller KE. Review article: the therapy of gastrointestinal infections associated with the acquired immunodeficiency syndrome. *Aliment Pharmacol Ther* 1997;11: 425–443.

11
CHAPTER

Diverticulitis

Kevin C. Oeffinger
University of Texas Southwestern Medical Center, Dallas, Texas 75235

DEFINITION

Diverticulosis of the colon is defined as one or more pseudodiverticuli or pouches of mucosa and submucosa that herniate between arcs of circular muscle. Uncomplicated diverticulitis is characterized by inflammation and subsequent peridiverticular infection of one or more diverticuli. Complicated diverticulitis is diverticulitis with large or distant abscess, free perforation, obstruction, fistula, or recurrence.

CAUSE

Diverticulosis is often referred to as a disease of the 20th century, a byproduct of industrialization, and it is the most common disease of the colon in the United States. Its epidemiology has been well characterized by several investigators, most notably N.S. Painter, who in

the 1960s hypothesized that a lack of dietary intake of fiber leads to the development of diverticulosis. In areas where the typical diet is still high in fiber, diverticulosis is uncommon.

There does not appear to be a familial predisposition in the development of diverticulosis.

COURSE OF DISEASE

Data from prospective studies suggest that between 10% to 25% of adults with diverticulosis progress to diverticulitis. Roughly 2% of adults with diverticulosis develop a complication each year. The incidence of diverticulitis in persons with diverticulosis increases with time. In patients with confirmed diverticulosis, diverticulitis developed in 10% by 5 years, 25% by 10 years, and 35% by 20 years. The average age at onset of diverticulitis is between 60 and 70 years. The age of presentation of diverticulitis is the same regardless of whether a few or many diverticula are present.

Diverticulosis

The number of diverticuli does not seem to increase significantly over time; therefore, a person with few diverticuli does not progress to have many diverticuli over the course of years. The prevalence of diverticulosis increases with age, approximated in the U.S. population based on autopsy specimens and barium enema studies (Table 11.1).

On gross examination, patients with diverticulosis have thicker taenia and circular muscle with a reduced luminal diameter. Whiteway and Morson described the microscopic progression of disease. As the colon ages, the amount of elastin increases along with a thickening of the colon wall. In patients with diverticulosis, the elastin content is markedly increased, and there is an alteration in the normal fascicular pattern of elastin fibers. The resulting dense mesh of fibers prevents the fasciculi from moving apart during relaxation of the muscle. These inelastic bundles lead to segments of intraluminal contraction and obstruction, resulting in a localized increase in intraluminal pressure, especially postprandially. A pulsion phenomenon occurs secondary to the increased pressure in the shortened and inelastic segments, weakening the bowel wall. The pressure follows the path of least resistance and projects through the area penetrated by the nutrient blood vessels that supply the mucous membrane. This process

Fraction of adult population (%)	Age (yr)
33	>45
50	>60
6	>85

TABLE 11.1. Prevalence of Diverticulosis by Age

results in a pseudodiverticulum: a pouch lined with mucosa, devoid of muscle fibers, that protrudes between the circular muscle layers (Fig. 11.1).

The sigmoid colon is the primary site; this is thought to be related to the smaller lumen diameter in the sigmoid colon, compared with the transverse and ascending colon. Typically, diverticuli are arranged in two longitudinal rows between the mesenteric and the antimesenteric taenia. Occasionally, a third row is found between antimesenteric taenia.

Diverticulitis

With slower transit times in the affected bowel and increased localized intraluminal pressure, an inspissated fecalith can wedge into a diverticulum. Because the diverticulum has lost its muscular layer, it cannot expel the fecalith. This situation leads to focal inflammation and, eventually, to necrosis and erosion of the mucosa. As the diverticulum perforates, fecal material extravasates into

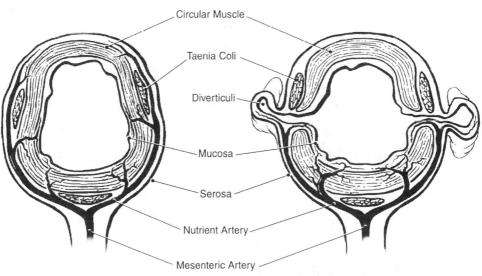

FIGURE 11.1.
An illustration of the pathogenesis of diverticulosis is presented.

the adjacent fat and mesentery, causing a peridiverticulitis. Depending on the size and location of the area involved, the perforation can result in a phlegmon (localized inflammation in the pericolic fat), a small pericolic abscess, a larger pericolic or mesocolic abscess, a distant abscess, or a pneumoperitoneum (free perforation into the peritoneum). Recurrent inflammation and infection may lead to formation of a fistula, as tracts are formed from the colon to nearby structures such as the bladder. Inflammation, either acute or chronic, can lead to a partial or total obstruction of the affected segment of colon.

PATIENT PRESENTATION

Acute diverticulitis is a clinical diagnosis and presumes the presence of diverticuli and the absence of other causes for regional infection or inflammation. The classic triad of presenting signs in a patient with acute diverticulitis consists of left lower quandrant tenderness, fever, and leukocytosis (Table 11.2). Patients generally develop left lower quadrant pain that is relatively abrupt in onset, colicky, or intermittent in character, without radiation, and unrelated to eating or activity. The pain may become continuous. Studies show a greatly varying presence of fever, ranging from half to all patients with acute diverticulitis. Nausea and vomiting are usually seen in sicker patients; they often have some element of obstruction. Patients with acute diverticulitis affecting the sigmoid colon adjacent to the bladder or with the presence of a colovesical fistula may complain of dysuria and urinary frequency.

The mean duration of symptoms before presentation for patients with acute diverticulitis is 48 hours (range, 1 hour to 80 days). Patients experiencing a free perforation generally have a much shorter duration of symptoms before presentation, but the symptoms may be prolonged in patients with a smaller perforation.

A grading system of the degree of perforation was devised by Hinchey and colleagues and is presented in Table 11.3.

Typically, patients with a complication of diverticulitis have either more pronounced or additional symptoms and signs. A patient with a larger abscess usually exhibits more systemic signs and symptoms and may have a palpable, tender mass. An individual with a pneumoperitoneum presents with sudden, severe abdominal pain, peritoneal signs, and, often, hypotension or septic shock. Obstruction secondary to diverticulitis is usually manifested by symptoms of nausea, vomiting, abdominal distention, and obstipation.

A fistula usually causes passage of colon air and feces through the fistula to the affected structure. For example, a patient with a colovesical fistula often notes pneumaturia or fecaluria; with a colovaginal fistula, a vaginal discharge with feces and gas is observed. The patient with a colocutaneous fistula often notes subcutaneous emphysema and soft-tissue infection.

In the United States, 90% to 95% of adults with diverticulosis have involvement of the sigmoid colon. An estimated 45% to 65% of persons have only sigmoid involvement. Diverticulosis of the right colon affects fewer than 10% of adults with diverticulosis in the United States. In contrast, 70% of persons with diverticulosis in Asian countries, notably Japan, have involvement of the right colon. The reasons for this difference are not well understood.

Patients 40 Years of Age or Younger

About 10% to 20% of patients with diverticulitis are younger than 40 years of age. The course of disease was previously thought to be more virulent in this patient group, but it is now recognized that the clinical presentation in younger patients is no different from that in patients older than 40 years of age. However, because of the lack of recognition of diverticulitis in this group,

---

TABLE 11.2.   **Frequency of Symptoms in Diverticulitis**

Sign or symptom	Frequency in presentation (%)
Pain in the left lower quadrant	93–100
Fever	57–100
Leukocytosis	58–83
Nausea	20
Fixed, tender mass in the left lower quadrant	20
Urinary symptoms	10

TABLE 11.3.   **Hinchey Grading System for Perforation of the Diverticulum**

Stage	Type of perforation
I	Diverticulitis associated with pericolic abscess
II	Diverticulitis associated with distant abscess
III	Diverticulitis associated with purulent peritonitis
IV	Diverticulitis associated with fecal peritonitis

younger patients often have a longer delay in diagnosis and a higher rate of surgical intervention.

Elderly or Immunocompromised Patients

Elderly and immunocompromised patients who develop diverticulitis often lack the typical signs and symptoms. The pain often does not localize to the left lower quadrant and may be absent. Fever and leukocytosis are often absent in these two groups of patients.

Patients with Right-Sided Diverticulitis

Patients with diverticulitis involving the right colon present with pain and tenderness in the right lower quadrant, rather than in the left lower quadrant. Otherwise, presenting symptoms and signs are similar to those seen in left-sided disease.

DIAGNOSIS

Laboratory Tests

If acute diverticulitis is suspected, a few laboratory tests can help make the diagnosis.

Complete blood count
A complete blood count (CBC) with differential should be ordered for all patients with suspected diverticulitis. In the majority of immunocompetent patients, a mild leukocytosis with a left shift is detected, although a normal CBC does not rule out diverticulitis. This is especially true for the elderly or the immunocompromised patient.

Urinalysis
The urinalysis may be abnormal, with the presence of white or red blood cells if the area of sigmoid colon involved is near the bladder. If bacteriuria is found, a colovesical fistula should be considered.

Other laboratory tests
Blood cultures should be obtained before parenteral antibiotic therapy is instituted. The erythrocyte sedimentation rate and C-reactive protein concentration are nonspecific and generally are not helpful in the evaluation.

Radiologic and Endoscopic Studies
Supine, upright, and lateral decubitus views of the abdomen
Plain films of the abdomen can help in the evaluation of a patient with signs and symptoms suggestive of acute diverticulitis. In a patient with acute diverticulitis, gas in

the bowel wall (or pneumatosis cystoides intestinalis) may be seen. If there is any question that the patient may have acute diverticulitis with a free perforation, evaluation with supine and upright (or lateral) views is essential. Free air within the peritoneal cavity can be seen as air under the diaphragm with an upright view or as air under the abdominal wall with a lateral view.

Free air can also be seen on a supine film, manifested by delineation of both the outer and inner wall of the bowel (Rigler's sign); an inverted "V" sign overlying the sacrum, representing air outlining the lateral umbilical ligament; delineation of the falciform ligament; and triangular-shaped collections of free air between loops of adjacent bowel.

Further studies
If the clinical presentation is consistent with acute diverticulitis and if systemic signs or symptoms of a complication of diverticulitis (obstruction, free perforation, or abscess or fistula formation) are absent, then further radiographs are unwarranted in the acute period and the patient can receive initial medical treatment. However, if either the diagnosis is in question or a complication is suspected, further evaluation with radiographic studies is important.

If the diagnosis is uncertain, three radiographic studies (contrast enema, computed tomographic [CT] scanning, and ultrasonography) or endoscopy may help. Selection and timing of tests are in part based on the availability and feasibility of the test and the physician's preference or expertise.

Although the question of which radiographic test should be ordered has generated much controversy, there are few prospective studies with adequate power to answer the question definitively. Nevertheless, CT scanning of the abdomen is generally considered to be superior, although perhaps the most important criterion in deciding which test to order is the expertise and experience of the imaging center in performing and interpreting the different tests. Tests can complement each other, and it is common to use two of the tests. The advantages and disadvantages of each are discussed below.

Computed tomographic scan From the findings of the few prospective studies that have been published, a CT scan of the abdomen is the preferred study when the diagnosis is in question and the patient is fairly ill. CT is particularly useful in revealing extracolonic disease and may stratify patients at risk for secondary complications. In three prospective studies, the specificity for diagnosis of acute diverticulitis was 100%, and the sensitivity ranged from 69% to 90%. A major advantage of the CT is its ability to identify both subtle changes suggestive of diverticulitis and extracolonic disease in a relatively noninvasive way. CT is especially preferred for patients who are very ill or are atypical in presentation. Also, a CT helps to distinguish right-sided diverticulitis from appendicitis.

Findings on a CT scan of the abdomen that are suggestive or positive for diverticulitis include infiltration or inflammation of pericolic fat (Fig. 11.2); colonic-wall thickening greater than 4 mm (Fig. 11.3); soft-tissue stranding; intraluminal gas (Fig. 11.3); diverticula; pericolic or distant abscess; extraluminal air; intramural sinus tracks; air in bladder (Fig. 11.4); and phlegmon or abscess (Fig. 11.4).

Contrast enema   If the diagnosis of acute diverticulitis is uncertain, a contrast enema may be indicated. Evaluation with a a contrast enema is less specific as a diagnostic test than is the CT scan of the abdomen, but it is more sensitive in finding changes. The contrast enema is probably best suited for the patient with early, milder disease or in whom obstruction is suspected. The main limitation of this test is the high rate of false-negative results (i.e., those in which disease is present but the contrast enema is unremarkable).

If used, the contrast enema must be single-contrast, without the addition of air, to avoid further distention of the colon. The use of barium as the contrast material should be avoided, because leakage through an undiagnosed free perforation may result in a severe peritonitis. Instead, a water-soluble contrast material, such as meglumine diatrizoate mixed with sodium diatrizoate (Gastrograffin) should be used. Because barium provides better contrast and mucosal detail, some institutions still use a gentle, single-contrast barium study in patients without evidence of pneumoperitoneum or peritonitis. Contrast enemas are particularly useful if obstruction secondary to acute diverticulitis is suspected.

Findings on contrast enema that are suggestive or positive for diverticulitis include segmental narrowing with thickening and tethering of the mucosa; "double tracking" of contrast material in the inflamed bowel wall, with the contrast agent extending along a longitudinal track in the submucosa (Fig. 11.5); marked irregularity with longitudinal strictures or obstruction; mural or extraluminal extravasation of contrast material; and sinus tract or fistula.

Ultrasound   Effective use of ultrasound depends on the hospital or institution and the examiner. Ultrasound can assist in the diagnosis of acute diverticulitis, but it is better suited for patients with suspected abscess. In one prospective study, the sensitivity of ultrasound in diagnosing acute diverticulitis was 84%, with a specificity of 80%; the false-negative rate was high, 15%.

Findings on ultrasound of the abdomen that are suggestive or positive for diverticulitis include focal-wall thickening (greater than 4 mm); pericolic-fat inflammation; intramural or pericolic mass; intramural fistula; and abscess.

Lower endoscopy   Generally, flexible sigmoidoscopy and colonoscopy are not recommended in the acute phase of diverticulitis. Insufflation with air can lead to an in-

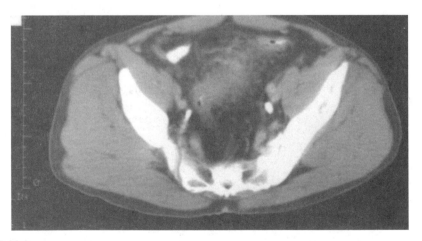

FIGURE 11.2.
Computed tomographic scan of the abdomen shows significant pericolic fat infiltration and inflammation in a patient with acute diverticulitis.

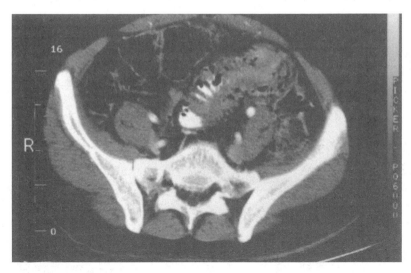

FIGURE 11.3.
Computed tomographic scan of abdomen shows intramural air with marked thickening of the colonic wall in a patient with acute diverticulitis.

creased localized intraluminal pressure and result in perforation. Carbon dioxide can be used as an alternate source of air for insufflation and is more quickly absorbed with a lower risk for perforation. If a physician has particular expertise and experience with endoscopy in patients with acute diverticulitis, endoscopic evaluation can aid in diagnosis while ruling out other potential causes of pain in the left lower quadrant.

There are two situations in which endoscopy may be preferred. In the patient with suspected sigmoid volvulus, endoscopy can be both diagnostic and therapeutic. Endoscopy is useful in evaluating a patient who has weight loss and progressive constipation and develops obstruction and left lower quadrant pain. Additionally, endoscopy may be helpful in identifying patients with inflammatory or ischemic bowel disease.

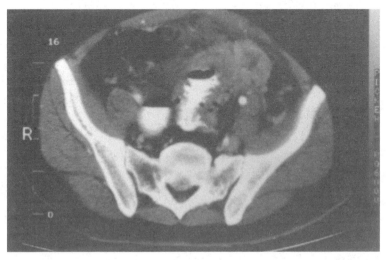

FIGURE 11.4.
Computed tomographic scan of abdomen shows air-fluid level in the bladder and phlegmon (thin arrow) in a patient with diverticulitis and a colovesical fistula.

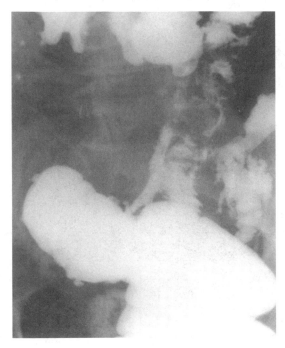

FIGURE 11.5.
Contrast enema shows "double tracking" of contrast material in the inflamed bowel wall (arrows) in a patient with acute diverticulitis.

Colonoscopy is superior to CT scanning for diagnosis of colon carcinoma.

The primary role of endoscopy is in the follow-up of patients with acute diverticulitis, as discussed later.

Differential Diagnosis

The diagnosis is straightforward in most patients who present with acute diverticulitis. However, as with many acute processes of the abdomen, other conditions must be considered.

Uncomplicated acute diverticulitis

Irritable bowel syndrome   In this syndrome patients may have left lower quadrant pain, but they do not have fever or leukocytosis and are generally younger.

Ischemic colitis   Ischemic colitis and acute diverticulitis occur in similar age groups, although persons with ischemic bowel disease often have diffuse, less localized abdominal pain and pass a large, bloody stool with the onset of pain. If uncertainty exists and ischemic colitis is suspected, colonoscopy usually distinguishes the two diseases. If uncertainty of diagnosis persists, patients with ischemic colitis can be identified

by CT scanning, which often reveals edematous or bloody bowel wall.

Other potential causes of left lower quadrant pain   Other causes that are less commonly confused with acute diverticulitis include herpes zoster, psoas abscess, ovarian abscess, torsion of the ovary, ectopic pregnancy, salpingitis, and ureterolithiasis.

Diverticulitis with obstruction

Adenocarcinoma of the colon   Usually, patients with obstruction secondary to malignancy have a history of weight loss and progressive constipation or a change in the caliber of stool. If a left lower quadrant mass is palpable on examination, it is usually tender with diverticulitis and nontender with colon cancer. Persons with colon cancer may also have a microcytic, hypochromic anemia secondary to iron loss. If the diagnosis is uncertain at presentation, a water-soluble single-contrast enema or colonoscopy/sigmoidoscopy without insufflation can be helpful.

Volvulus of the sigmoid   Sigmoid volvulus usually occurs in the sixth or seventh decade of life. Patients typically present with sudden onset of nausea, vomiting, obstipation, and colicky abdominal pain that may be more prominent in the left lower quadrant. Fever, hypotension, and sepsis may develop if gangrenous changes occur. Changes on plain-film radiographs are characteristic in patients with sigmoid volvulus; it usually is not difficult to distinguish the two diseases. Contrast enema can help if the diagnosis is in question. Lower endoscopy can be both diagnostic and therapeutic.

Diverticulitis with fistula

Crohn's disease   A patient with a single or recurrent episodes of acute diverticulitis may develop a fistula and needs to be distinguished from patients with Crohn's disease. If a patient with Crohn's disease develops a fistula, anorectal disease (rectal fissure, perirectal abscess, or cutaneous fistula) is usually present on examination. This is an uncommon site for a fistula tract associated with diverticulitis. Likewise, colovesical fistula is the most common site in diverticulitis but is fairly uncommon in patients with Crohn's disease. Colonoscopy or contrast enema is diagnostic in patients with Crohn's disease, but in patients with diverticulitis it generally shows other extracolonic disease, such as abscess formation.

Ulcerative colitis   Patients with ulcerative colitis uncommonly present with fistulas; however, ulcerative colitis and diverticulitis rarely coexist.

Summary of Diagnosis

- Uncomplicated diverticulitis
  Pain in the left lower quadrant
  Fever
  Leukocytosis
- Complicated diverticulitis
  Large, multiple, or distant abscesses
      Generally "sicker" patients, often with
        systemic signs and symptoms
      Pericolic abscess may be palpable as a tender
        mass in the lower left quadrant
      Abscesses visualized on CT scan of abdomen
  Pneumoperitoneum
      Abrupt, severe abdominal pain with
        peritoneal signs
      Clinical presentation and plain films of the
        abdomen are usually diagnostic
  Obstruction
      Signs and symptoms of acute diverticulitis
      Obstipation, abdominal distention, and
        decreased or absent flatus
      Diagnostic studies include contrast enema or
        colonoscopy
- Fistula
      Colovesical fistula: pneumaturia and pyuria
      Colovaginal fistula: feculent vaginal discharge
        with air bubbles
      Colocutaneous fistula: subcutaneous air and
        soft-tissue infection
      Diagnostic studies: CT scan of abdomen or
        contrast enema

Diverticulitis with pneumoperitoneum

Several underlying diseases can result in a perforation of the colon and subsequent peritonitis. Pneumoperitoneum is a surgical emergency, and the underlying cause is usually determined at the time of surgery. Perforation may occur secondary to obstruction; therefore, the causes already described should be considered if there is a history of obstructive symptoms. If the perforation is spontaneous, inflammatory and vascular conditions should be considered, including Crohn's disease, ulcerative colitis, ischemic colitis, sigmoid volvulus, and adenocarcinoma of the colon.

Diverticulitis in right colon

The most common preoperative diagnosis for patients with right-sided diverticulitis is acute appendicitis. Both groups present with right lower quadrant pain and progress to peritoneal signs. Patients with right-sided diverticulitis tend to be older and have less nausea and vomiting than do those with appendicitis.

Diverticulitis in the elderly or mmunocompromised

As with other abdominal diseases, diverticulitis can be very difficult to diagnose in elderly or immunocompromised patients, necessitating a high index of suspicion on the part of the physician. Often these two populations of patients have a more rapid progression of illness, less localizing pain, and a normal CBC. For this reason, further radiographic studies (e.g., CT, contrast enema) and early surgical intervention are often warranted.

MANAGEMENT

The overall mortality rate of patients with diverticulitis is 5%. Patients with acute diverticulitis have a mortality rate of 1.3%, whereas those with diverticulitis who undergo surgery for a complication have a mortality rate of 18%. These high rates reflect the age of the patient population at risk for diverticulitis, compounded by the frequent comorbid medical conditions. Risk factors for an increased mortality rate include a concurrent medical illness, shock on admission, and an American Society of Anesthesiologists' Physical Status Classification of 3 or higher (patient with a severe systemic disease that limits activity but is not incapacitating).

Treatment

The Hinchey grading system is useful in the management of diverticulitis.

Outpatient medical management

In selected patients, diverticulitis can be successfully treated with outpatient management and close follow-up. Generally, these are patients with a phlegmon who present early in the course of illness. To date, there are no published data concerning the percentages of cases in which resolution is achieved with outpatient treatment. Accepted criteria for outpatient management include the following:

    Milder clinical presentation without systemic or
      peritoneal signs or symptoms
    Patient with a high likelihood of response (excludes
      elderly and immunocompromised persons)
    Reliable and compliant patient

Patient who can take fluids and medications by mouth
Patient who can return for frequent follow-up visits

Patients should be prescribed bowel rest with clear liquids until the pain has resolved, followed by a slow progression of the diet. A broad-spectrum antibiotic that covers gram-negative enteric aerobes, combined with an antibiotic effective against anaerobic organisms, is recommended for 7 to 10 days of therapy. Choices include ampicillin, trimethoprim-sulfamethoxazole (Bactrim), or ciprofloxacin (Cipro) in combination with metronidazole (Flagyl) or clindamycin (Cleocin). The newer quinolones, such as levofloxacin (Levaquin) have moderate anaerobic coverage and may become an option for single antibiotic therapy. The patient should be instructed to call or go to the emergency department for any increase in fever or abdominal pain or inability to drink fluids, and follow-up should occur within 24 to 36 hours. If the patient does not improve within 48 hours, hospitalization for parenteral antibiotic therapy and further evaluation is warranted.

Inpatient medical management

Eighty-five percent of hospitalized patients with their first episode of Hinchey stage I acute diverticulitis respond to medical therapy. Patients should be placed at bowel rest and rehydrated intravenously. As the patient improves, clear liquids can be started and slowly advanced to a low-residue diet. Morphine should not be used as an analgesic because it can cause an increase in intraluminal pressure.

Mild-to-moderate disease In community-based episodes of uncomplicated diverticulitis, infection is usually with normal bowel flora, so parenteral antibiotic therapy should be directed to cover gram-negative enteric organisms such as *Escherichia coli* and anaerobes such as *Bacteroides fragilis*. In mild-to-moderate community-acquired infections, monotherapy has been shown to be as effective as an aminoglycoside in combination with clindamycin. Recommended choices include cefoxitin, cefotetan, and ticarcillin–clavulanic acid. The choice should be based on local resistance patterns and formulary options that generally provide a lower cost.

In the past, patients with acute diverticulitis were treated for 10 to 14 days. However, no change in outcomes was seen with a much shorter duration of therapy in randomized clinical trials. Patients with mild-to-moderate infections should be treated with a parenteral antibiotic until the bowel is functioning and any associated ileus has resolved, usually 4 to 5 days, and then changed to an oral route for 5 to 7 days.

Severe disease In severe infections, *Enterococcus* and *Pseudomonas aeruginosa* must be considered. These organisms are more commonly encountered in elderly, debilitated patients and in those with a nosocomial or postoperative infection. Recommended antibiotic choices include a β-lactam antibiotic combined with a β-lactamase inhibitor, a carbapenem, or a combination therapy that includes an antibiotic effective against the gram-negative enterics and *Enterococcus* plus an antibiotic that is effective against enteric anaerobes. Clinical trials have shown the following combinations to be effective: ciprofloxacin with metronidazole, aztreonam with clindamycin, and aminoglycoside with clindamycin. Aminoglycosides have been shown to be more effective in abdominal infections when administered on a once-daily schedule, as opposed to three times a day. Because of the potential for renal toxicity, aminoglycosides should be avoided in elderly, critically ill patients and in those with renal insufficiency.

Recommendations for severe infection include a β-lactam/lactamase inhibitor, piperacillin/tazobactam (Zosyn), ampicillin/sulbactam (Unasyn), carbapenem, imipenem/cilastatin (Primaxin), combination therapy, ciprofloxacin (Cipro) combined with metronidazole (Flagyl), aztreonam (Azactam) combined with clindamycin (Cleocin), and an aminoglycoside combined with clindamycin (Cleocin). The choice of antibiotic is based in part on local resistance patterns of suspected pathogens and in part on the availability and cost of the antibiotic. As with mild-to-moderate infections, the duration of therapy depends on clinical response and return to normal bowel function and is usually 4 to 5 days. Oral administration of antibiotic can then be instituted. Because of the ease of changing to the same antibiotic in oral form, ciprofloxacin plus metronidazole are a popular combination.

Computed tomography–guided percutaneous drainage

Patients with Hinchey stage I or II disease (Table 11.3) and a large intraabdominal abscess that is near the abdominal wall are often amenable to CT-guided percutaneous drainage and parenteral antibiotics, with a success rate of 70% to 90%. Selection of patients for percutaneous drainage depends on location of the abscess. Drainage of deep or inaccessible abscesses is contraindicated.

Surgical treatment

Surgery is required by 20% and 30% of patients with diverticulitis who are admitted to a hospital, including acute cases with or without complications and recurrence.

Surgery is indicated for patients whose condition is unresponsive to medical therapy or CT-guided percutaneous drainage. It is also indicated in patients with intra-abdominal, pelvic, or multiple abscesses (Hinchey stage II); obstruction; pneumoperitoneum (Hinchey stages III and IV); fistula; or recurrent disease. Additionally, surgical intervention should be considered if there is a high index of suspicion of cancer or if that possibility cannot be excluded.

The Standards Task Force of the American Society of Colon and Rectal Surgeons recommends a primary sigmoid resection with anastomosis for patients who meet criteria for a safe anastomosis: adequate bowel preparation, healthy bowel, adequate blood supply, and no tension on the anastomosis. Most patients with Hinchey stage I or II disease that fails to respond to parenteral antibiotic therapy or that is unamenable to or does not respond to CT-guided percutaneous drainage can be surgically treated with a single-stage primary anastomosis.

Patients with a free perforation and Hinchey stage III or IV disease and most patients with large-bowel obstruction require emergency surgical intervention, fluid resuscitation, and parenteral antibiotics. A two-stage Hartmann's resection procedure is performed. In the first stage the affected segment is resected, an end-colostomy is performed, and a Hartmann's pouch is created. Re-anastomosis is performed 6 to 8 weeks later.

Patients with a diverticular fistula should have resection of the diseased segment of colon and repair of the affected organ. A primary resection and anastomosis can be performed in most patients.

Patients with a second episode of Hinchey stage I or II diverticulitis should undergo elective primary resection. After the first episode, a patient has a 40% to 45% chance of recurrence, and the likelihood of recurrence increases with each episode. Only 6% of patients with a third episode respond to medical management, so surgery is recommended after the second episode. In the past, patients who were 40 years of age or younger were treated with surgical intervention after the first episode because it was thought that their rate of recurrence was higher and their response rate to medical therapy lower. More recent studies suggest that younger patients respond the same as older patients, and surgical intervention can be postponed until after the second episode.

Prevention

A diet with increased fiber should be recommended to most patients as primary prevention. A high-fiber diet is used as secondary prevention after the onset of diverticulitis. The following are recommended:

1. Eat five servings of fruits and vegetables each day. Fruits and vegetables high in fiber include apples, oranges, berries, pears, figs, prunes, broccoli, cauliflower, Brussels sprouts, lettuce, carrots, beans, and potatoes.
2. Replace white bread with whole-grain breads and cereals.
3. Eat bran cereal for breakfast.
4. Consider daily use of psyllium.

Follow-Up

The increasing incidence of diverticulitis associated with age mirrors the rise in the incidence of adenocarcinoma of the colon. Regardless of testing during the acute phase, the colon must be evaluated after inflammation has resolved. The follow-up evaluation serves two purposes. For patients who did not undergo further radiographic or endoscopic examination during the acute period, follow-up testing helps to verify the presence of diverticulosis, thus supporting the diagnosis. In addition, a follow-up evaluation is used to identify the 10% to 20% of patients who have coexisting colon cancer.

As discussed earlier, colon cancer can mimic the symptoms of diverticulitis, manifesting with left lower quadrant pain and obstruction. CT scanning identifies many of these cancers but has a high rate of false-negative results. Single-contrast enemas and endoscopy without insufflation can be inadequate to rule out colon cancer. It is standard to recommend either an air-contrast barium enema and flexible sigmoidoscopy or colonoscopy for follow-up testing. As with testing in the acute phase, there are few data concerning the most cost-effective method of follow-up, and the decision should be based in part on the available expertise and technology.

Patients should be counseled with regard to a high-fiber diet and early evaluation for any symptoms suggestive of recurrence or development of a complication.

REFERRAL

Patients who have an unclear diagnosis or whose condition fails to respond to therapy should be referred to a surgeon or gastroenterologist.

There are various indications for a surgical referral: complication or failure of CT-guided percutaneous drainage of abscess, obstruction, pneumoperitoneum, fistula, recurrent disease, and suspicion of or an inability to exclude cancer.

KEY POINTS

- The classic triad can be seen on presentation: left lower quadrant pain, fever, and leukocytosis.

- Elderly and immunocompromised patients often have fewer signs and symptoms and more severe illness. A high index of suspicion must be maintained in the evaluation of these patients.

- Most patients with acute diverticulitis, Hinchey stage I, respond to conservative, medical therapy with parenteral antibiotics and bowel rest.

- All patients should be evaluated for coexisting colon cancer after the acute inflammation has resolved. The recommended procedure is either colonoscopy or an air-contrast barium enema combined with flexible sigmoidoscopy.

- Between 20% and 30% of hospitalized patients with diverticulitis eventually need surgery, either for a complication or for recurrence.

COMMONLY ASKED QUESTIONS

What is diverticulitis?
It is a small pocket, like a cul-de-sac, that forms along the wall of the colon.

Is diverticulosis the same as diverticulitis?
No. Most people with diverticulosis never have any symptoms. Diverticulitis is an infection of one of the diverticuli, somewhat like a "mini-appendicitis."

How can I prevent diverticulosis?
Talk with your physician and discuss increasing the fiber in your diet.

If I have diverticulitis, can I be treated as an outpatient?
Generally, outpatient treatment can be given for patients with local inflammation in the fat around the colon who go to the doctor early in the course of illness or who have a milder clinical presentation without signs or symptoms in other parts of the body. Patients who do well with outpatient treatment include those who are likely to respond well to medical treatment and reliable patients who can take fluids and medications by mouth and are able to return for frequent follow-up. Usually, elderly and immunocompromised patients are hospitalized for treatment.

SUGGESTED READINGS

Classic Readings on Etiology, Epidemiology, and Natural History
Painter NS. Diverticular disease of the colon. *BMJ* 1968;3: 475–479.
Parks TG. Natural history of diverticular disease of the colon: a review of 521 cases. *BMJ* 1969;4:639–645.
Whiteway J, Morson BC. Pathology of ageing: diverticular disease. *Clin Gastroenterol* 1985;14:829–845.
Mendeloff AI. Thoughts on the epidemiology of diverticular disease. *Clin Gastroenterol* 1986;15:855–877.

Radiologic Studies in Diverticulitis
Johnson CD, Baker ME, Rice RP, Silverman P, Thompson WM. Diagnosis of acute colonic diverticulitis: comparison of barium enema and CT. *AJR Am J Roentgenol* 1987; 148:541–546.
Shrier D, Skucas J, Weiss S. Diverticulitis: an evaluation by computed tomography and contrast enema. *Am J Gastroenterol* 1991;86:1466–1471.
Stefansson T, Nyman R, Nilsson S, Ekbom A, Pahlman L. Diverticulitis of the sigmoid colon: a comparison of CT, colonic enema and laparoscopy. *Acta Radiologica* 1997;38: 313–319.

Treatment of Diverticulitis and Abdominal Infections
Duma RJ, Kellum JM. Colonic diverticulitis microbiologic, diagnostic, and therapeutic considerations. *Curr Clin Top Infect Dis* 1991;11:218–247.
The Standards Task Force American Society of Colon and Rectal Surgeons. Practice parameters for sigmoid diverticulitis. *Dis Colon Rectum* 1995;38:125–132.
Bohnen JMA. Antibiotic therapy for abdominal infection. *World J Surg* 1998;22:152–157.

Right-Sided Diverticulitis or Diverticulitis in Young Patients
Spivak H, Weinrauch S, Harvey JC, Surick B, Ferstenberg H, Friedman I. Acute colonic diverticulitis in the young. *Dis Colon Rectum* 1997;40:570–574.

CHAPTER 12

Ischemic Colitis

Kevin C. Oeffinger
University of Texas Southwestern Medical Center, Dallas, Texas 75235

DEFINITION

Ischemic colitis is a pathologic condition of the colon that results from inadequate blood flow into the mesenteric vascular system. Ischemic colitis, the most common form of gastrointestinal ischemia, can be divided into gangrenous and nongangrenous colitis. The latter can be further subdivided, depending on the depth of involvement and chronicity. Table 12.1 shows the generally accepted classification of ischemic colitis.

Fifty percent of all patients with ischemic colitis have a transient, reversible colitis, whereas 15% to 20% develop gangrenous colitis. About 10% of patients develop strictures of the colon. The condition, ischemic colitis, is generally considered a disease of the left colon, with about 75% of patients having involvement of the left colon, including 25% of all patients with ischemic colitis affecting the splenic flexure. The right colon is involved in only 8% to 12% of cases.

Mild transient ischemia of the colon results in edema of the mucosa and submucosal hemorrhage. If the ischemic insult resolves, the mucosa returns to normal in 2 to 3 weeks. However, if the hypoxia affects the mural layers, fibrosis occurs and the healing time is slower. Patients with mural hypoxia are likely to have a recurrence in the form of segmental colitis or to develop strictures of the colon. Severe ischemic injury results in transmural infarction and the development of gangrenous colitis.

CAUSE

Circulation to the colon is supplied by branches from three main sources, the superior mesenteric artery, the inferior mesenteric artery, and the internal iliac arteries. A vast network of collaterals exists among the branches, with the two most important collaterals being the mesenteric and marginal arteries. Various branches and collaterals may be absent or poorly developed in some persons, leading to areas that are more susceptible to ischemia. Notably, the marginal artery, which provides collateral communication between the superior and inferior mesenteric arteries in the area of the splenic flexure, is absent in about 5% of the population. In persons without a marginal artery, the splenic flexure has little collateral circulation, and as a result this watershed area is particularly susceptible to ischemic injury.

TABLE 12.1. Classification of Ischemic Colitis

Gangrenous colitis (transmural)
Nongangrenous colitis
  Transient or reversible (mucosal)
  Chronic or irreversible (mural)
    Chronic ulcerative ischemic colitis
    Ischemic colonic stricture

TABLE 12.2. Causes of Ischemic Colitis

Vascular occlusion
  Large artery embolism or thrombosis (SMA and
    branches, IMA and branches)
  Small-artery disease (diabetes mellitus, vasculitis,
    radiation)
  Venous thrombosis (hypercoagulable syndromes,
    pancreatitis, portal hypertension, sickle cell
    disease)
Mechanical obstruction
  Cancer of the colon
  Volvulus
  Stricture
  Adhesions
"Low flow" states
  Cardiogenic shock or failure
  Sepsis
  Anaphylaxis
Miscellaneous
  Spontaneous, idiopathic
  Sequela of abdominal aortic repair
  Medications
    Digitalis preparations
    Estrogen preparations, including including oral
      contraceptive pills
    Nonsteroidal antiinflammatory medications
    Catecholamines
    Psychotropic medications
    Diuretics
    Danazol
  Illicit drugs (cocaine, methamphetamine)
  Long-distance running

Interruption of the circulation to the colon can lead to ischemic changes, depending on the size and location of the vessel and the integrity of the collateral circulation. A wide array of problems can result in ischemic colitis, but most causes for inadequate circulation to the colon fall in three primary groups: vascular occlusion, mechanical obstruction, and decrease in flow, as in hypotension and shock. Additionally, there are a number of poorly understood causes, including vasoconstriction secondary to a wide array of medications.

Causes of ischemic colitis are displayed in Table 12.2. Ischemic colitis is a disease generally associated with older adults (average age, 60 years). Almost 90% of patients with ischemic colitis have widespread atherosclerosis involving the vessels supplying the colon. In the elderly population, men are more frequently affected, by a ratio of 1.5:1. Incidence does not depend on ethnic background. However, ischemic colitis can affect younger patients, especially those who use oral contraceptive pills or cocaine or who are long-distance runners.

PATIENT PRESENTATION

A careful history and a thorough examination are necessary in evaluating patients with suspected ischemic colitis. This is especially true in the elderly patient with insidious abdominal pain and few other symptoms or signs.

Patients with ischemic colitis can present with a wide array of signs and symptoms. Presentation depends, to a degree, on the size and location of the involved vessels and can range from an insidious, indolent process to a very abrupt, fulminant course.

The great majority of patients are older and have evidence of atherosclerosis, such as cardiovascular or peripheral vascular disease. Usually, the patient complains of abdominal pain that is insidious in onset, mild to moderate in severity, colicky in nature, and either localized to the left lower quadrant or poorly localized. Often the patient experiences a change in bowel habits and bloody diarrhea or hematochezia. Passage of dark blood within 24 hours of onset of abdominal pain is a typical presentation. If an ileus is present, the patient notes nausea, abdominal distention, and occasionally vomiting. Most patients do not have a significant fever. The onset can also be abrupt, followed by an urgent desire to defecate and a large, bloody stool.

In contrast, in 15% to 20% of patients, transmural necrosis of the colon results from the vascular compromise, and signs and symptoms of shock and sepsis develop. This group of patients experience a much more abrupt and fulminant course.

Less commonly, young patients develop abrupt onset of poorly localized abdominal pain and rectal bleeding. Often the younger patient notices preceding constipation. The physical examination is variable. Patients may exhibit signs of shock or sepsis. Pain with abdominal palpation is common and usually is poorly localized.

Patients should be questioned about use of illicit drugs, particularly cocaine and methamphetamine, and other potentially predisposing medications (digitalis preparations, catecholamines, oral contraceptives, estrogens, nonsteroidal antiinflammatory medications, psychotropic medications, diuretics, and danazol).

DIAGNOSIS

Laboratory Tests

Laboratory tests are generally not very helpful in the evaluation of a patient with suspected ischemic colitis. The leukocyte may be normal or increased. Serum markers (e.g., lactate dehydrogenase) are nonspecific and have little value in the evaluation of a patient with ischemic colitis.

Radiologic Studies

Colonoscopy

The gold standard for diagnosis is lower endoscopy, preferably colonoscopy. Changes seen with colonoscopy are well described and depend on the depth and progression of involvement of the bowel wall. Early in the process, the mucosa is pale and edematous, with interspersed areas of petechial hemorrhage or hyperemia. Multiple superficial, small ulcerations may be seen scattered in the hyperemic areas. Figure 12.1 displays the submucosal hemorrhage and ulcers that are typically seen in a patient with transient ischemic colitis. Examination of a biopsy of the affected mucosa shows a loss of the normal crypt architecture and surface epithelial cells. A mild inflammatory cell infiltrate of the lamina propria and vascular congestion can be seen.

As the ischemia progresses in extent and depth, a blue-to-black discoloration of the mucosa, representing mucosal necrosis and submucosal hemorrhage, can be seen on colonoscopy. If ulceration is present, a biopsy can distinguish ischemic colitis from other causes of ulceration, such as colon carcinoma, Crohn's disease, ulcerative colitis, and pseudomembranous colitis.

If the changes become chronic, colonoscopy may show the development of a colon stricture with a scarred mucosa and poor distensibility of the bowel. Biopsy of the mucosa in a stricture shows fibrosis in the lamina propria, submucosa, and circular muscle layers, with a lack of an inflammatory cell infiltrate.

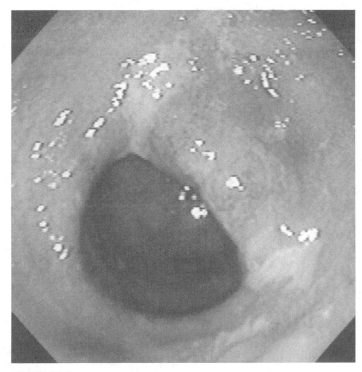

FIGURE 12.1.
Colonoscopy showing ulceration and submucosal hemorrhage in a patient with ischemic colitis.

Abdominal radiographs

Plain films of the abdomen are nonspecific and are not helpful in the diagnosis of ischemic colitis. Barium enema, once the diagnostic test of choice, can be useful in the evaluation if lower endoscopy is unavailable. Thumbprinting of the colon, a classic feature with ischemic colitis, is visualized as a scalloped appearance of the bowel wall, resulting from submucosal hemorrhage and mucosal edema. Discrete or multiple small ulcers and strictures can be seen on barium enema.

Computed tomography

CT scanning of the abdomen is not very sensitive or specific in ischemic colitis. However, if the patient is exhibiting signs and symptoms of progressive obstruction, CT scanning can be useful to distinguish between an obstruction caused by ischemic colitis and one caused by colon carcinoma.

Differential Diagnosis

Various diseases should be considered depending on the extent and chronicity of ischemic colitis.

Acute reversible ischemia

Patients with acute, reversible ischemic colitis need to be distinguished from those with other causes of abdominal pain or colitis. Diseases causing abdominal pain, especially in elderly patients, include acute mesenteric ischemia, diverticulitis, and obstruction of the colon.

Acute mesenteric ischemia   Patients with acute mesenteric ischemia experience an abrupt onset of pain that is usually much more severe than in ischemic colitis. The patients appear seriously ill and often have a precipitating factor, such as dysrhythmia, myocardial infarction, or congestive heart failure.

Diverticulitis   A person with diverticulitis usually has fever and leukocytosis as well as more localized pain in the left lower quadrant than a patient with ischemic colitis.

Obstruction of colon   A patient with ischemic colitis may present with obstructive signs and symptoms, necessitating the consideration of other causes for colon obstruction, such as volvulus and carcinoma of the colon.

VOLVULUS   Patients with a sigmoid volvulus experience sudden onset of nausea, vomiting, obstipation, and colicky abdominal pain. Plain films of the abdomen are generally diagnostic.

COLON CARCINOMA   Patients who develop obstruction secondary to carcinoma usually have a history of weight loss and progressive constipation or a change in the caliber of stool. Colonoscopic examination with biopsy should distinguish between obstruction secondary to ischemic colitis and that resulting from colon carcinoma. CT scans of the abdomen may be helpful in distinguishing tumor infiltration from ischemic segments in patients with ischemic colitis proximal to a colon carcinoma.

Other types of colitis

Other causes of colitis should be considered in the evaluation of a patient with suspected ischemic colitis.

Ulcerative colitis   Ulcerative colitis, rather than ischemic colitis, usually affects younger patients, although there is a growing recognition of young patients with ischemic colitis. Ischemic bowel disease can be distinguished from ulcerative colitis by colonoscopy with biopsy.

Infectious colitis   In contrast to patients with ischemic colitis, those with infectious colitis usually present with fever and leukocytosis.

Pseudomembranous colitis   A history of recent or current antibiotic use is found in patients with pseudomembranous colitis. If there is any question, colonoscopy should distinguish among the causes of colitis.

Chronic disease with stricture formation

Patients with chronic ischemic colitis may develop strictures of the colon, which need to be distinguished from

Summary of Diagnosis

- Acute, transient ischemic colitis
  Abdominal pain, poorly localized or in left lower quadranteukocytosis
  Bloody diarrhea or hematochezia
  Usually, absence of fever
  Nonspecific laboratory test results
  Diagnostic test of choice: colonoscopy
- Chronic ischemic colitis
  Persistent or recurrent abdominal pain with bloody diarrhea
  Stricture formation
  Diagnostic test of choice: colonoscopy
- Gangrenous ischemic colitis
  Signs and symptoms of peritonitis and sepsis
  Emergency surgical intervention

other causes of stricture formation, such as Crohn's disease or carcinoma of the colon. Again, colonoscopy with biopsy should provide the necessary information to make the diagnosis.

Gangrenous ischemic colitis

Patients with gangrenous ischemic colitis present with progressive signs and symptoms of peritonitis and sepsis, necessitating emergency surgical intervention. Other causes of peritonitis and sepsis can usually be distinguished at the time of surgery.

MANAGEMENT

Treatment

Mild transient episode

A mild episode of transient ischemic colitis can be treated on an outpatient basis. Patients should be restricted to clear liquids for 1 to 2 days, followed by a slow reinstitution of the diet. Close follow-up is recommended, necessitating a reliable and compliant patient. Potentially predisposing medications should be stopped.

Moderate to severe transient episode

Patients with moderate to severe transient ischemic colitis should be hospitalized, prescribed bowel rest, and rehydrated with intravenous fluids. Parenteral broad-spectrum antibiotics with coverage of gram-negative enteric organisms (e.g., *Escherichia coli*) and anaerobes (e.g., *Bacteroides fragilis*) should be used because of the potential for bacterial invasions after the loss of mucosal integrity and subsequent development of gangrene or sepsis. Other comorbid diseases that may affect the splanchnic circulation should be aggressively managed. The episode of ischemic colitis usually resolves in one week.

Gangrenous colitis or transmural necrosis

If the patient manifests signs and symptoms of gangrenous ischemic colitis or if colonoscopy shows evidence of transmural necrosis, emergency surgical intervention is necessary to resect the affected bowel. The mortality rate of patients requiring surgery for gangrenous colitis is higher than 50%.

Follow-Up

Reevaluation with colonoscopy is recommended, although this practice has not been evaluated in a prospective study. Follow-up colonoscopy is intended to evaluate for the presence of strictures or persistent ischemic changes. Elective colon resection with primary anasto-

mosis is recommended for patients with chronic strictures or evidence of chronic segmental colitis. Follow up includes long-term management of underlying causes.

REFERRAL

Surgical referral is recommended for patients with gangrenous ischemic colitis, stricture of the colon, or chronic segmental colitis.

Consultation with a gastroenterologist or a general surgeon is suggested for patients with ischemic colitis who require hospitalization.

KEY POINTS

- Generally, this is a disease of elderly persons with underlying atherosclerotic disease.
- Ten percent of patients are young; these cases are usually secondary to use of certain medications or illicit drugs.
- A high index of suspicion for ischemic colitis is needed, especially in elderly patients.
- It is predominantly a disease of the left colon.
- Colonoscopy is the primary diagnostic tool.
- Transient ischemic colitis is treated conservatively.
- Gangrenous ischemic colitis is a surgical emergency.

COMMONLY ASKED QUESTIONS

What is ischemic colitis?
The word colitis means "inflammation of the colon," and ischemic means "lack of oxygen." If the walls of the colon do not receive enough blood flow to deliver oxygen to the tissues, then the wall begins to become inflamed. This usually occurs because of atherosclerosis, or hardening of the arteries that supply the colon. If the blockage is severe enough, some of the colon wall dies, leading to a medical emergency.

Will my ischemic colitis go away?
Half of the patients with ischemic colitis experience a transient, reversible episode, which may last up to 1 week.

What can I do to prevent ischemic colitis?
Because atherosclerosis is the cause of ischemic colitis in most patients, keeping a lifelong eye on reducing one's cardiovascular risk is important. This includes regular exercise, prudent eating habits, and periodic examination for cholesterol screening.

SUGGESTED READINGS
General Reading
Boley SJ. Colonic ischemia: 25 years later. *Am J Gastroenterol* 1990;85:931–934.
Bower TC. Ischemic colitis. *Surg Clin North Am* 1993;73: 1037–1053.

Gadhi SK, Hanson MM, Vernava AM, et al. Ischemic colitis. *Dis Colon Rectum* 1996;39:88–100.

Reeders JWAJ, Tytgat GNJ, Rosenbusch G, et al: *Ischemic colitis.* The Hague: Martinus Nijhoff, 1984.

Reinus JF, Brandt LJ, Boley SJ. Ischemic diseases of the bowel. *Gastroenterol Clin North Am* 1990;19:319–343.

Colonoscopy

Dawson MA, Schaefer JW. The clinical course of reversible ischemic colitis: observations on the progression of sigmoidoscopic and histologic changes. *Gastroenterology* 1971;60:577–580.

Habu Y, Tahashi Y, Kiyota K, et al. Reevaluation of clinical features of ischemic colitis: analysis of 68 consecutive cases diagnosed by early colonoscopy. *Scand J Gastroenterol* 1996;31:881–886.

Scowcroft CW, Sanowski RA, Kozarek RA. Colonoscopy in ischemic colitis. *Gastrointest Endosc* 1981;27:156–161.

Medication and Illicit Drug–Related Ischemic Colitis

Deana DG, Dean PJ. Reversible ischemic colitis in young women: association with oral contraceptive use. Am J Surg Pathol 1995;19:454–462.

Gurbuz AK, Gurbuz B, Salas L, et al. Premarin-induced ischemic colitis. J Clin Gastroenterol 1994;19:108–111.

Niazi M, Kondru A, Levy J, Bloom AA. Spectrum of ischemic colitis in cocaine users. Dig Dis Sci 1997;42:1537–1541.

CHAPTER 13

Perianal Disorders

Clifford L. Simmang,* Jay A. Crockett,** and Philip J. Huber, Jr.†
*University of Texas Southwestern Medical Center, Dallas, Texas 75235
**Greenville Colon and Rectal Associates, Greenville, South Carolina 29605
†University of Texas Southwestern Medical Center and St. Paul Medical Center, Dallas, Texas 75235

DEFINITION

Perianal disorders are very common conditions for which patients seek the advice of their primary care physicians. Patients may delay consultation because they are embarrassed to be seen and evaluated. Three common symptoms with which patients present to the physician are anorectal bleeding, anorectal pain, and anal and perianal itching (pruritus ani).

Virtually all patients and many physicians attribute anorectal symptoms to various manifestations of hemorrhoidal disease. Although all people have hemorrhoidal vessels that can manifest in a variety of conditions, it is important to distinguish those conditions are not a manifestation of hemorrhoidal disease, because the treatment and the need for referral depend on an accurate diagnosis.

PATIENT EVALUATION

The cornerstone in the evaluation of patients with anorectal complaints is a detailed and thorough history and physical examination. The diagnosis can often be made on the basis of history and confirmed by the physical examination.

Patient Presentation

Rectal bleeding is often the predominant reason that patients consult a physician. Most patient visits to the colon and rectal surgeon involve the symptom of blood per rectum. Patients may present with bright red blood per rectum, blood in the stool, or blood on the toilet paper or in the toilet water, or they may have been referred for occult bleeding.

History

The duration and severity of bleeding and its relation to bowel movements are important to elicit.

A thorough history should include questions about alteration of bowel habits and degree of continence. There is a great variation in normal bowel habits, with normal function varying from three bowel movements per day to one bowel movement only every 3 to 4 days. Questions about changes in the number, consistency, and relative ease of passing a stool should be asked. A change in medications or dietary habits or even surgery may result in altered bowel habits.

Physical Examination

Body position

Most patients are very apprehensive about undergoing an examination of the anorectal area. To minimize embarrassment, exposure should be limited and the patient should remain covered. The examination can be performed with the patient in any of several positions. The prone jackknife position is frequently used, but many patients feel more comfortable if they are examined while in the left lateral (Sims') position. This allows the patient to curl up on the left side, as if going to sleep. It is helpful to position the buttocks slightly over the side of the examination table with the patient's head near the opposite side of the table.

When the anorectal examination is performed in conjunction with pelvic examination, the patient is already in a lithotomy position and no change of position is required.

Components of the Examination

The two primary components of the anorectal examination are inspection and palpation.

Inspection   Inspection is a key element. Inspection should begin with examination of the perianal skin and anal margin. Areas of erosion, excoriation, evidence of masses, external hemorrhoids, scarring, and prolapse can all be readily observed. Gentle retraction close to the anal verge also allows inspection of the distal anal canal lining and permits visualization of an anal fissure when present. If this eversion is not performed, an anal fissure can be missed.

The standard physical examination of a patient complaining of blood per rectum involves direct inspection of the anus for lesions, ulcers, skin tags, and fistulous openings.

Digital rectal examination The digital rectal examination (DRE) is performed with a well-lubricated, gloved index finger. Insertion should be slow and not jerky or quick. Jerky motions result in discomfort for the patient, which causes squeezing of the sphincters and limits the clinician's ability to perform a thorough examination. In particular, the clinician should palpate for sphincter tone, ability to squeeze, palpable sphincter defects, and masses. Return of stool or mucous from the gloved finger may be examined for evidence of occult blood. Anteriorly, the prostate is palpated in men, and in women the cervix can often be detected. The DRE is completed by rotation of the examining finger circumferentially above the anorectal ring.

DRE is paramount in the diagnosis of patients who present with anorectal bleeding. Although the examination is uncomfortable and potentially embarrassing for the patient, failure to perform a DRE is not defensible. Any patient who does not receive a DRE and has rectal bleeding written off as "hemorrhoids" has been done a potentially tragic disservice by the physician.

Invasive diagnostic techniques

When bleeding is the presentation, DRE is followed by anoscopy and rigid or flexible sigmoidoscopy, which can identify the cause of the most colorectal conditions that produce visible rectal bleeding.

Anoscopy Anoscopy permits evaluation of the distal several centimeters of the anal canal. The slotted anoscope is particularly useful in assessing the degree and protrusion of internal hemorrhoids. It can also identify the internal opening of an anal fistula and distal rectal tumors, anal canal tumors, and hypertrophied anal papilla can be seen.

RIGID PROCTOSIGMOIDOSCOPY The proctosigmoidoscopy yields the most accurate measurement of the distance between the anal verge and a carcinoma, and this technique is recommended for measurement of all rectal cancers. The rigid sigmoidoscope requires less maintenance and cleaning, making it useful in a busy office practice. Premedication is not necessary, and a single Fleet enema is adequate for preparation. This technique can readily be learned by all primary care physicians.

FLEXIBLE SIGMOIDOSCOPY This examination has gained popularity, especially for the screening of colorectal cancer or polyps. Several preparations can be used before flexible sigmoidoscopy; two commonly used preparations are a laxative followed by a single Fleet enema, and two Fleet enemas. The examination may be performed without premedication. Usually, a sigmoidoscope of 60 to 65 cm is used.

Flexible sigmoidoscopy can be used to examine the sigmoid and descending colon; it allows detection of up to two thirds of colon cancers. If a polyp is detected, it should be biopsied. If the polyp returns hyperplastic tissue, then no further examination is required. If the pathology result shows adenomatous tissue, then colonoscopy should be performed. Flexible sigmoidoscopy is well tolerated and has very few complications. Perforation has been reported in fewer than 1 of 1,000 examinations, and bleeding is rare. Bacteremia can be caused by endoscopic examinations, and antibiotic prophylaxis should be used as indicated.

DIFFERENTIAL DIAGNOSIS

Anorectal Bleeding

There are multiple causes for rectal bleeding and it is important not to attribute all anorectal pathology to either hemorrhoids or cancer.

Hemorrhoids

Bright red rectal bleeding that drips into the toilet bowel and streaks the stool is frequently caused by bleeding internal hemorrhoids.

Fissures

Blood seen on the toilet tissue after a painful bowel movement is often the result of an anal fissure or abrasion.

Pruritus ani

Occasional spotting of blood on the tissue may be seen in pruritus ani.

Gastrointestinal source

Melena results from enzymatic action of bacteria on the blood and usually represents an upper gastrointestinal source of bleeding.

Other causes

Blood mixed with the stool may indicate a proximal colon lesion, and a total colonic evaluation should be performed. Although blood mixed with mucus is typically found in patients with inflammatory bowel disease, it may also be seen in association with large colonic polyps and carcinoma. Again, total colonic evaluation should be performed.

Anorectal Pain

A significant portion of the pain generated in anorectal conditions is secondary to spasm of the sphincter muscle. The sphincter muscle, like any muscle when injured, responds by going into spasm. This is particularly true with an anal fissure.

The three most common causes of anorectal pain are anal fissure, abscess, and thrombosed external hemorrhoid.

Anal fissure

Classically, the complaint of pain associated with a large or constipated stool and blood on the tissue paper is caused by an anal fissure. When this history is elicited, the diagnosis is an anal fissure until proven otherwise.

Anal abscess

An abscess usually manifests with a continuous, throbbing pain along fever and possibly the presence of a tender mass.

Thrombosed hemorrhoid

Sudden onset of a throbbing pain is the usual history for a patient with a thrombosed external hemorrhoid. The pain is severe for 1 to 2 days and then gradually resolves.

Proctalgia fugax

Sharp rectal pain that is often described as knife-like and fleeting is more likely to result from proctalgia fugax or levator muscle spasm.

Coccygeal pain

Coccygeal pain is a frustrating problem for both the patient and the physician. This type of pain is infrequently a result of anorectal disease. Surgical treatment (e.g., coccygectomy) usually should be reserved for the rare patient who has a demonstrable anatomic abnormality of the coccyx, such as a fracture.

Tenesmus

This sensation of incomplete evacuation may be associated with distal colonic or rectal lesions or with colitis.

Cancer

Other causes for anorectal pain include neoplasms. As in most other areas of the body, it is unusual for a malignancy to produce pain unless it is fairly extensive and invading the neuroplexes. Rare cases, including carcinoma of the anal glands involving the sphincter complex, may occur. Therefore, it is important, if the cause cannot accurately be determined, to perform an examination with the patient under anesthesia.

Summary of Diagnosis

- Anorectal bleeding is a symptom most commonly caused by a benign condition of the anal canal; many causes are possible.
- Patients with anorectal bleeding must have a thorough anorectal and colonic evaluation before this symptom can be definitively attributed to an anorectal condition.
- Physical examination for anorectal bleeding is very important and includes the following components:
  Inspection for external hemorrhoidal tissue, anal fissures, and mass lesions; discoloration should be noted.
  DRE is mandatory, and the following findings should be described:
  Pain on digital insertion.
  Sphincter tone (inability to squeeze).
  Rectal masses and the location of the quadrant.
  Prostrate enlargement or nodules in a male patient.
- Laboratory tests include fecal occult blood testing and a hematocrit to evaluate for anemia.
- Anoscopy is used to best visualize findings in the anal canal; some conditions can be treated within the clinic using an anoscope (hemorrhoidal banding).
- Flexible sigmoidoscopy is used to evaluate the rectum and distal colon; this modality is primarily used for screening of asymptomatic persons.
- Colonoscopy is the diagnostic procedure of choice for the evaluation of patients with rectal bleeding; it allows complete colonic visualization and the ability to diagnose and/or treat discovered lesions.
- Barium enema may be combined with flexible sigmoidoscopy for colonic evaluation; however, it has the disadvantage of not allowing direct visualization of the mucosal changes of colonic abnormalities nor treatment of discovered lesions.

CLINICAL PRESENTATIONS

ANAL FISSURE

A common cause of rectal bleeding and pain is an anal fissure. A fissure is a superficial linear tear of the distal rectum at the anal verge. The passage of a hard stool may tear the distal mucosa. Repetitive tearing from subsequent bowel movements results in a chronic inflammatory state, internal sphincter spasm, and higher anal canal pressures, setting the stage for a vicious cycle.

Cause

The cause is unclear, and many theories have been proposed. Fissures encountered laterally are likely to be associated with inflammatory bowel disease.

Patient Presentation

History

An anal fissure typically is precipitated by an episode of constipation, associated with a hard bowel movement, and the sensation of a tearing or burning pain. Blood is often noted on the tissue paper. When this history is present, a diligent search for an anal fissure must be performed.

Physical examination

An anal fissure can be identified on external examination of the anus. A skin tag or sentinel pile can usually be identified in the posterior midline as an enlarged, fleshy fold of anal skin. This edematous skin tag is secondary to the chronic inflammation and is not an external hemorrhoid.

When the buttocks are separated, inspection is often normal (Fig. 13.1); mucosal eversion must be performed to identify a fissure (Fig. 13.2). If this eversion is not performed, an anal fissure may be missed. By gently spreading the anal verge, the clinician can inspect the area, which often reveals a tear or raw area of the anoderm. Close inspection may reveal the white, circular fibers of the internal sphincter at the wound base.

In women, 90% of fissures are located posteriorly and 10% are located anteriorly. In men, 99% of fissures are located posteriorly, and only 1% are located anteriorly.

DRE and anoscopy can be very uncomfortable and are not necessary when the classic findings of anal fissure are identified. Even if no obvious abnormalities are noted on inspection, during insertion of the distal tip of the finger pressure should first be applied laterally, then anteriorly, and finally posteriorly. This is because the majority of fissures are located posteriorly. Severe pain noted on insertion of just the distal tip of the finger is consistent with an anal fissure.

For patients with significant anal pain whose anal canal is palpably normal, no additional studies are required at that time. If the patient's pain is too severe to allow DRE, then examination under anesthesia should be performed. No radiologic or laboratory evaluation is required for diagnosis.

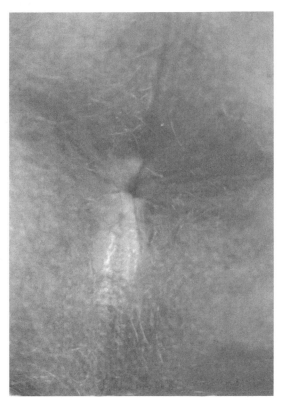

FIGURE 13.1.
Anorectal inspection is demonstrated. The buttocks have been separated, and the area appears normal. No fissure is seen.

Multiple fissures

Multiple fissures, especially those that occur laterally or have shaggy edges, should generate prompt consideration of other diagnoses besides a typical anal fissure. Such diagnoses include the chancre of condyloma latum (syphilis), human immunodeficiency virus (HIV) infection, and inflammatory bowel disease (especially Crohn's disease). Other sexually transmitted diseases, especially viruses, including herpes simplex virus and cytomegalovirus, may occasionally be found in atypical fissures or anal ulcers and may be very painful.

Management

Initial management is conservative; resolution of symptoms is the goal. Approximately 70% to 80% of patients with anal fissures are expected to heal with a conservative bowel management program.

Conservative treatment

Bulking agents and stool softeners are given to prevent tearing of the anoderm. Hydrocortisone creams may be

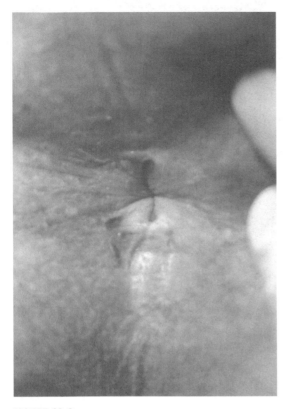

FIGURE 13.2.
Anorectal inspection is demonstrated. The buttocks have been separated and mucosal eversion performed by gentle retraction near the anal verge, revealing synchronous anterior and posterior anal fissures.

placed on the fissure to decrease inflammation and aid in pain relief. Sitz baths keep the area clean and give symptomatic relief.

Nitroglycerin ointment

The percentage of anal fissures responding to therapy may be increased by adding nitroglycerin ointment. Approximately 85% to 90% of patients with acute fissures heal, and even up to 50% to 65% of patients with chronic fissures have demonstrated healing with nitroglycerin ointment. It is well known that nitropaste produces relaxation of smooth muscles, such as the internal sphincter of the anal sphincter complex.

Currently, this preparation must be compounded. It is important that this ointment be placed in either a dark glass jar or tube or a nonplastic dark jar, because nitroglycerin is broken down by light and absorbed by plastic.

A 0.2% ointment of nitroglycerin may be prescribed, consisting of 2% nitroglycerin paste diluted to 0.2% in petrolatum. The recommended application, 0.25 g twice a day, is achieved by applying a pea-sized bead of ointment on the perianal skin with a cotton swab. This can be performed up to three or four times daily and is often required for 4 to 6 weeks. If healing is not present by 6 weeks, it is unlikely to occur.

Sphincterotomy

When conservative measures have failed, a lateral, internal sphincterotomy is the procedure of choice. This can be performed by either an open technique or a closed technique. In the open technique, a small incision (approximately 1 cm in length) is made, and the internal sphincter is clearly identified and divided, usually with electrocautery. No closure is required. A closed technique is performed by placing either a no. 11 scalpel blade or a Beaver blade through a stab incision in the intersphincteric groove and dividing the internal sphincter by feel. In both situations, closure of the incised mucosa is not required.

Although a closed technique can be performed in the office, the open technique is often selected. It is common for the fissure to heal before the operative stab incision heals. Most patients notice that their pain is markedly decreased by the second or third bowel movement after surgery.

The bowel management regimen and warm tub baths (sitz baths) should be prescribed postoperatively and until the pain has resolved. Warm tub baths are often recommended three to four times daily and after each bowel movement.

Prevention

Prevention centers on a proper bowel management program. The mainstay of bowel management is a high-fiber diet, with 25 to 30 g of fiber as the recommended daily dosage. This is difficult to achieve with food alone. Fiber supplements in the form of psyllium are often recommended. The initial dose is often 6 g twice a day, which provides approximately 50% of the recommended daily dose of fiber. The goal is to avoid straining. Although an initial push is usually required to initiate evacuation, with proper bowel management colonic peristalsis should complete the evacuation. This requires a stool large enough to allow the colon to assist. A very soft but small and mushy stool requires straining just to squeeze the contents out and does not solve the problem. Reading materials should be removed from the bathroom. Merely sitting on the toilet promotes repetitive straining episodes.

Follow-Up

Depending on the accuracy of the initial diagnosis, follow-up may consist of a return to the clinic if the symptoms do not resolve. If the diagnosis was not definitively established during the first visit, follow-up or referral must take place to ensure an accurate diagnosis and avoid a missed or overlooked condition.

Referral

It is important both to understand the causes of anorectal pain and to develop a relationship with either a colorectal surgeon or a general surgeon with a special interest in anorectal disorders.

If an anal fissure is acute, conservative treatment can be instituted and referral performed if the condition fails to respond to the initial therapy. If the lesion fails to heal, the patient should be referred to a endorectal surgeon to discuss surgical options. The standard procedure performed in the United States is a lateral interval sphincterotomy, as discussed previously.

HEMORRHOIDS

Hemorrhoids are prevalent in the population. In fact, all patients have them. They are the vascular complexes lining the anal canal just proximal to the dentate line (internal hemorrhoids) and at the anal verge (external hemorrhoids). Although often referred to as veins, hemorrhoids have arterial pH and oxygen tension, demonstrating an arterial component; this explains why hemorrhoidal bleeding is bright red. They are commonly referred to as vascular cushions and, when symptomatic (bleeding, itching, protuberant), may require treatment.

Patient Presentation

History

The most common presentation of a symptomatic hemorrhoid is bleeding. The blood is frequently bright red and may be found on the toilet paper or dripping into the toilet water. It is also seen streaking the stool. Severe hemorrhoidal bleeding may cause anemia or even massive lower gastrointestinal bleeding.

Patients may describe a sensation of protrusion that can require manual reduction after a bowel movement or straining. In this instance, the internal hemorrhoid has enlarged, allowing prolapse through the anal opening. This sensation may also be attributable to a large external hemorrhoid or skin tag. Neither of these entities reduces, because they are located in the external anal canal.

Pain may also be associated with hemorrhoids. Acute onset of pain is frequently caused by a thrombosed hemorrhoid (see later discussion).

Physical examination

The diagnosis of hemorrhoids is made by physical examination. There is little need for laboratory evaluation.

By DRE the physician may be able to detect large internal hemorrhoids, although the examining finger is better suited to find masses or tumors.

Anoscopy is the most useful portion of the anorectal examination for the diagnosis of hemorrhoids. The patient is most easily examined in the prone jackknife position, although the left lateral position may be more comfortable and allows the patient to feel less exposed. The lubricated anoscope is gently inserted after the DRE has been completed. It is rotated 360 degrees to inspect the anal canal. Generally, an anoscope with a scalloped end gives the best view. As the instrument is rotated, the hemorrhoidal columns (located in the left lateral, right anterior and right posterior aspects of the anal canal) fall into view.

Grades of prolapse

The degree of prolapse associated with internal hemorrhoids has been graded 1 through 4. Grade 1 is the presence of internal hemorrhoids without prolapse. In grade 2 internal hemorrhoids, prolapse occurs along with bowel movements but reduction is spontaneous. Grade 3 hemorrhoids prolapse, and manual reduction is required to reduce the prolapse. In grade 4 hemorrhoids, reduction cannot be performed (Fig. 13.3).

Management

Treatment

The initial therapy for symptomatic, nonprolapsing hemorrhoidal disease is usually nonsurgical. The goal of nonsurgical therapy is to soften and increase the bulk of the patient's stool. This decreases the need to strain and prevents hard stool from abrading the friable hemorrhoidal tissue. Patient are encouraged to drink 6 to 8 glasses of water a day and to increase the amount of fiber in their diets. Twenty-five grams of dietary fiber per day is recommended. This may be achieved by supplemental fiber (psyllium) intake or by changing dietary habits. Stool softeners (docusate) can also be given. This therapy is continued for 4 weeks.

Many over-the-counter products are available to patients for symptomatic relief. These creams, pads, and lotions have not been shown to shrink or resolve hemorrhoids. Although their use need not be discouraged, they are not definitive treatment; because hemorrhoidal symptoms often improve in a self-limited fashion, it is difficult to know whether the treatment helped or the condition merely improved.

Prevention

The best way to prevent recurrence of hemorrhoids is to keep the stool soft and bulky, usually with fiber supple-

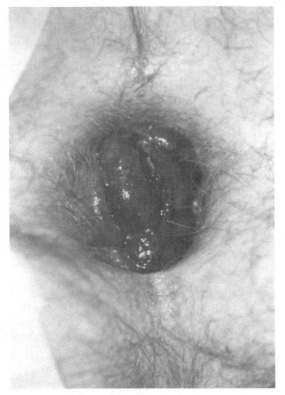

FIGURE 13.3.
Grade 4 hemorrhoids are shown. Incarceration has resulted in thrombosis, followed by gangrenous changes.

mentation. It is important to avoid straining at stool and to avoid sitting on the commode for an extended period after the call to stool.

Follow-up
Patients older than 50 years of age should receive colonic screening (barium enema or flexible sigmoidoscopy) to rule out neoplastic lesions. In the older population, merely finding hemorrhoids does not rule out other diagnoses that may cause blood per rectum.

Referral
Patients whose hemorrhoids continue to be symptomatic after an adequate trial of nonsurgical therapy should be referred for surgical treatment. There are many surgical options, but the most common are surgical excision, rubber band ligation, sclerotherapy, and cryotherapy.

Both injection of sclerosing agents and rubber band ligation are ambulatory procedures, but multiple visits may be required for adequate treatment. Excision, which can be performed on an outpatient basis in the operat-

ing room, is generally reserved for patients with prolapsing large internal hemorrhoids or with a significant external hemorrhoidal component, and for patients who prefer excision to banding. When the hemorrhoid is incarcerated and gangrenous (Figure 13.3), emergency hemorrhoidectomy should be considered.

CANCER
When patients present to the doctor with a history of rectal bleeding, their worst fear is likely to be "Is it cancer?" In patients younger than 50 years of age, the chance that their bleeding is secondary to cancer is very small. However, there are syndromes in which young people are found to have colon or rectal cancers.

Patient Presentation
History
In the family history, it is important to identify relatives who had colon cancer (especially before 50 years of age), familial polyposis, cancer, ulcerative colitis, or hereditary nonpolyposis syndromes (HNPCC or Lynch). A patient may present with a history of stool mixed or streaked with blood, anemia, or occult blood in the stool.

Physical examination
Suspicion of cancer should be foremost in the practitioner's mind when the patient presents with blood per rectum. A standardized history and physical examination, including DRE, anoscopy, and rigid sigmoidoscopy, can detect the majority of benign anorectal disease that can cause rectal bleeding.

Diagnosis
Laboratory examination
There are no tumor markers that can confirm or deny the presence of colorectal cancer, and none is useful for screening. However, the assay for carcinoembryonic antigen (CEA) may be of benefit in detecting recurrent disease, and a baseline measurement is routinely obtained at the time of diagnosis.

Endoscopic studies
One must be careful not to end the search for sources of rectal bleeding as soon as a column of hemorrhoids is seen on examination. This is especially true for patients older than 50 years of age and for those who have a family history that places them at higher risk.

To rule out a malignant lesion, inspection of the entire colon is necessary. This can be accomplished with either barium enema or colonoscopy. For the evaluation of bleeding, colonoscopy is preferred, because if a lesion is identified, it can be biopsied immediately and the diagnosis can be confirmed histologically (see Chapter 8).

Management

Treatment

A complete discussion of colorectal cancer and its management is beyond the scope of this chapter. Surgery followed by adjuvant chemotherapy in advanced disease is the standard of care for patients with colon carcinoma. Radiation plays little role. Patients with advanced metastatic disease are still candidates for palliative surgical therapy (for either excision or diversion).

Patients with rectal cancer have a multitude of treatment options. Surgical options range in scope from local excision to excision of part or all of the rectum, with or without resection of the anus. Transanal excision is possible for small lesions that are close to the anal verge. Depending on the depth of invasion and other histologic findings (vascular or lymphatic invasion), some patients require no further surgical intervention. Although there is some controversy as to the timing of adjuvant therapy, chemotherapy and radiation either preoperatively or postoperatively are useful adjuncts in the treatment of rectal cancer.

Prevention

The discussion of prevention of anal fissures provides further information about a proper bowel management program and the use of fiber. The benefits of fiber therapy include increased colonic transit time and dilution of potential carcinogens that may be present in the stool. In Africa, where diets are very high in fiber, colon cancer is relatively uncommon. Therefore, not only does an increase of fiber in diet promote the prevention of anorectal problems, but it may also decrease the incidence of colorectal cancer.

Follow-up

Follow-up after treatment is important, but its efficacy in terms of overall survival is in question. There is no standardized follow-up protocol for patients with colon or rectal cancer. However, general guidelines are as follows. Patients are seen in the office for physical examination and determinations of CEA level every 3 months for 2 years. These visits may then extend to biyearly for 3 more years and then yearly after that. Postoperatively, if no recurrent disease is identified, colonoscopy is performed every 3 to 5 years.

Referral

All patients diagnosed with colon or rectal cancer should be referred for surgical evaluation. For patients with rectal cancer, referral to a specialist in colon or rectal surgery who has the training to perform advanced operative techniques for sphincter preservation should be obtained.

RECTAL PROLAPSE

Patient Presentation

Rectal prolapse, or procidentia, may occasionally manifest with rectal bleeding. More commonly, it manifests in an elderly female patient as a sense of protrusion from the rectum that may or may not manually reduce after evacuation of a stool. A physical examination of the patient elicits the correct diagnosis.

Types of prolapse

A chronically prolapsed rectum may become friable and bleed. The patient may also present with incontinence as a result of chronic sphincter stretching.

Mucosal prolapse   Simple mucosal prolapse is differentiated from procidentia by the amount of prolapse: Mucosal prolapse does not involve the full thickness of the rectal wall. A mucosal prolapse is unlikely to protrude much further than a few centimeters from the anal verge. Also, in mucosal prolapse, the mucosal folds are aligned in a radial fashion.

Rectal prolapse   Complete rectal prolapse usually extends at least 6 or more centimeters from the anal verge. In direct contrast to mucosal prolapse, with complete rectal prolapse concentric folds of mucosa are seen around the central opening of the bowel (Fig. 13.4).

Internal prolapse   Internal prolapse, or rectal intussusception, is a variant of rectal prolapse that may also manifest with blood per rectum. In this circumstance, bleeding is usually the result of a solitary rectal ulcer. This lesion may be confused with a rectal carcinoma on anoscopy or proctoscopy, because the gross appearance may be either as an ulceration or a mass.

Diagnosis

Body position

It is very helpful to examine the patient while he or she is sitting on a commode. This straightens the anorectal angle and promotes prolapse of the rectum. The prone, jackknife position is suboptimal when examining a patient for this disease because some patients are unable to reproduce their prolapse in this position.

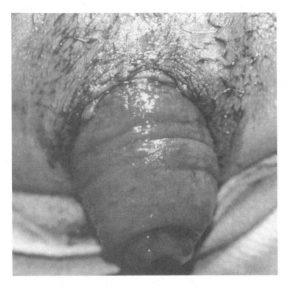

FIGURE 13.4.
Rectal prolapse is shown. Note the concentric folds of rectal mucosa seen with complete procidentia.

Diagnostic tests

Defecography is the radiologic examination of choice in this group of patients, although it is not mandatory. This examination reveals a redundant sigmoid colon and a lax pelvic floor. It is essential in patients with suspected internal prolapse, because rectal intussusception can be demonstrated.

Patients older than 50 years of age should have a complete colonic examination before definitive therapy is undertaken, to rule out other lesions. For this condition, a barium enema is usually preferred, because the contour of the redundant sigmoid colon is better demonstrated.

Management

Patients with true rectal prolapse who are in adequate general medical health should be referred for surgery. Surgical treatments vary from intraabdominal procedures, both open and laparoscopic, to perineal resections of the rectosigmoid colon. Most currently employed procedures involve either resection of the redundant sigmoid colon with rectal mobilization and rectopexy or rectal mobilization with mesh fixation to suspend the rectum. Although the risk of recurrence is higher, older patients generally tolerate the perineal approach better. A non-resectional approach involves the subcutaneous placement of a Silastic sling around the anal verge in an attempt to tighten the rectal outlet, thus preventing prolapse. Symptomatic internal prolapse should be managed by one of the abdominal operative approaches.

Referral

All patients with rectal prolapse should be referred for surgical evaluation.

PROCTITIS

Cause

Inflammation of the rectum has many causes, including infectious disease, radiation, and ulcerative proctitis. Radiation proctitis is not an uncommon complication after treatment for rectal, prostatic, or gynecologic cancers.

Patient Presentation

Patients may present with grossly bloody stool mixed with mucus. They may also complain of tenesmus, loose stools, and/or abdominal pain.

Ulcerative proctitis

Ulcerative proctitis is a variant of ulcerative colitis. In a significant portion of patients with ulcerative colitis, the disease is isolated to the rectum (see Chapter 7). They complain of grossly bloody bowel movements mixed with mucus. Physical examination, including DRE, anoscopy, and proctoscopy with biopsy, confirms the diagnosis.

Radiation proctitis

Diagnosis is by physical examination, history, and proctoscopy. An irradiated rectum appears pale yellow-white, telangiectatic, and noncompliant. Acute radiation proctitis may be difficult to distinguish from acute ulcerative proctitis in appearance. The rectal area appears acutely inflamed, edematous, friable, and ulcerated. Early lesions are likely to be inflammatory in nature and to involve the distal few centimeters of the rectum. Isolated bleeding lesions usually occur secondary to telangiectases found in the rectal mucosa.

Infectious proctitis

There are many causes of infectious proctitis. Most patients contract the infection as a sexually transmitted disease, and the coexistence of the acquired immunodeficiency syndrome must be considered. Most patients present with pain, rectal discharge, and possibly ulcerations. Diagnosis is made by performing the appropriate culture. Occasionally, biopsy of an anorectal lesion is helpful.

Management
Treatment
Ulcerative proctitis   Initial therapy is medical in nature. Steroid retention enemas of 10% hydrocortisone

twice a day for 14 days may control the inflammation. Steroid enemas may be exchanged for steroid foams, although the foam may not reach as far proximally as the enemas. As symptoms resolve, the twice-daily enemas are decreased in frequency to daily and ultimately discontinued.

Acetylsalicylic acid in oral or enema form has been shown to be effective in the treatment of ulcerative proctitis in some patients who have had a poor response to steroid therapy.

Radiation proctitis Medical treatment for radiation proctitis is similar to that for ulcerative proctitis. Steroid enemas or foams have been recommended to reduce the acute inflammation; however, complete resolution often is not achieved. Chronic inflammation and bleeding from telangiectases can be treated with cautery or laser ablation in an outpatient setting. For the few patients with severe ulceration and bleeding from radiation proctitis, fecal diversion with a colostomy ameliorates the symptoms.

Infectious proctitis Treatment is with specific antibiotic, antiviral, or antifungal therapy for the identified organism.

Follow-up

There is no increased incidence of colorectal neoplasia among patients with ulcerative proctitis, and routine screening guidelines are recommended. In many patients, this condition regresses and resolves completely in 2 to 3 years. In up to 50%, however, the inflammatory process extends proximally, evolving into ulcerative colitis.

Referral

Referral to a colon and rectal surgeon should be made if initial treatment fails, diagnosis remains elusive, or sophisticated diagnostic evaluation beyond the general clinic is required.

ANORECTAL ABSCESS

Patient Presentation

An anorectal abscess is often associated with gradually increasing pain and possibly a low-grade fever. There may also be a history of purulent drainage. An anorectal abscess manifests as an erythematous, tender, fluctuant mass (Fig. 13.5). When a DRE is performed, the perirectal abscess is found to be fluctuant and tender. At times, palpation of the abscess produces purulent discharge from the anal canal, demonstrating that, in addition to the ab-

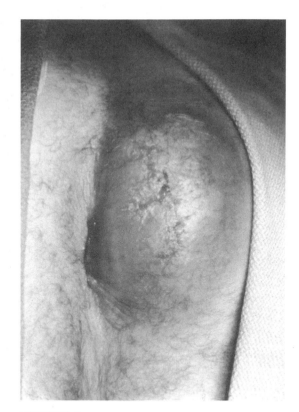

FIGURE 13.5.
Anorectal abscess is shown. Note the bulging mass, which is very tender and fluctuant on examinatioin.

scess, a fistula is probably present through which the discharge occurs.

If a diagnosis can not be reached, an examination under anesthesia should be performed.

Management

Treatment

Drainage of the abscess should be performed. Several techniques have been used to perform simple drainage. The most common follows the simple stab incision; however, the abscess often recurs because the skin edges heal before obliteration of the abscess cavity is complete.

Another option is to place a mushroom catheter through a simple stab incision; this minimizes the skin defect and maintains drainage by keeping the skin open. A no. 10, 12, or 14 French mushroom catheter is often selected. A Malecot catheter should not be used. The Malecot catheter has thin bridges to maximize the open lumen; these bridges become incorporated in the scar tissue, which may prevent removal. It is imperative that the physician choose a mushroom catheter, which is primarily solid with small holes. The catheter should exit about 1 inch outside of the skin to maintain its position.

Another option is to excise an ellipse of skin; this leaves the skin edges separated and prevents early sealing of the skin.

The abscess cavity is often packed at the initial drainage; the packing is removed the following morning or at the time of the first bowel movement. It is not necessary to repack the wound.

Complications

After simple incision and drainage of an abscess, approximately 50% of patients present with a fistula, which represents a continued open, internal passage through the cavity. Therefore, it is important to place the initial incision as close to the anal canal as possible, so as to minimize the extent of the fistula that might occur. This technique minimizes the incision required to perform a fistulotomy at a later date.

Prevention

The discussion of prevention of anal fissures provides further information about a proper bowel management program and the use of fiber in the diet.

Follow-up

Only a single follow-up visit may be needed after drainage of a perirectal abscess if the incision completely heals without drainage, tenderness, or question of a fistula.

Referral

Referral should be performed when the anorectal abscess is noted, unless the clinic office is particularly well suited for performing drainage of an abscess in this location. The clinician should develop a close working relationship with a colorectal surgical colleague and a thorough understanding of the causes of anorectal pain.

THROMBOSED HEMORRHOID

Patient Presentation

A thrombosed hemorrhoid occurs suddenly and is associated with a firm, painful, perianal lump. Although it may occur after an episode of straining, it may also appear spontaneously. A thrombosed hemorrhoid manifests as a firm, tender, ecchymotic, or blue mass and can usually be diagnosed by inspection. A thrombosed hemorrhoid usually involves the external component of the hemorrhoidal plexus; internally, the rectal examination is often normal. An examination under anesthesia is recommended if a diagnosis cannot be reached.

Management

Hemorrhoidectomy

If a thrombosed hemorrhoid is encountered in a patient who presents within the first 24 to 48 hours after onset of pain and the pain has not diminished, a hemorrhoidectomy is offered. This provides definitive treatment for the thrombosed hemorrhoid. The patient is already in severe pain, and little additional pain is caused by the hemorrhoidectomy, which can often be performed under local anesthesia in a surgeon's office.

Conservative management

If the patient presents 2 to 4 days after the onset of pain, the pain is often beginning to diminish. At this point, a hemorrhoidectomy would increase the pain. Also, this condition is likely to continue to resolve, with the thrombosis being reabsorbed and disappearing. Therefore, continued conservative management is indicated.

The mainstay of conservative management is a bowel management program based on the use of stool softeners in the form of fiber. Stool softeners such as docusate do not necessarily provide enough bulk to assist with evacuation. A small, soft, mushy stool still requires straining for evacuation. A larger stool, which is also soft, allows colonic peristalsis to complete the evacuation and avoids straining. Mild analgesics may also be used to relieve pain. In addition, soaking in a warm tub of water and use of mild soap for cleansing helps relieve pain.

Prevention

The discussion of prevention of anal fissures provides further information about a proper bowel management program and the use of fiber.

Follow-up

Depending on the accuracy of the initial diagnosis, follow-up may consist of returning to the clinic if the symptoms of discomfort or perianal lump do not resolve.

Referral

Key elements in the decision to refer are a close working relationship with a colorectal surgical colleague and a thorough understanding of the causes of anorectal pain. If pain from a thrombosed hemorrhoid is decreasing, conservative treatment can be instituted. Referral should be performed for failure to respond to the initial therapy.

PRURITUS ANI

Pruritus ani, or perianal itching, is an almost uncontrollable sensation of perianal itching that has many possible causes. Usually, simple procedures are available for cure or relief. Itching can be profound, particularly at night. Patients characteristically think they have hemorrhoids or malignancy. Despite significant efforts for diagnosis, no cause is established in almost half of the cases of pruritus.

Cause

Pruritus ani usually is a secondary problem. A good understanding of the variety of simple problems that can create pruritus ani is extremely helpful in giving the patient relief. Fundamentally, a wet anus is a generic invitation to pruritus ani. The following causes are described from most to least likely.

Perianal hygiene is a common problem that leads to itching and follows two scenarios: too little cleansing with residual stool left on the perianal skin, and stool contact. On the other hand, too fastidious cleansing with vigorous rubbing to eradicate stool can lead to skin injury and tearing of hair elements, with serous exudate, wet bottom, and an itching problem. This can lead to further redoubled attempts to "clean" the skin. These patients, and patients with large buttocks, are prone to a deep-seated anus outlet that can be continually moist if not frankly wet. This body habitus is another important factor in predisposing patients to pruritus ani.

Excessive intake of certain foods must be carefully ascertained. Coffee, tea, and colas (caffeinated and non-caffeinated), chocolate, spicy foods, and milk products have been shown to cause itching when large amounts of these materials are eaten. Many patients do not consider many quarts of coffee or colas, or other excessive diet fads, to be problematic or related to their itching bottom.

Systemic illnesses (e.g., renal failure, diabetes, collagen vascular diseases) have also been related to severe perianal itching. A thorough review of systems is critical.

Obvious diarrheal conditions related to Crohn disease, ulcerative colitis, or irritable bowel syndrome predispose to itching or irritation, not unlike diaper rash.

Rarely, dermatologic conditions, particularly *Monilia* but also perineal rashes, can be obviously appreciated as the cause for pruritus.

Drug reactions, psychogenic difficulties, and infections are more subtle causes but nonetheless important to check.

Patient Presentation

History

Patients present with the complaint of recurring perianal itching. They scratch to the point of causing pain to get transient relief. They acknowledge that they have a wet anus, but this is most often caused by excoriation from the scratching. Stools can exacerbate, if not precipitate, itching. Cleaning becomes a real concern and effort. Patients rarely note changes in bowel habit or stool consistency, unless diarrhea is a precipitating cause.

Physical examination

The perianal skin is excoriated, reddened, or noticeably absent of hair elements. In the perianal skin, there are frequently superficial skin ulcer lesions, 1 to 2 mm in size. In chronic cases, the pigmented epithelium is replaced with epidermis that appears whitish or (in black skin) gray, again with typical shallow, punched-out ulcers.

Routine anorectal examination, including visual inspection of the perianal skin, DRE with a stool guaiac test, anoscopy, and flexible sigmoidoscopy, is the standard. With rare exceptions, this examination reveals no pathologic lesion, although hemorrhoids, prolapsing anal papilla, and fistula can result in a wet anus and lead to pruritus ani. This usually is not a coexistent disease with these lesions. Nevertheless, if these lesions are found coexistent with pruritus, they can be considered contributory and managed accordingly.

Diagnosis

Laboratory studies might include biopsy if neoplasia or a dermatologic condition is suspected.

The cellophane-tape test for pinworm, *Enterobius vermicularis,* should be done if this organism is suspected. In such cases, patients characteristically itch only at night when the worms come out. Most of the time, pets sleeping in bedclothes are implicated in this infection.

Management

Routine attention to diet modification and perianal skin care should correct most of the cases of pruritus ani that are encountered. Most pruritus ani can be controlled with simple local measures.

Dietary modification

Dietary advice is usually the first item of management. Patients should be screened for excessive intake of the foods noted previously that can trigger pruritus. Cessation of these foods, at least for a 7 to 10 days, is an excellent start. Permanent banning of foods is not realistic; patients need to be cautioned to be moderate in their intake if the foods have a correlation with pruritus.

Hygiene

Hygiene needs review. The emphasis of treatment and prevention is to encourage thorough, but not excessive, cleansing of the anal area after defecation.

Gentleness with cleansing, using medicated hemorrhoidal pads (Tucks) or lotion (Balneol), can greatly ameliorate itching. Encouraging the patient to wipe carefully with blotting rather than rubbing as a way of removing stool is important. Tub bathing with warm water daily or twice daily is helpful, provided that extra care is exercised during drying; the patient should not rub, only blot gently.

Daily use of powder prevents chaffing and wetness. Use of powders without sweet-smelling esters (Ammens or Micatin), applied in the morning after defecation, helps keep the anus dry and soothe the skin. Rarely, a small cotton pledget must be placed next to the anus to "wick" moisture away from the skin.

Referral

Follow-up for a referral should take place when persistent symptoms continue. Cutaneous lesions at variance with the usual punched-out, superficial ulcers should generate a biopsy request or referral to a dermatologist or colon and rectal surgeon.

HIDRADENITIS SUPPURATIVA

The term *hidradenitis suppurativa* is derived from the Greek words *hydros* ("sweat") and *aden* ("gland"). This condition represents a chronic infection of the apocrine glands and subcutaneous tissue and is confined to those areas that contain apocrine glands. The most commonly affected areas are the axilla and groin, followed by the perineum in about 30% of patients.

Cause

The predominant organisms cultured from these wounds are staphylococci and streptococci. Hidradenitis has been associated with obesity, poor hygiene, and hyperhidrosis.

Patient Presentation

On physical examination, the diagnosis is based on the observation of multiple small furuncles in the appropriate distribution with clustering in the axilla, groin, or perineum. Most commonly, patients are between the ages of 16 and 40 years, and there is a two-to-one male predominance.

Management

Initial therapy is conservative, with improved hygiene, warm compresses, and broad-spectrum antibiotics. In the initial phases, when there are few furuncles, treatment may consist of simple incision and drainage for isolated abscess.

Patients who progress to chronic or recurrent disease despite appropriate treatment require excision of all affected tissue. The physician may need to pack the wound that was created by the excision, and secondary healing or coverage with skin grafts or skin flaps may be needed.

Referral

Patients who have extensive or chronic hidradenitis should be referred for surgical evaluation.

PILONIDAL DISEASE

The term *pilonidal* was first associated with this condition in 1880; it is derived from the Latin words *pilus* ("hair") and *nidus* ("nest"). This term emphasizes the frequent finding of hair trapped within a cyst.

Patient Presentation

There are three common presentations for pilonidal disease. Most patients have an episode of acute abscess formation. When this abscess resolves, either spontaneously or with medical assistance, a pilonidal sinus often develops. Most sinus tracts resolve; however, some patients continue to have chronic disease or recurrence of the pilonidal cyst associated with the sinus tract after the initial treatment. The treatment depends on which presentation of pilonidal disease is being treated.

Diagnosis is made by inspection and palpation of an abscess, cyst, or sinus located in the upper gluteal cleft or in the skin area posterior to the sacrum. This condition is not associated with perirectal or anal canal fistulas.

Management

Treatment

For patients who present with an acute pilonidal abscess, simple incision and drainage is all that is indicated initially. Incision and drainage of acute abscesses is usually performed in an office setting with local anesthesia. This simple treatment relieves the symptoms; in about 60% of patients, the condition does not recur. When incision and drainage is performed, a shaggy gray lining is often noted inside the cavity. This represents the lining of the cyst wall; it should be removed to further improve the chances of complete healing without recurrence.

The hair surrounding the area should be shaved or removed with a depilatory to facilitate hygiene and healing. It has been well demonstrated that shaving of the hair is associated with an increased rate of healing.

The wound is loosely packed to prevent premature closure of the skin over the cavity. Hygiene involves washing the area two to three times per day with either a warm shower or soaking in a warm tub.

Because cellulitis and sepsis are uncommon, antibiotics are rarely required.

Follow-up

In up to 40% of patients, a chronic sinus develops after incision and drainage of an abscess. Many of these sinuses resolve by the age of 40 years; regular shaving of this area to keep the hair removed promotes healing.

Other patients develop a recurrent cyst or intermittent drainage from the sinus tract. For these symptomatic recurrences, simple local excision is often effective in curing the disease.

For the small subgroup of patients who are left with persistent nonhealing wounds, several more complex procedures are available. Most of these techniques require hospitalization, and many require skin flaps for wound coverage after excision. Satisfactory treatment of complex or recurrent disease is possible with good results, but it often requires an aggressive approach. The use of asymmetric incisions or skin flaps that obliterate the gluteal cleft results in reliable primary healing and a low recurrence rate but a high rate of flap complications.

Referral

If the condition does not respond to antibiotics and simple abscess drainage, referral to a colon and rectal surgeon should be sought.

CONDYLOMA ACUMINATUM

Condylomata acuminata (anal and perianal warts) is the most common sexually transmitted disease seen by the colorectal surgeon. There has been a marked increase in this disease over the past 20 years.

Cause

The cause of condyloma acuminatum is the human papilloma virus (HPV). More than 40 subtypes of HPV have been isolated. Type 6 is the subtype most often isolated from perianal condylomata; however, types 16 and 18 have been associated with more aggressive behavior of dysplasia and malignant transformation to squamous cell carcinoma.

The usual mode of transmission is by anal intercourse, although autoinoculation from genital warts may occur.

Patient Presentation

The most common presenting symptom is a perianal mass; the most common complaint is that of "hemorrhoids." Other symptoms include pruritus, bleeding, discharge, persistent perianal wetness, and occasionally pain.

The lesions are wart-like; they can arise alone but are more frequently seen in groups (Fig. 13.6). They may range in size from a few millimeters to a cauliflower-like Buschke-Löwenstein lesion (Fig. 13.7). They are often seen on the perianal skin or in the anal canal; however, in nonimmunocompromised patients, the condylomata do not extend proximal to the dentate line.

Anal condylomata may occur in combination with genital condylomata.

Management

Treatment may consist of chemical destruction by local application of podophyllin or bichlorocetic acid in the office. These treatments are toxic to normal skin, and the application must be precisely on the warts. After application, talcum powder is often applied, and the patient is instructed to shower approximately 4 hours after the application. Treatments can be performed at either weekly or biweekly intervals, with resolution in about three fourths of patients treated. Recurrence is common and occurs in 50% to 65% of patients by 12 months.

Referral

For extensive warts that require surgical therapy, referral should be made. Excision under local anesthesia may be performed in the office for isolated condylomata; however, if they are multiple, this is better performed in the operating room. The goal is to excise or destroy the

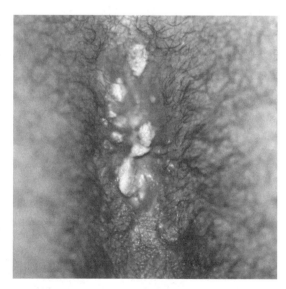

FIGURE 13.6.

Condylomata acuminata are shown. Note the multiple, small, diffuse, wart-like lesions.

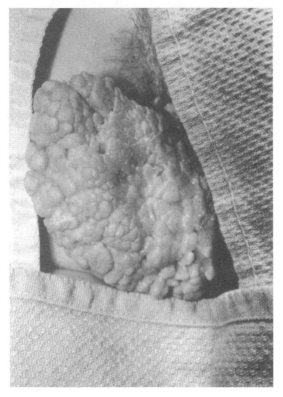

FIGURE 13.7.

Condylomata acuminatum is shown. Note the large, cauliflower-like appearance of giant Buschke-Löwenstein condyloma.

condyloma and preserve the surrounding skin. This is performed by precise excision, electrical coagulation, or laser therapy directed to each individual wart, preserving the skin islands in between. After surgical treatment, more than 90% of patients experience resolution; even in this group of patients, however, up 30% have recurrence within the 1 to 2 years.

ANAL INCONTINENCE

Anal incontinence is the inability to control passage of stool or flatus.

Patient Presentation

Anal incontinence is a common complaint that increases in frequency with increasing age. Minor degrees of fecal incontinence with primarily seepage are extremely common.

Physicians examining patients with major incontinence (loss of control of a formed stool) must obtain a thorough history of associated medical conditions, med-

ications, and prior surgeries that may have involved a sphincter injury.

Management

For minor cases, other than use of dietary bulking agents, hygiene, and a pad, there is often little that can be done.

Patients with major incontinence and prior anorectal surgery, anal trauma, or obstetric injuries may be found to have an anatomically correctable defect.

Referral

Patients with severe incontinence should be referred to a colon and rectal surgeon associated with an anorectal physiology laboratory. Sophisticated testing with anal manometry, anal ultrasound for sphincter mapping, and pudendal nerve terminal motor latency testing can detect those patients who will benefit from sophisticated reconstruction, including anal sphincter reconstruction, repair of defects, or muscle transposition or artificial sphincter implantation for neurogenic incontinence.

KEY POINTS

- Thorough evaluation must be performed before symptoms can be attributed to hemorrhoids.

- Rectal bleeding with blood on the tissue paper and painful bowel movements is almost always caused by a fissure.

- Interventional treatment for hemorrhoids is required only for the symptomatic patient requesting therapy.

- Bowel management with fiber supplementation is the foundation for successful treatment and prevention of many anorectal conditions.

COMMONLY ASKED QUESTIONS

Does rectal bleeding mean that I have cancer?

Although one of the warning signs for colon and rectal cancer is rectal bleeding or blood mixed with the stool, most people who notice rectal bleeding do not have cancer. The most common cause for rectal bleeding is hemorrhoids. Bright red blood that drips into the toilet bowel after a bowel movement is typical for bleeding associated with hemorrhoids. However, when bleeding is present, evaluation should be performed to confirm the cause and to ensure that there is not an associated malignancy. For patients who are younger than 40 to 45 years of age, flexible sigmoidoscopy is appropriate for those patients when there is bleeding typical for hemorrhoids. For older patients who have a positive result on a fecal occult blood test or have conditions that place them at higher risk for cancer, colonoscopy is the preferred diagnostic evaluation to ensure that there is no associated malignancy.

If there is no blood in the stool, does that mean that I can feel comfortable that I do not have colon or rectal cancer?
No. Approximately 50% patients who are diagnosed with cancer of the colon or rectum have had no associated bleeding. Routine screening guidelines are established, and all patients should be encouraged to follow these guidelines even if they are asymptomatic.

What are hemorrhoids?
Hemorrhoids represent the blood vessels that line the inside of the anal canal. All people have hemorrhoids. They tend to coalesce in three areas. It is these areas that tend to enlarge when patients become symptomatic. Hemorrhoidal symptoms are exacerbated by straining. Valsalva-type straining places pressure across the top of the anal canal, similar to putting a tourniquet on your arm and observing the veins enlarge because the return of flow is impeded. Repetitive episodes can cause the hemorrhoids to enlarge over time. Occasionally they may markedly enlarge after a severe episode of straining. When they are enlarged and the stool passes across the hemorrhoids, it scrapes the lining and produces bleeding. The best way to avoid symptoms from hemorrhoids is to avoid straining. This is most commonly accomplished by adding fiber supplementation to the diet.

Do all treatments for hemorrhoids hurt?
The density of free nerve endings in the area of the anal canal approximates that near the fingertips. Excisional procedures to remove hemorrhoids are painful. For external hemorrhoids that are covered by skin, excisional procedures are required. The pain of this procedure can be reduced by the addition of local anesthesia for postoperative pain and use of ketorolac (Toradol) for analgesia. Although some hemorrhoids require surgery, most hemorrhoidal conditions (primarily internal hemorrhoids) can be treated in the clinic. Internal hemorrhoids are covered by the lining of the colon and rectum and are not sensitive to the same pain. Several techniques, including the use of rubber bands, injection therapy for sclerosis, cryotherapy, and infrared therapy, can be performed in the clinic without anesthesia and with minimal discomfort for the patient. The primary reason treatment is performed for hemorrhoids is for the alleviation of symptoms. Just because hemorrhoids are present does not mean that treatment has to be performed.

Why do perianal abscesses occur?
The overwhelming majority of perianal abscesses result from a cryptoglandular cause. About 15 to 20 anal glands are located at the base of crypts of Morgagni. If the crypt becomes plugged, then the gland can swell as the infection enlarges because of blocked drainage. This results in an abscess. About half of such abscesses heal after simple drainage. The other half result in a fistula because the initial tunnel from the crypt to the gland remains open. Fistulas will not heal without treatment. The majority of the treatments require an operative procedure.

What is a fissure and why does is hurt so much?
*A fissure is a tear in the lining of the anal canal. Most of the pain is secondary to spasm of the internal sphincter, which forms the base of the fissure. This is why soaking in a warm tub, which helps promote muscle relaxation, provides relief of pain for fissures and other anal condi-*tions. *The most common cause of a fissure is a very large, constipated bowel movement that creates a tear during evacuation. Fissures can also occur in patients who have diarrhea, probably as a result of the trauma of frequent wiping, which creates an irritated and tender spot.*

SUGGESTED READINGS

Abcarian H. Surgical correction of chronic anal fissure: results of lateral internal sphincterotomy vs. fissurectomy-midline sphincterotomy. *Dis Colon Rectum* 1980;23:31–36.

Allen-Mersh TG. Pilonidal sinus: finding the right track for treatment. *Br J Surg* 1990;77:123–132.

Bascom J. Pilonidal disease: origin from follicles of hairs and results of follicle removal as treatment. *Surgery* 1980;87:567–572.

Bascom JU. Repeat pilonidal operations. *Am J Surg* 1987;154:118–122.

Brown SCW, Kazzazi N, Lord PH. Surgical treatment of perineal hidradenitis suppurativa with special reference to recognition of the perianal form. *Br J Surg* 1986;73:978–980.

Eusebio EB, Graham J, Mody N. Treatment of intractable pruritus ani. *Dis Colon Rectum* 1990;33:770–772.

Guyuron B, Dinner MI, Dowden RV. Excision and grafting in treatment of recurrent pilonidal sinus disease. *Surg Gynecol Obstet* 1983;156:201–204.

Hanley PH. Acute pilonidal abscess. *Surg Gynecol Obstet* 1980;150:9–11.

Jensen SL, Harling H. Prognosis after simple incision and drainage for a first-episode acute pilonidal abscess. *Br J Surg* 1988;75:60–61.

Lewis P, Bartolo DCC. Treatment of trans-sphincteric fistulae by full thickness anorectal advancement flaps. *Br J Surg* 1990;77:1187–1189.

MacLeod CAH, Balcos EG, Buls JG, Goldberg SM. Seton management of anorectal fistulas: a study of incontinence. *Dis Colon Rectum* 1990;33:P10.

Parks AG, Thomson JPS. Intersphincteric abscess. *Br Med J* 1973;2:537–539.

Pearl RK, Andrews JR, Orsay CP, et al. Rose of the seton in management of anorectal fistulas. *Dis Colon Rectum* 1993;36:573–579.

Perez-Gurri JA, Temple WJ, Ketcham AS. Gluteus maximus myocutaneous flap for the treatment of recalcitrant pilonidal disease. *Dis Colon Rectum* 1984;27:262–264.

Ramanujam PS, Prasad ML, Abcarian H, Tan AB. Perianal abscesses and fistulas. *Dis Colon Rectum* 1984;27:593–594.

Ravikumar TS, Sridhar S, Rao RN. Subcutaneous lateral internal sphincterotomy for chronic fissure-in-ano. *Dis Colon Rectum* 1982;25:778–801.

Read DR, Abcarian H. A prospective study of 474 patients with anorectal abscesses. *Dis Colon Rectum* 1979;22:566–569.

Rosen L, Abel ME, Gordon PH, et al. Practice parameters for the management of anal fissure. The Standards Task Force, American Society of Colon and Rectal Surgeons. *Dis Colon Rectum* 1992;35:206–208.

Rosen L. Anorectal abscess-fistulae. *Surg Clin North Am* 1994; 74:1293–1308.

Schouten WR, van Vroonhoven TJMV. Treatment of anorectal abscess with or without primary fistulectomy: results of a prospective randomized trial. *Dis Colon Rectum* 1991; 34:60–63.

Scoma JA, Salvati EP, Rubin RJ. Incidence of fistulas subsequent to anal abscesses. *Dis Colon Rectum* 1974;17:357–359.

Toubanakis G. Treatment of pilonidal sinus disease with the Z-plasty procedure (modified). *Am Surg* 1986;52: 611–612.

Vasilevsky CA, Gordon PH. The incidence of recurrent abscess or fistula-in-ano following anorectal suppuration. *Dis Colon Rectum* 1984;27:126–130.

Vasilevsky CA, Gordon PH. Results of treatment of fistula-in-ano. *Dis Colon Rectum* 1984;28:225–231.

Index

Index

thrombosed, 192
treatment, 187–188
Hepatitis
A
causes, 57
characteristics, 73
clinical features, 58
complications, 58–59
diagnosis, 56, 59
incidence, 57–58
infection sources, 57–58
prevention, 59–60
B
causes, 59–60
characteristics, 73
chronic, 63
complications, 63–64
diagnostic serology for, 56, 64–65
incidence, 61–62
prevention, 65–67
risk factors, 62–63
stages, 61–62
symptoms, 63
treatment, 74–75
C
characteristics, 73
diagnostic serology for, 56, 69
incidence, 66–67
prevention, 70
risk factors, 67–68
symptoms, 68
transmission, 66
treatment, 75–76
D
characteristics, 73
clinical course of, 70–71
diagnosis, 56, 71
incidence, 70
transmission, 70
treatment, 76
differential diagnosis, 55–56
E
characteristics, 71–73
diagnosis, 56–57
with HIV infection, 159
incidence, 54
injury patterns, 55
treatment, 72–76
Hepatocellular carcinoma, hepatitis B and, 63, 64
Hepatotropic viruses, types, 54
Herpes simplex virus (HSV)
in HIV-infected patients, 150–151
ulcers caused by, 22
Hiatal hernia, lower esophageal sphincter affected by, 3
Hidradenitis suppurativa, 194
Highly active antiretroviral therapy (HAART), 147
Hinchey grading system, for diverticulum perforation, 166, 171–173
Histamine receptor antagonists, for gastroesophageal reflux, 11–12
HPV (human papilloma virus infections), 195–196
HSV. *See* Herpes simplex virus
Human immunodeficiency virus infection (HIV)
comorbid conditions
biliary tract disease, 161
diarrhea, 154–156
enteropathy, 156

esophagitis, 151–153
gastrointestinal disease, 148
liver disease, 159–161
mortality decrease, 147
oral complications of
aphthous ulcers, 150
candidiasis, 148–150
gingivitis, 150
herpes simplex virus, 150–151
malignancies, 151
oral hairy leukoplakia, 150
xerostomia, 150
pancreatic involvement, 153
pathogens associated with, 156–159
Human papilloma virus infections (HPV), 195–196
Hyoscyamine, for irritable bowel syndrome, 142–143
Hyperamylasemia
causes, 82
in pancreatitis, 81
Hypergastrinemia, *H. pylori*-related, 20–21
Hypertriglyceridemia, gallstone risk and, 37

I
IBD. *See* Inflammatory bowel disease
IBS. *See* Irritable bowel syndrome
Ileum, terminal, Crohn's disease involving, 107
Imipramine, for irritable bowel syndrome, 144
Immunomodulators, for inflammatory bowel disease, 112–113
Immunosuppression, inflammatory bowel disease and, 106
Induction therapy, for CMV-related diarrhea, 159
Inflammatory bowel disease (IBD)
causes, 106
clinical features, 107–108
complications
extraintestinal, 116–117
intestinal, 115–116
definition, 105
diagnosis, 108–110
genetic predisposition to, 106
initiating events of, 106
management
nutritional, 113
pharmacologic, 110–113
surgical, 113
prognosis, 117
with sclerosing cholangitis, 117
types
Crohn's disease. *See* Crohn's disease
Ulcerative colitis. *See* Ulcerative colitis
Interferon
for chronic hepatitis B, 74–75
for chronic hepatitis C, 75–76
Intravenous drug use
gallstone risk and, 62
hepatitis C from, 68
hepatitis D from, 70
Intravenous therapy, for diarrhea, 99
Iritis, with inflammatory bowel disease, 116
Irritable bowel syndrome (IBS)
causes
altered pain perception, 135–136
luminal irritants, 136
motility abnormalities, 134–135
psychiatric illness, 136
classification, 140
clinical features, 136–138